RENAL TRANSPLANTATION

Theory and Practice

Second Edition

RENAL TRANSPLANTATION
THEORY AND PRACTICE
Second Edition

Edited by
JEAN HAMBURGER, M.D.
JEAN CROSNIER, M.D.
JEAN-FRANÇOIS BACH, M.D.
HENRI KREIS, M.D.

Renal Transplantation Unit and Transplantation Immunology Laboratory
(I.N.S.E.R.M., C.N.R.S., Association Claude Bernard)
Hôpital Necker, Paris

WILLIAMS & WILKINS
Baltimore/London

428 E. Preston Street
Baltimore, MD 21202, U.S.A.

Made in the United States of America

First Edition, 1972

Library of Congress Cataloging in Publication Data

Main entry under title:

Renal transplantation.

Translation of La transplantation rénale.
Includes index.
1. Kidneys—Transplantation. I. Hamburger, Jean.
[DNLM: 1. Kidney—Transplantation. WJ368 R393]
RD575.T6812 1981 617′.4610592 80-19012
ISBN 0-683-03872-9

Composed and printed at the
Waverly Press, Inc.
Mt. Royal and Guilford Aves.
Baltimore, MD 21202, U.S.A.

Preface to the Second Edition

Writing successive editions of a book is a good way to evaluate progress in the field. In the case of renal transplantation, the rate of progress is striking—almost nothing could be retained from the first edition published in 1972. We were then speaking of some 5000 transplantations; the number now exceeds 50,000. Advances in the understanding of graft immunology have been impressive, but some believe that clinical results have not shown similar improvement. Indeed, general procedures have not changed dramatically, but the multiple technical and tactical improvements that have been made in the years since 1972 lead us to take the opposite opinion. That opinion is reflected in this book.

Preface to the First Edition

Young men and women die every day because their kidneys are destroyed by disease, although the rest of their body is perfectly sound. Faced with this situation, it is hardly surprising that nephrologists have been preoccupied with the idea of saving these young lives by kidney transplantation. But a mere 20 years ago, this seemed no more than a hopeless dream.

The problem did not lie in the actual surgery. The operative technique had been established by surgeons such as René Küss and Jean Vaysse in France, David Hume and Joseph Murray in the United States, but it was known that the transplant was inevitably recognized as foreign and as such rejected. This immunologic obstacle appeared insurmountable, apart from the special case of identical twins, who are, so to speak, two examples of the one individual. In 1956, a Boston team headed by John Merrill achieved the first successful kidney transplantation between identical twins and so proved the validity of the surgical technique.

Four years earlier, in December 1952, a young carpenter aged 16 years, Marius R., had fallen from a scaffolding and ruptured his right kidney. The kidney had to be removed but after the operation it was discovered that he had congenital absence of the left kidney. He was now anephric. Repeated dialysis with the artificial kidney had not been developed at that time. Because we at the Necker Hospital had for several years been carrying out experiments in kidney grafting, the question of renal transplantation was put to us. The boy's mother pleaded that we should attempt to transplant one of her kidneys to her son. It had already been established in animals that genetic factors played an essential role in graft tolerance. The close immunologic relationship between mother and son seemed, in our ignorance at that time, to be confirmed when we found that they shared the same major and six minor red blood groups.

Our doubts and hesitation can be imagined, but finally we decided that to turn a deaf ear on the pleas of the family would be no less reprehensible than to agree. On Christmas night 1952, Louis Michon, Nicolas Oeconomos and Jean Vaysse took the mother's left kidney and transplanted it to the right iliac fossa of her son. The grafted kidney functioned immediately. In the following week we had high hopes of success. The blood urea fell to normal and the boy's general condition improved to the point that he was able to be up and about. On the 22nd day rejection set in with sudden arrest of kidney function. This may have been, to start with, only a transplant crisis (such as we described later) that can be reversed with suitable treatment, but this knowledge lay in the future. The length of time that the graft was tolerated was, however, at variance with all previous experience. We were confirmed in the hypothesis that, in man as in animals, genetic relationship could favor tolerance. We went on to consider the possibility of achieving indefinitely prolonged tolerance in similar cases by depressing to some degree the immunologic reaction of the recipient.

In that same year, 1952, Frank Dixon and his collaborators published, in the *Journal of Immunology* evidence that immune reactions could be depressed in rabbits by using x-rays. French experts in radiotherapy, such as Claude M. Lalanne, Maurice Tubiana and many others, had acquired considerable experience in the techniques of total body radiation for certain malignant disorders of the blood. It was tempting to apply this method to the problem of transplantation and indeed this was suggested by W. J. Dempster in London. Animal experiments, however, gave very inconstant results and we might never have gone on to attempt the procedure in man but for the influence of John P. Merrill.

He had come to spend a sabbatical year in Paris and we soon fell under the spell of this patrician Bostonian with the inquiring mind, who was firmly convinced that desperate diseases called for daring remedies. One day, during a discussion on the new and difficult ethical problems of kidney transplantation in man, he said: "Your fears and hesitant attitude seem wrong to me. Think of all the patients who may die in the future because you have not had the courage to do what was necessary to add to our knowledge and open the way to new methods of treatment." But in France, as elsewhere, the idea was and, indeed, still is deeply rooted that no treatment is acceptable unless it benefits the patient himself as an individual, and it can never be justified merely to further medical knowledge.

Early in 1959, John Merrill tried a kidney graft between nonidentical twins after irradiating the recipient. One of our patients in terminal renal failure, George S., also had a nonidentical twin who had volunteered to donate a kidney. We decided that our scruples were no longer justified in view of the good immediate result of the Boston case. So we in turn performed a graft on George S., using cobalt therapy for immune depression. Although it chanced that our case was published during that year, 1959, 4 months after the operation, whereas the Boston case did not appear in print until 1960, the initiative of John Merrill was not only first in point of time, but was the determining factor in our own case.

It was, however, suggested that these two initial successes might be due to some peculiarity of the nonidentical twins. It was known from the work of Owen that, in animals, it is not uncommon for binovular twins to acquire during fetal life a reciprocal tolerance so that they can form "chimera" in which two types of red blood cells, those of the animal itself and those of its nonidentical twin, are found side by side. It was suggested that something of the sort might have happened in the two cases described above. Were these mere curiosities or did they point the way to a solution of the problem of organ grafting in general?

For many reasons, particularly the absence of any detectable blood chimerism and the rejection by one of the binovular twins of a skin graft from the other, we concluded that the real reason for the success was the close genetic relationship of donor and recipient. From this followed the necessity of discovering means of donor selection and of assessing the degree of immunologic similarity between donor and recipient. This was the parting of the ways between us and the Boston group. The latter turned all their efforts to the discovery of new methods of immunosuppression while we concentrated on immunologic selection of the donor. In our case this led to collaboration with a man who was to play a decisive part in the orientation of our thinking, Jean Dausset.

Jean Dausset was, at that time, in the same hospital group, attached to the service of Professor Jean Bernard. With admirable intelligence and tenacity, he had established that the white blood cells carry "isoantigens" which differ from one individual to another; it was tempting to suppose that this might provide a method of comparing the immunologic charactersitics of the donor and recipient of a graft. The remarkable development of this line of research is described in Chapters 2 and 3. After our first attempts at kidney transplantation between nonidentical twins, we decided to apply the technique developed by Jean Dausset in making the choice of donor. Knowing what we do today, it is reasonable to think that the first successful nontwin kidney transplantation (the patient, transplanted by our group on February 12, 1962, is in good health more than 9 years later) owes much to the fact that comparison of leukocyte antigens was used to select the donor at a time when the very principle of immunologic donor selection was regarded elsewhere with great skepticism.

Developments in organ grafting were very rapid. In 1960, Schwartz and Dameshek demonstrated a remarkable prolongation of graft survival using immunosuppressive drugs of the 6-mercaptopurine series prepared by Gertrude B. Elion in the Burroughs Wellcome Laboratories. The English surgeon, Roy Calne, working in Merrill's laboratory in Boston, used these drugs successfully in kidney transplantation in dogs. Many other centers took up kidney transplantation in man. Küss and Legrain were among the first in France, while another important center was set up in Lyon by Traeger and Perrin; in the United States, in addition to the Boston pioneers, centers were set up in Richmond by Hume, in Denver by Starzl, and in Los Angeles by Goodwin. Centers were founded in Great Britain by Woodruff, father of antilymphocyte serum; in Belgium by Alexandre, in Australia by Kincaid-Smith, and in Ireland by Walsh. Many more centers followed throughout the world and at the same time immunologists the world over were making great contributions to the problems of transplantation, doubtless stimulated by the clinical implications. The International Transplantation Society originated in New York in 1965, thanks mainly to the efforts of John Converse and Felix Rapaport. The memberhsip now covers 34 countries. The number of kidney transplantations in man is now well over 5000.

Kidney transplantation has reached a crossroads. From the stage of tentative experiment, it is passing to the stage of routine therapeutics. Yet there are many problems still to be solved. The methods of selection of living donors are fairly clearly established, but the same cannot be said for cadaver donors. Current methods of immunosuppression have many drawbacks; the monitoring of the grafted patient still depends on clinical and biochemical data rather than on the study of the immunologic situation, although this latter must, in the last analysis, provide the only true criteria for the intelligent direction of therapy.

Analysis of the immunologic situation of the grafted patient was, until now, impossible because we knew far too little about the mechanisms of rejection. This is no longer so. One of the chief purposes of this book is to suggest that from our current knowledge of the reaction of the host against the graft, and more particularly from models which reproduce to varying degrees *in vitro* the stages of this immunologic reaction, it should be possible to evolve a range of clinical tests which would allow the physician to evaluate the immunologic situation at any moment. Until now we have been able to detect rejection only when the damage has been done. In the future we should be able to detect the immunologic events in time to prevent the damage. This critical advance in organ transplantation demands the total destruction of the artificial barriers often erected between basic transplantation immunology and clinical transplantation practice. Transplantation is not practicable without a full appreciation of all the problems, ranging from the immunology laboratory to the operating room. It is for this reason that we have thought it necessary, in this book, to consider both theory and practice.

It would in any case be a pity to separate these two extraordinary adventures in human experience, the one a therapeutic adventure transforming the horizons of medicine, the other a scientific adventure that is making us revise our concept of personality by revealing the secrets of the complex, subtle and wonderful system which constantly defends our individual self from any deviation from our biologic originality.

Contributors

Jean-François Bach, M.D.,
Associate Professor of Immunology, Université René Descartes, Department of Nephrology, Hôpital Necker, Paris

Marie-Anne Bach, M.D.,
Chargé de Recherche, I.N.S.-E.R.M. Unité 25, Hôpital Necker, Paris

Jean Crosnier, M.D.,
Professor of Nephrology, Université René Descartes, Director, Department of Therapeutics in Nephrology, Hôpital Necker, Paris

Monique Debray-Sachs, Ph.D.,
Maître de Recherche, C.N.R.S., I.N.S.E.R.M. Unité 25, Hôpital Necker, Paris

Béatrice Descamps, M.D., D.Sc.,
Maître de Recherche, I.N.S.E.R.M. Unité 25, Hôpital Necker, Paris

Dominique Droz, M. D.,
Department of Nephrology, Hôpital Necker, Paris

Michel Dy, D.Sc.,
Chargé de Recherche, C.N.R.S., I.N.S.E.R.M. Unité 25, Hôpital Necker, Paris

Catherine Fournier, Ph.D.,
Chargé de Recherche, I.N.S.-E.R.M. Unité 25, Hôpital Necker, Paris

Jean Hamburger, M.D.,
Professor of Nephrology, Université René Descartes, Director, Department of Nephrology, Hôpital Necker, Paris

Jacques-Henri Hors, M.D.,
Associate Professor of Immunology, Hôpital Saint-Louis, Paris

Henri Kreis, M.D.,
Associate Professor of Nephrology, Université René Descartes, Department of Therapeutics in Nephrology, Hôpital Necker, Paris

Michel Lacombe, M.D.,
Professor of Surgery, Université Paris VII, Chief, Department of Surgery, Hôpital Beaujon

Michel Leski, M.D.,
Professor of Nephrology, Chief, Division of Nephrology, Hôpital Cantonal Universitaire, Geneva

Jean-François Moreau, M.D.,
Associate Professor of Radiology, Hôpital Necker, Paris

Toong See Ngeh, M.D.,
Department of Radioisotopes, Hôpital Necker, Paris

Anh Thu N'Guyen, M.D.,
Department of Nephrology, Hôpital Necker, Paris

Laure-Hélène Noël, M.D.,
Department of Nephrology, Hôpital Necker, Paris

Patrice Rioux, M.D.,
Attaché de Recherche, I.N.S.-E.R.M. Unité 88 (Professor F. Grémy), Hôpital de la Pitié-Salpêtrière, Paris

Technical assistance in preparing manuscripts and index: Doreen Broneer

Contents

CHAPTER EIGHT

Extrarenal Complications

APPENDIX I

Surgical Techniques

APPENDIX II

Immunologic Techniques

APPENDIX III

Other Techniques

CHAPTER ONE

Transplantation Immunology

Jean Hamburger

Terminology—Immunologically competent cells—Sequence of events following allografting—Mixed lymphocyte reaction—Actual in vivo reaction against an allogeneic transplant.

TERMINOLOGY

The words graft and transplant are used synonymously. It was formerly suggested that the term transplantation should be reserved for the connection of organs to the host vessels and that the word grafting should be used when tissue fragments were implanted without vascular suture. But usage, which is overriding in matters of terminology, has not upheld this distinction and many authorities now talk of grafting a heart or a kidney.

Autotransplantation or *autograft* signifies that the organ is reimplanted in the same body from which it was removed. Donor and recipient are one and the same person. It may be necessary, for example, to carry out kidney autotransplantation to the iliac fossa when there is an irreparable vascular lesion in the part of the aorta which normally gives rise to the renal arteries. There are no immunologic problems in autotransplantation.

Isotransplantation or *isograft* signifies that donor and recipient have identical antigenic determinants. This is exemplified in man by transplantation between identical twins who, as far as *basic antigenic structure* is concerned, are but two examples of one individual. Grafts between inbred animals are another example. These will be discussed in detail in Chapter Two, "The Graft Antigens." The term isogenic has now generally been replaced by the term *syngeneic*. Like autografts, grafts between syngeneic individuals usually pose no immunologic problem.

Homotransplantation or *allografting* is carried out between individuals of the same species, for example from rat to rat or from dog to dog or from man to man. This is the usual form of kidney transplantation, and it is with this that the present work is mainly concerned.

Heterotransplantation or *xenografting* implies that donor and recipient belong to different animal species. The first efforts at renal transplantation in man were xenotransplants. In 1906, Jaboulay[36a] tried to connect goat and pig kidneys to the arm vessels of uremic patients. More recent attempts to transplant kidneys from monkeys to man also fall into this category of xenotransplantation, although some authors point out that this is a special case because both donor and recipient are primates, and as such undoubtedly share some antigenic determinants.[6, 23]

* * *

All higher animals are equipped to recognize allografts as foreign. Any allograft triggers an immunologic conflict leading to graft rejection. The protagonists in the conflict are the antigenic structures of the graft and the immunologically competent cells of the host.

The graft antigens will be considered in Chapters 2 and 3. Meanwhile, suffice it to say that they are characteristic of the individual as a whole and their complexity is such that there are probably no two persons in the world with absolutely identical antigenic structures, except, of course, identical twins.

The immunologically competent cells of the host must now be considered in detail because it is their reaction that causes rejection of an allografted organ.

It is generally held that the immune response to an allograft essentially belongs to the class of immune reactions known as cell-mediated and thus related to delayed hypersensitivity reactions such as the tuberculin reaction. This cell-mediated response is distinguished from humoral responses (in which cells are in fact involved but act by releasing circulating antibodies into the blood). It will be seen later, however, that the role of circulating antibodies is far from negligible in the process of rejection of allotransplanted organs. But there is no doubt that the cell-mediated immune response is a predominant factor in allograft rejection.

IMMUNOLOGICALLY COMPETENT CELLS

Research on cell-mediated immunity and in particular on graft immunity has gradually brought to light a remarkable system whereby the molecular personality of the individual is protected.

This system provides information on all surface antigenic structures in every part of the body open to the vascular system. With information obtained from cell surfaces, these sources can detect any structure which is, or appears to be, foreign. When foreign invasion (such as the massive invasion represented by the presence of an allograft) is recognized, a specialized machinery for the destruction and elimination of the elements regarded as foreign is set in motion. The principal vigilante agent, both for information and for action, is the lymphocyte, or, more precisely, the lymphocyte subsets. Although one lymphocyte looks very much the same as another, lymphocytes are in fact a very mixed population, varying in function, longevity and specialization. In addition, lymphocytes are not the only cells involved in the reaction to an allograft. Macrophages and polymorphs also interfere. Finally, the whole machinery appears as a complex system where the various types of cells either cooperate or, on the contrary, act as antagonists.

The natural history of the various populations of lymphocytes has come to light only very recently and it is much too soon to attempt a definitive account. In addition, many of the facts have been discovered in small rodents, and caution should be exercised in extrapolating all data to man. It is, however, already certain that in man, as in other animals, allograft rejection (or tolerance) results from the intricate action of different cell types.

Lymphocytes

The first distinction between lymphocyte subpopulations was between T and B lymphocytes. T lymphocytes are those whose maturation depends on the thymus. B lymphocytes are bone marrow-derived cells whose maturation is not thymus-dependent. In transplantation immunology T lymphocytes are responsible for the alloantigen recognition and for the generation of cytotoxic cells specifically directed against the graft. B lymphocytes are responsible for the generation of circulating antibodies (the "humoral" response). Although B and T lymphocytes have no unambiguously demonstrated morphologic difference, they may be distinguished by surface markers and by functional tests. B lymphocytes are characterized by much more readily detectable surface immunoglobulins than T lymphocytes, as demonstrated for example by immunofluorescent techniques. T lymphocytes have various surface markers: the best known in mice is the theta antigen, but the list also includes TL (thymus-leukemic) and Ly antigens (Lyt, T lymphocytes; Lyb, B lymphocytes).[11] In humans similar markers exist (for example, Hu-TLA, or human thymus lymphocyte antigen) but are not as conveniently used as in mice. Recent data obtained by using monoclonal anti-T cell antibodies (produced by hybridomas issued from spleen cells of mice immunized by human T cells) indicate, however, that good T cell antigen markers will be available in man in the near future. Functional tests also differentiate human T from B lymphocytes: human T lymphocytes form rosettes with sheep erythrocytes (termed E Rosettes), and they undergo blast transformation when stimulated by phytomitogens such as Concanavalin A (Con A) or phytohemagglutinin (PHA).

This preliminary classification of lymphocytes into T and B subpopulations has been greatly refined during the last 10 years. In particular, T lymphocytes are now subclassified into various populations that should be clearly distinguished for the understanding of transplantation immunology (Fig. 1.1). At least three main subsets may be considered separately: 1) "*Cytotoxic T cells*," responsible for the cytolysis of allogeneic target cells; 2) "*Helper T cells*," responsible for enhancing both cell-mediated and humoral response, particularly for cooperating with B cells in antibody formation but also essential in the cell-mediated response; and 3) "*Suppressor T cells*," which may inhibit the response, for example, suppressing antibody synthesis by B cells. The relationships among these various subsets of T cells are not yet clear. It is commonly accepted that they take place in the natural history of lymphocyte maturation under the local or peripheral (through a circulating thymic hormone) influence of the thymus. Immature T cells give rise to several T cell subsets with different functional capacities, whose differentiation perhaps also depends on stimulation by antigen.

Several T cell subsets have been described in the mouse and more recently in man. Mature T cells can be divided into two subsets: Lyt 1^+ cells, which include helper T cells and T cells involved in delayed type hypersensitivity; and Lyt 2.3^+ cells, which include cytotoxic and suppressor T cells.[11, 12] Both cell types derive from a common precursor (Lyt $1.2.3^+$) which is depleted by adult thymectomy and already itself exerts important regulatory functions. In particular, the Lyt $1.2.3^+$ cell contributes to the suppressive effect of the Lyt 2.3^+ cell. Data obtained in man in in vitro lymphocyte cultures and by use of anti-T cell monoclonal antibodies have confirmed the existence of similar T cell subsets as described in the mouse.

Lymphocytes recognize antigens by means of antigen specific receptors, and in particular, lymphocytes possess specific receptors for alloantigens.

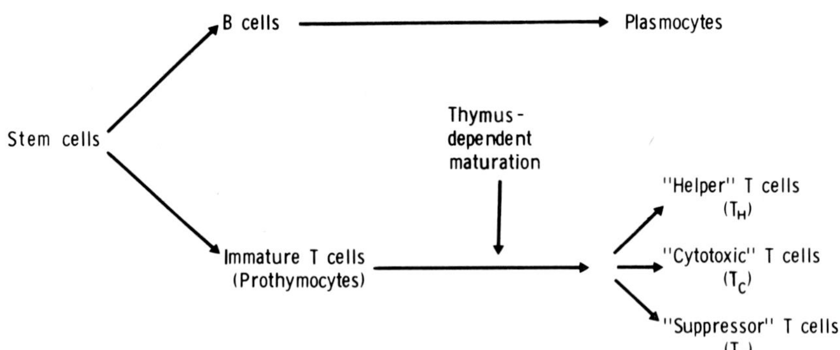

Fig. 1.1. Simplified diagram of lymphocyte development. The maturation of bone marrow-derived B cells is not dependent on the thymus, while the thymus-dependent maturation of prothymocytes gives rise to cytotoxic, helper and suppressor T cells.

It has already been shown that such receptors share idiotypes with the antibodies directed against the same alloantigens.[9] Anti-idiotypic antibodies specifically bind to the T cell clone specialized in the recognition of the alloantigens corresponding to the idiotypic specificity. Incubated with T cells, they inhibit their capacity to react in mixed lymphocyte reaction and graft-versus-host reaction. When their production is induced in vivo by autoimmunization, they delay skin graft rejection. The presence of common idiotypes on B and T cell receptors and on humoral antibodies indicates that specificity for alloantigens is coded for by the same genes in B and T cells. It opens a new field of immunomanipulation (anti-idiotypic immunization) that we shall treat in more detail in Chapter Five.

Problem of "K Cells"

In addition to the two classical modes of attack of the graft, cell-mediated (cytotoxic T cells invading the graft) and antibody-mediated (complement-dependent circulating antibodies), a third mechanism of cytotoxicity has been described. It involves the participation of both antibodies and effector cells. This phenomenon is commonly referred to as antibody-dependent cell cytotoxicity, or ADCC, as opposed to the above mentioned complement-dependent cytotoxicity, or CDC. Antibodies involved in ADCC (of the IgG class) are not cytotoxic by themselves. But, when incubated with the target cells, they make them vulnerable to nonspontaneously cytotoxic cells.

These effector cells are not common B or T lymphocytes. They are generally termed K cells (K for Killer). There is a possibility that several types of cells may act as effector cells in ADCC, including T cells. But the most characteristic K cell has a lymphocyte-like appearance, with an Fc receptor (that may explain the fixation of the cell by the Fc end of the antibody whose Fab end(s) are fixed on the target cell) but with neither the features of B cells nor the markers of T cells (K cells belong to the category of cells sometimes termed "null" cells). It has been hypothesized that K cells might be promonocytes.[22] Treatment with steroids greatly depresses K cells in patient blood, while treatment with azathioprine does not.[20]

Natural Killer Cells

In normal subjects, the peripheral blood contains mononuclear cells spontaneously cytolytic for a wide range of target cells. These *Natural Killer (NK) cells* have mainly been studied in cancer immunology. Their possible role in allograft rejection is not yet clearly demonstrated. The nature and origin of NK cells are also debated.

Interestingly enough, NK cells are deeply depressed in patients receiving immunosuppressive drugs such as those used in allograft recipients.[39] This observation may be important in view of the increased number of viral and cancer complications in these patients, including malignant lymphoma, whose development is greatly enhanced by NK deficiency.

Macrophages

The participation of macrophages in the allograft reaction has long been overshadowed by the lymphocyte. Recent observations, both in the human and in experimental models, have suggested that macrophages may also be of crucial importance for the recognition of alloantigens, the rejection process and the overall regulation of the immune response against the graft.

The role of macrophages in the initial step of the response, i.e., *recognition* of the graft as a foreign, "nonself" body, is mainly suggested by the observation of an in vitro model of the allogeneic response that will be described hereafter, the mixed lymphocyte culture (MLC). Elimination of all macrophages from the culture may suppress the reaction of the responding lymphocytes against the allogeneic cells. This has been compared to the well known effect of macrophages in the processing and effective presentation of antigens to lymphocytes at the initial phase of many immune reactions. For example, hapten-protein conjugates or sheep red blood cells are far more immunogenic when bound to macrophages than when unbound. However, in the case of allografted cell recognition by the host lymphocytes, the role of macrophages is not yet completely clarified.

Macrophages may also act as auxiliary *effector cells* in allograft destruction. Here again, however, evidence is based on in vitro experiments rather than undebatable in vivo demonstration.

In vitro models have demonstrated that lymphocytes of animals sensitized by an allograft produce "lymphokines" when placed in contact with cells from the graft donor. Some of these lymphokines act on macrophages. The *macrophage inhibition factor* (MIF), first described in delayed hypersensitivity models by David,[17] is also produced by lymphocytes in allograft immunity.[36] Thus a local release of MIF within the graft could retain macrophages in situ. The *macrophage activating factor* (MAF) has the capacity of "arming" macrophages, i.e., making them nonspecifically cytotoxic against any allogeneic target cell.* This

* The terminology of macrophage "activation" is unfortunately confusing. The term

phenomenon has in fact been mainly demonstrated with tumoral target cells,[27] but it is now also well substantiated with normal, nontumoral targets.[36] If these results obtained in vitro are once more extrapolated to what actually occurs in vivo within the graft, it may be hypothesized that macrophages locally activated by lymphocytes releasing MAF could exert an auxiliary lytic effect on graft cells already damaged by cytotoxic lymphocytes. There is no direct evidence that this actually occurs in allografted organs, but a number of in vivo observations and experiments are in favor of such an interpretation.[26]

Still another function of macrophages in the allograft reaction may concern the *regulation* of the response. It is now well established that macrophages can inhibit the immune responses of T and B lymphocytes in some conditions,[45] while in other conditions a stimulatory effect has been described.[60]

It has been suggested that human monocytes enhance lymphocyte proliferation in MLC, while mature human macrophages rather suppress the response.[50] In fact, the word macrophage probably covers several subsets of cells whose functions are not perfectly identical. This regulatory role of macrophages is probably exerted via the secretion of soluble mediators such as the lymphocyte activating factor (LAF) or substances inhibiting the lymphocyte response, for example prostaglandins secreted in large amounts by "activated" macrophages.[25]

SEQUENCE OF EVENTS FOLLOWING ALLOGRAFTING

We may now try to reconstruct the sequence of events provoked by an allogeneic transplant from the recognition of the histocompatibility antigens carried by the graft to the initiation of hostilities against the graft. Rapid progress in understanding the sequence of events is largely due to the use of a simplified in vitro model of antiallogeneic reaction, the mixed lymphocyte reaction (MLR). This reaction has been so extensively used in recent research that a brief description of the phenomena observed in this in vitro model seems necessary before discussing the actual in vivo sequence.

Mixed Lymphocyte Reaction

The study of MLC with lymphocyte populations of two different individuals in the same test tube was first suggested in 1964 by Fritz Bach

---

"activated macrophage" was introduced by Mackaness in the 1960s to describe the enhanced microbicidal activity of macrophages from animals with acquired immunity to infection. But it is now employed extensively in the most varied situations in the study of inflammation and immunology.[44] It should be underlined here that the phenomena accompanying macrophage activation in graft immunology are by no means identical to those observed in other circumstances.[33]

and Kurt Hirschhorn in the United States[2] and by Barbara Bain and coworkers in Canada.[5] They showed that the contact of one population with the other triggers profound transformation of the lymphocytes. In order to study separately the reaction of population A against population B, and vice versa, the reaction of one of the two lymphocyte populations (the "stimulator" cells) was inhibited by submitting it to x-rays or mitomycin before introducing it into the mixed culture; this procedure was termed one-way MLC.[2] Practical details concerning the MLR technique will be found in another section of this book (Appendix II).

The first stage of the reaction is *the recognition* of the histocompatibility antigens of the stimulator cells by responding cells. These responding cells are T lymphocytes, as demonstrated by the absence of any MLR if lymphocytes are taken from T cell-deprived animals (for example, animals thymectomized at birth) or if they have been pretreated with an antiserum directed against T cell antigens and with complement. The presence of cells from the monocyte-macrophage series in the medium is also necessary for this initial step of allogeneic recognition, as already mentioned above.

Not all T lymphocytes are involved in the phenomenon of recognition. For one given allogeneic cell population to be recognized, approximately 1 to 3% of the potentially responding lymphocytes actually react. Elimination of these 1 to 3% lymphocytes (one procedure consists of adding highly tritiated thymidine that will be incorporated into these reacting lymphocytes and will specifically kill them; see the following paragraph) suppresses any further reaction to this specific strain of stimulator cells, without suppressing the reaction to other allogeneic cells. This is to be compared with the classical clonal selection theory attributing to different lymphocyte clones the response to different antigens. However, in the usual immune response to one given antigen, involving the production of antibodies, the commonly accepted figure for specifically responding lymphocytes does not exceed 0.01%, a much lower percentage of committed lymphocytes than the 1 to 3% committed in allogeneic reactions. It is interesting to note that the percentage of lymphocytes binding anti-idiotypic antibodies corresponding to a given allogeneic combination is of the same order.[1, 64]

The second stage of the reaction is *the transformation and proliferation* of the stimulated lymphocytes. The transformation is often termed blastogenesis because the transformed cells are similar to immature lymphoblasts: after 6 or 7 days in the human, or 4 or 5 days in mice, many lymphocytes are metamorphosed into large cells of the blast type, with abundant basophilic cytoplasm and a nucleus that synthesizes considerably increased amounts of DNA, easily measured by the incorporation of tritiated thymidine. Many mitotic figures are visible in the culture.

Another element of the mixed lymphocyte reaction is *the production of cytotoxic lymphocytes* whose cytotoxicity is specific, in other words, directed only against cells bearing histocompatibility antigens of the stimulator cells. The acquisition of these cytotoxic properties is commonly evaluated by the "cell-mediated lympholysis" (CML) test (see Appendix II). Cytotoxic lymphocytes have the capacity of releasing a cytotoxic factor, a protein fraction of a molecular weight of approximately 35,000 to 55,000, termed lymphotoxin; however, lymphotoxin is hardly detectable in supernatants of MLR but rather when cells are stimulated with mitogens such as phytohemagglutinin or ConA. Hence, its actual role in T-lymphocyte cytotoxicity against grafted cells is still debatable.

It should be noted that the proliferation of effector cells in MLC is remarkably rapid, with cell multiplication occurring every 6 to 12 hours, a time which in terms of ordinary cell multiplication is extraordinarily short.[40] Few other cells are known to multiply as rapidly except those producing humoral antibody.[10]

The above described sequence of the MLR is under the double control of regulatory cells and of various substances released in the culture medium.

Some cells can *enhance* the reaction. The T cell subset hereabove described as T helper cells may considerably increase the development of cytotoxic cells. This effect was particularly studied by Cantor and Boyse in the mouse, a species in which helper and cytotoxic cells may be distinguished by the Ly 1 and Ly 2.3 surface markers, respectively.[11] Once sensitized by a first allogeneic contact, helper cells (Ly 1^+) may produce a "secondary cytotoxic T lymphocyte inducing factor" that may even be released under nonspecific influences such as stimulation of these sensitized helper cells by a phytomitogen, Con A.[61]

Other cells, on the contrary, *inhibit* the reaction. Suppressor T cells may be found in MLC from the very first days. They probably act both by depressing the intervention of helper cells and later by preventing antibody formation by B lymphocytes. Here again, it has been suggested that the suppressing effect may be due to the release of soluble mediators.

Such mediators and other soluble substances released by cells during the allogeneic immune response have been extensively studied during recent years.[62] They have been mainly sought in supernatants of MLC. It soon became apparent that they play an important role in cell-to-cell interaction and in the overall regulation of the response.

So many mediators have been described in recent years that we shall purposely omit many of them and retain only a few major ones, unanimously recognized as important. Some are released by lymphocytes and others by macrophages.

Mediators produced by lymphocytes are termed lymphokines.[15] They include factors acting on macrophages (chemotactic factor, attracting macrophages; MIF, inhibiting macrophage migration; and MAF, inducing a nonspecific cytotoxicity of macrophages against allogeneic target cells) and factors acting on lymphocytes ["helper" factors, specific or nonspecific, such as the blastogenic or mitogenic factor, enhancing blast transformation and cell proliferation; and "suppressive" factors, again specific or nonspecific, the best known nonspecific factor being SIRS, or soluble immune response suppressor, described in the mouse and probably similar to a suppressive factor described in the human by Sasportes et al[52]. The latter factor is not specific for the stimulating cell (the donor) but is specific for the stimulated cell (the recipient); it suppresses the response of the sensitized cell, and only that cell, against any allogenic stimulating cell. A specific suppressive factor has also been described in the mouse by Rich and Rich[49]].

Mediators produced by macrophages and/or monocytes may also be responsible for either effect, activating or suppressing. Among activating factors, one of the best studied is the lymphocyte activating factor, or LAF, a nonspecific factor potentiating the responses of T cells.[60] Suppressive mediators are still poorly defined. Their study is made more complex because macrophages may also release many commonplace organic substances, some of which are powerful depressors of the immune response.

Prostaglandin (PG) may be cited first. PGE_2 and prostacyclin, in particular, are found in the supernatants of mixed lymphocyte cultures. The amount found is greatly increased if the lymphocyte populations are those of a donor and a recipient of an allograft (secondary or presensitized MLC).[25] This extra production of PG in a presensitized MLC is for a large part produced by macrophages, perhaps under the influence of the MAF released by the sensitized lymphocyte in the presence of the stimulator cell. PGs thus released may modulate the eventual immune response, since they exert a suppressive effect on almost all steps of the lymphocyte response. They are not, however, the only suppressive substances released by activated macrophages in the supernatant of MLC: *arginase, polyamine oxidase* and some *complement factors* should also be mentioned, as well as *thymidine,* which may interfere with the incorporation of tritiated thymidine used for measuring the proliferative response, leading to falsely low evaluations.[1]

Other substances released in MLC supernatants include type II *interferon* and *histamine.*[24] Clearly enough, the mixed lymphocyte culture appears to be a very complex process, intermingling many types of cell subsets and a large number of soluble factors released during the reaction. Some factors enhance and others depress the reaction. The final result depends on a delicate balance between opposite forces. This image, suggested by the most typical in vitro model of the allogeneic immune response, is important, since we shall find this concept of a balance between rejection and antirejection forces throughout the whole story of allograft destruction or tolerance.

Actual in Vivo Reaction Against an Allogeneic Transplant

To what extent do the above phenomena described in in vitro models actually occur in vivo in the allograft recipient? Here again, a series of successive stages may be studied: recognition of the graft antigens, stimulation of the host immunocompetent cells, production and proliferation of cytotoxic lymphocytes, possible intervention of circulating antibodies and finally destruction of the graft. The auxiliary role of macrophages, polymorphs and platelets will also be mentioned.

Recognition of the Graft Antigens

T lymphocytes of the recipient are the main cells responsible for alloantigen recognition. This has been suggested by the discovery that animals thymectomized at birth become poorly armed for allograft rejection.

Current concepts suggest that circulating T lymphocytes of the recipient penetrate into the graft, where the recognition stage takes place locally. This stage implies close contact between the allogeneic and host cells. A classical in vitro image of such a contact accompanying recognition is given by the phenomenon of spontaneous rosettes.[4] We shall briefly describe this phenomenon since the technique is widely used in transplantation immunology.

When an animal of species A is immunized against the red blood cells of species B, the lymphocytes of A in the presence of red cells from B tend to form a rosette by adherence of a group of red cells on the circumference of the lymphocyte (Fig. 1.2). This phenomenon has long been studied by immunologists under the name of immunocytoadherence.[10] An animal that has not been preimmunized may form similar rosettes, but in much smaller amounts. These *spontaneous rosettes* probably represent a model for studying primary recognition of alloantigens. Indeed, depleting a spleen cell population of rosette forming cells formed toward a given antigen induces unresponsiveness of this population, as demonstrated by transferring the depleted cells into an irradiated host.[3] It has even been shown that T lymphocytes may form "autorosettes" with the animal's own red blood cells.[29] This has been considered evidence that an individual actually recognizes its own antigens, as well as foreign antigens, and that tolerance to the "self" is not due to nonrecognition but rather to the absence of subsequent immune reaction when the recognized antigens are those of the individual itself.

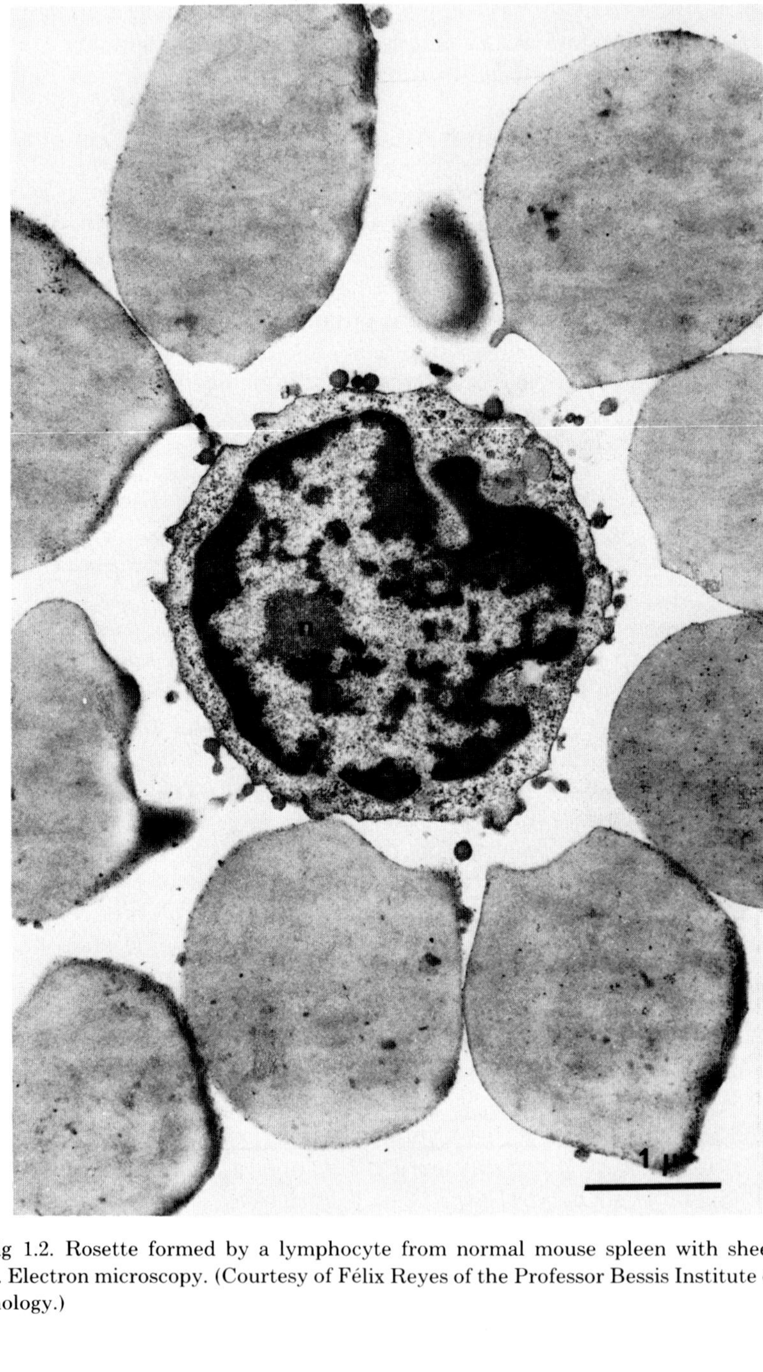

Fig 1.2. Rosette formed by a lymphocyte from normal mouse spleen with sheep red cells. Electron microscopy. (Courtesy of Félix Reyes of the Professor Bessis Institute of Cell Pathology.)

The graft antigens recognized by the recipient T lymphocytes will be discussed in the following chapter. They are mainly "histocompatibility antigens," present on the surface of practically all nucleated cells, including—if the grafted organ is a kidney—cells forming the renal parenchyma of the donor. It has been claimed, however, that donor lymphocytes present within the graft could play a major role by promoting recognition and reaction of alloantigens by the recipient lymphocytes. As early as 1957, Snell suggested that "passenger leukocytes" might be involved as a source of antigen in skin grafts. This hypothesis has been confirmed in experiments using mouse radiation chimera. Skin from a CBA mouse, whose leukocytes have been replaced by those of a C3H mouse, loses much of its immunizing capacity when grafted to a C3H mouse.[54] Guttmann and Lindquist have produced evidence that the same phenomenon may be involved in kidney grafts.[31] Experiments, again using radiation chimera in rats, suggest that the most immunogenic cells in the renal allograft are the passenger leukocytes. In the following chapter we shall describe the special role of the so-called Ia (in the mouse) or DR (in man) histocompatibility antigens in the induction of allogeneic recognition by the recipient. These antigens, which are essentially present on B lymphocytes, might represent one of the most important elements recognized by host immunocompetent cells within the grafted kidney.

Reaction of the Recipient's Lymphocytes

In the same manner as observed in vitro in MLC, allogeneic recognition in vivo is followed by a *blast transformation* of the recipient lymphocytes and the appearance of specifically *cytotoxic lymphocytes* whose activity is directed against any cell bearing the donor alloantigens.

Blast transformation takes place in vivo in allografted animals, as described above in the in vitro model of MLC. Evidence for this has been produced in kidney allografts in sheep by the Australian research workers Pedersen and Morris[46] and in dogs in our own laboratory by D. Dimitriu and D. Pavel.[32] Lymphocytes leaving an allografted kidney can be collected by catheterizing the renal lymphatics; when the collected renal lymph is examined during rejection, it is found that normal cells have been transformed into numerous blast cells with frequent mitoses, so that the collected lymph resembles in every way a MLC examined on the 6th or 7th day. We have also shown that this lymph is capable of incorporating up to 50 times as much labeled thymidine as lymph from control kidneys.

We have confirmed this finding in man.[35] In five allografted patients, a catheter was placed in an efferent lymphatic from the kidney at the time of transplantation and was brought out the abdominal wall. In this way we were able to collect lymph from the graft for 7 days after transplantation. One of these patients had received a cadaver kidney (Fig. 1.3). The lymph contained only normal lymphocytes for the first few days, but on the 5th day there was transformation exactly like that found in MLC culture in vitro. Up to 16% of the cells underwent blast transformation and the incorporation of tritiated thymidine increased from 165 to 2258 cpm. A few hours later, there was a similar rise in the incorporation of thymidine in the leukocytes of the circulating blood. Three other patients received allografts from related living donors. In one of these cases, the MLC in vitro showed no significant stimulation before transplantation (1.6% of cells transformed), and no blast transformation was found in the lymph from the grafted kidney; in another case, there was stimulation in vitro before transplantation (28.5% of cells transformed), and the transformation was equally evident in vivo in the lymph. This seems to show that the phenomena observed in culture in vitro are an accurate model of what happens in vivo in the lymphocytes of the lymph from the human allografted kidney. When the sex of donor and

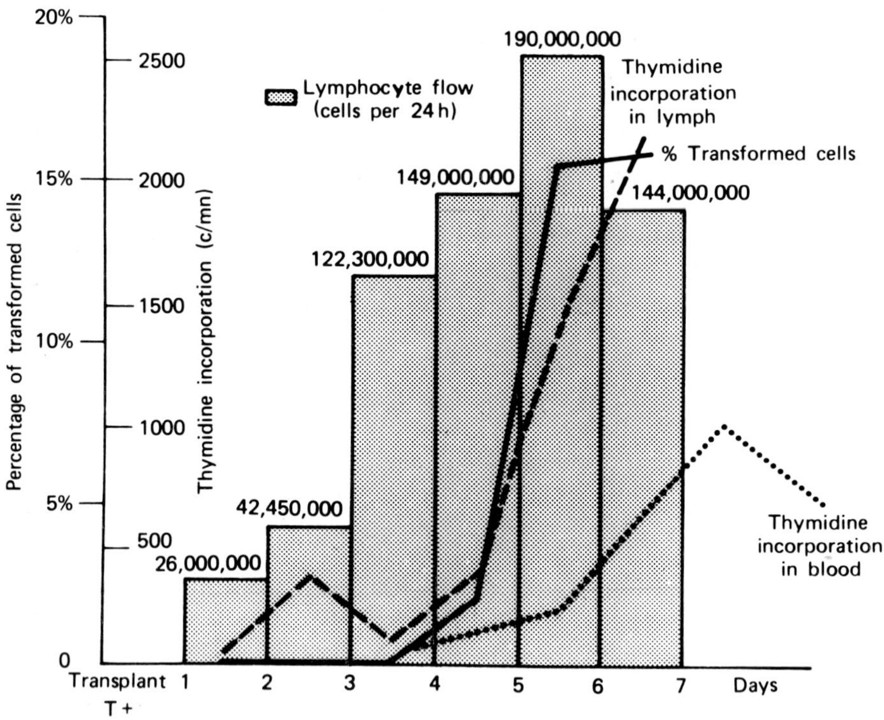

Fig. 1.3. Drainage of a lymphatic from an allografted human kidney. Output of lymph cells, percentage of transformation of lymphocytes and degree of incorporation of tritiated thymidine in the lymph collected and in the blood. (Redrawn from Hamburger et al.[35])

recipient was different, the study of sex chromatin showed that apparently all transformed lymphocytes found in the renal lymph belonged to the recipient.

Appearance of cytotoxic cells, specifically directed against the donor, has been demonstrated by many authors. Following skin allografting in rats, cytotoxic lymphocytes are found in lymph nodes as early as the 4th day, with a maximum on day 7 and a slow subsequent diminution once the skin has been rejected (solid line on Fig. 1.4). Allogeneic transplantation of kidneys in rats induces a similar phenomenon, with spleen or lymph node lymphoid cells acquiring specific cytotoxicity which appears at day 3 or 4, reaches a peak at 5 days (the very time of rejection in the donor-recipient combination studied) and declines sharply to low levels 3 weeks after renal grafting.[8] Within human renal allografts undergoing rejection, specifically cytotoxic lymphocytes have also been found.[56] The cytolytic effect of these lymphocytes recovered from rejected human renal allografts, measured on ^{51}Cr labeled peripheral blood lymphocytes bearing donor antigens, was closely correlated with the histologic grade of rejection. This correlation would suggest that cytotoxic lymphocytes are an important element in cellular rejection.

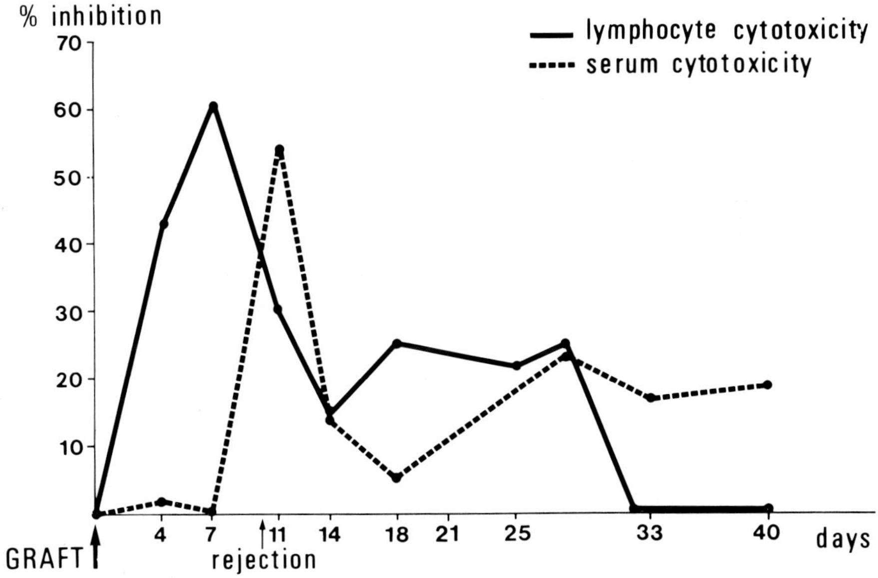

Fig. 1.4. Kinetics of cytotoxic activity of lymph node lymphocytes (——) and serum CDC (– – –) of Lewis rats after allografting skin from (Lewis × August) F_1 rats. Cytotoxicity is evaluated by inhibition of growth of August rat fibroblasts. (Reprinted by permission from: J. Hamburger. The immunological basis of transplantation. Proceedings of the Fifth International Congress on Nephrology, Mexico, vol. 1, p. 86. Karger, Basel, 1972.)

Humoral Response: Role of Circulating Antibodies

It was long believed that allograft rejection depends on cell-mediated immunity and not on humoral immunity. Circulating antibodies directed against donor antigens were said to be absent from the blood of transplanted subjects at the time of rejection. Allograft immunity could be transmitted to a third animal by transferring lymphocytes from the recipient but was not transmitted by plasma injections.

After closer study, however, it now seems certain that humoral antibodies may have an important role in the fate of a transplant, such as an allografted kidney. In fact, several types of antibodies may be involved: antibodies leading to local activation of complement (complement-dependent antibodies, or CDA), antibodies rendering the target vulnerable to nonsensitized cells (antibody-dependent cell-mediated cytotoxicity, or ADCC) and enhancing or blocking antibodies exerting, contrary to the first two types, a protective effect on the graft.

Complement-dependent antibodies are found in the blood of animals following skin (dotted line on Fig. 1.4) or kidney allografting.[8, 18] In human recipients of renal allografts these antibodies are found only with sensitive methods such as that of Rogentine and Plocinik[51] modified by Descamps et al.[19] With the latter technique, we have found CDA in 4% of sera when patients had a well functioning renal graft and in 50% of cases when the graft function was mediocre or poor.[19] Positive results were frequently observed during rejection crises, especially at the beginning of the rejection episode.

The absence of detectable CDA in the circulating blood of recipients rejecting their allograft may sometimes be explained by an immediate fixation of such antibodies on the grafted organ, behaving as a target. We shall see that immunoglobulin deposits may be demonstrated in such kidneys by immunofluorescent techniques, even when no circulating antibodies have been found. It may even happen that circulating antibodies become detectable only after the removal of a transplanted kidney destroyed by rejection.[21, 63]

The deleterious effect of CDA is underlined by the phenomenon of hyperacute rejection observed when the recipient has preformed antibodies against the donor antigens before transplantation. We shall see that the search for such preformed antibodies must imperatively be checked before any decision of transplantation. The mechanism of these very rapid rejections may be a hyperacute vasculitis with accumulation of platelets and polymorphs on the vascular endothelium reacting to circulating antibodies, with the possible participation of complement.[41, 43, 53, 63)]

Antibodies inducing the ADCC phenomenon may also be found with a similar sensitive technique. Contrary to the preceding findings, these antibodies were observed by Descamps et al[19] in cases with excellent graft function as frequently as in patients with mediocre or poor graft function (positive test in 31% of sera in the former case versus 18% in the latter). These results suggest that this type of antibody may be less deleterious than the CDA. Confirmation of the data observed in our group has now been reported by several authors.[55] It is now clear that the appearance of antibodies detected by the ADCC test and appearing *after* organ transplantation may be seen in successful as well as in unsuccessful cases.

The case of the same antibodies discovered *before* transplantation is not yet as clear. Initially this was considered as potentially responsible for acute rejection, exactly like the finding of CDA before transplantation. The ADCC technique was nothing but a much more sensitive method than the CDA technique. Both represented evidence for a dangerous specific presensitization, and a positive "cross-match" test with donor cells with either method in the prospective recipient led to abandoning the proposed graft.[59] It remains true that a positive ADCC test before transplantation may be followed by rejection,[58] but several cases have been reported where a positive pretransplant test (positive ADCC with negative CDA) did not prevent excellent graft survival.[37] It may be provisionally concluded that a positive ADCC test with donor cells in the prospective recipient is not as imperative a contraindication as is a positive CDA test.

Enhancing antibodies are those that may exert a protective action on graft survival. This effect can easily be demonstrated in some experimental models. In rats, for example, the serum obtained from the recipient strain immunized against the donor strain cells may prolong skin allografts by several days.[14, 18, 64] The survival of allografted kidneys may even be indefinite in rats treated by such methods of "passive enhancement"[30] or by mixed protocols of passive and active enhancement.[57] "Active enhancement" relates to cases in which prolonged allograft survival has been observed following injection of donor antigens to the recipient prior to transplantation; this effect is interpreted as being due to enhancing antibodies produced by the recipient animal itself instead of being passively received by the animal in the form of enhancing sera. Here again some species like the rat have been found remarkably well suited to successful active enhancement.[13]

In man, some authors using an in vitro "cell-inhibition" test suggested that "blocking antibodies" were frequently found in the blood of renal allograft recipients with a long-term successful course.[48] These results, however, were not confirmed by other authors, including in our own laboratory. The role and significance of immunologic enhancement in the well tolerated human renal allograft is still, in fact, a matter of debate.

The question is of such importance that we shall discuss it in more detail in Chapter Five.

* * *

In the preceding pages we have described the various types of antibodies without discussing the type of antigens against which they are specifically directed. As will be seen in Chapter Two, "The Graft Antigens," at least three classes of antigens should in fact be considered separately: classical histocompatibility antigens, mainly controlled in the human by the regions A, B and C of the main histocompatibility complex located on chromosome 6; histocompatibility antigens controlled by the D region of that same complex and mainly found on B lymphocytes, monocytes and vascular endothelia; and finally, tissue specific antigens that, contrary to histocompatibility antigens, are characteristic of some given cells or tissues rather than of the individual as a whole. In recent years antibodies directed against the second of these three classes (antigens depending on the D genetic region and termed DR) were extensively studied by both the CDA and the ADCC tests. The search for and the role of these anti-DR antibodies now appear to be of great importance. For the purpose of clarity, however, they will be discussed subsequently, after the description of the corresponding graft antigens.

Auxiliary Role of Macrophages, Polymorphs and Platelets

Macrophages. The reader may remember that in vitro studies suggest a triple role of macrophages in the allogeneic reaction: they may facilitate antigen recognition by T lymphocytes; they acquire a nonspecific cytotoxicity under the effect of MAF released by sensitized lymphocytes in the presence of graft antigens; and finally they may control to some extent the intensity of the lymphocyte reaction.

The possibility that macrophages also play an important role in vivo is suggested by the high percentage of host macrophages invading allografts during rejection. Experimental heart allografts in the rat contain 26±3 macrophages per 100 infiltrating cells.[28] In human renal allografts, no less than 23.4 ± 4.6% of infiltrating cells are macrophages.[42] Indirect evidence has been presented for the following interpretation[26]: host macrophages are retained within the graft by the release of MIF inhibiting their migration; they may locally exert the various effects described in in vitro models, including a complementary destructive effect on graft cells by macrophages rendered cytotoxic by a local release of MAF.

Other Effector Cells. There is not yet enough data concerning the role of *granulocytes* in the antiallograft reaction to know whether they are important in rejection. A few of these cells are usually found in the cellular infiltrate of allografted organs. In human renal transplant biopsies, a mean proportion of 2.5 ± 1% of infiltrating cells are granulocytes.[42] Some authors believe that the IgE-basophil system may intervene in allograft immunology,[16] in particular by releasing certain factors such as the platelet-activating factor (PAF) which alter vascular permeability.[7] Histamine production by basophils or mastocytes may also be important.[24] The role of *platelets* is suggested by their presence together with fibrin and PMNs in glomerular capillaries during rejection crises.[34, 38, 47] They might act both by inducing local intravascular coagulation and by releasing vasoactive amines.

REFERENCES

1. Allison, A. C. Mechanism by which activated macrophages inhibit lymphocyte responses. Immunol. Rev., *40:*3, 1978.
2. Bach, F. H., and Voynow, N. K. One-way stimulation in mixed leukocyte cultures. Science, *153:*545, 1966.
3. Bach, J. F., Dardenne, M., and Muller, J. Y. In vivo specific antigen recognition by rosette-forming cells. Nature, *227:*1251, 1970.
4. Bach, J. F., Reyes, F., Dardenne, M., Fournier, C., and Muller, J. Y. Rosette formation, a model for antigen recognition. In *Symposium on Cellular Interactions in Immune Responses.* Academic Press, Helsinki, 1970.
5. Bain, B., Vas, M. R., and Lowenstein, L. The development of large immature mononuclear cells in mixed leucocyte cultures. Blood, *23:*108, 1964.
6. Balner, H., Van Leeuwen, A., Dersjant, H., and Van Rood, J. J. Defined leukocyte antigens of chimpanzees: Use of chimpanzee isoantisera for leukocyte typing in man. Transplantation, *5:*624, 1967.
7. Benveniste, J. Platelet-activating factor, a new mediator of anaphylaxis and immune complex deposition from rabbit and human basophils. Nature, *249:*581, 1974.
8. Biesecker, J. L. Cellular and humoral immunity after allogeneic transplantation in the rat. Transplantation, *15:*298, 1973.
9. Binz, H., and Wigzell, H. Shared idiotypic determinants on B and T lymphocytes reactive against the same antigenic determinants (I and II). J. Exp. Med., *142:*197, 218, 1975.
10. Biozzi, G., Stiffel, C., Mouton, C., Bouthillier, Y., and Decreusefond, C. A kinetic study of antibody producing cells in the spleen of mice immunized intravenously with sheep erythrocytes. Immunology, *14:*7, 1968.
11. Cantor, H., and Boyse, E. A. Functional subclasses of T lymphocytes bearing different Ly antigens. J. Exp. Med., *141:*1376, 1390, 1975.
12. Cantor, H., and Weissman, I. Development and function of subpopulations of thymocytes and T lymphocytes. Prog. Allergy, *20:*1, 1976.
13. Chavez-Peon, F., Monchik, G., Winn, H. J., and Russell, P. S. Humoral factors in experimental renal allograft and xenograft rejection. Third International Congress of The Transplantation Society, The Hague, 1970. Transplant. Proc., *3:*573, 1971.
14. Cohen, I., Brautbar, H., and Nelken, D. Passive immunological enhancement of skin allografts in rats. Transplantation, *11:*135, 1971.
15. Cohen, S., Pick, E., and Oppenheim, J. J. (Eds). Biology of the Lymphokines. Academic Press, New York, 1979.
16. Colvin, R. B., and Dvorak, H. F. Basophils and mast cells in renal allograft rejection. Lancet *i:*212, 1974.
17. David, J. R. The elusive humors of the lymphocyte mediators of delayed hypersensitivity. J. Allergy, *47:*237, 1971.

18. Debray-Sachs, M., Soucy, P. E., and Hamburger, J. A lymphocyte cytotoxicity rebound phenomenon induced by enhancing sera. J. Immunol., *110:*661, 1973.
19. Descamps, B., Gagnon, R., Debray-Sachs, M., Barbanel, C., and Crosnier, J. Lymphocyte-dependent and complement-dependent antibodies in human renal allograft recipients. Fifth International Congress of the Transplantation Society, Jerusalem, 1974. Transplant. Proc., *7:*635, 1975.
20. Descamps, B., Gagnon, R., Van Der Gaag, R., Meyer, O., and Crosnier, J. Influence of azathioprine and prednisone in vivo treatment on lymphocyte-dependent antibody-mediated cytotoxicity (LDAC) in 57 human renal allograft recipients. Transplant. Proc., *9:*981, 1977.
21. Dixon, F. H., McPhaul, J. J., and Lerner, R. A. The contribution of kidney transplantation to the study of glomerulonephritis. The recurrence of glomerulonephritis in renal transplants. Transplant. Proc., *1:*194, 1969.
22. Domzig, W., and Lohmann-Matthes, M.-L. Antibody-dependent cellular cytotoxicity against tumor cells. II. The promonocyte identified as effector cell. Eur. J. Immunol., *9:* 267, 1979.
23. Dorf, M. E., and Metzgar, R. S. Serological relationships of human, chimpanzee and gorilla lymphocyte isoantigens. In *Histocompatibility Testing*, edited by P. I. Terasaki. Munksgaard, Copenhagen, 1970.
24. Dy, M., Lebel, B., Kamoun, P., and Hamburger, J. Histamine production during the antiallograft response. Demonstration of a new lymphokine enhancing histamine synthesis. J. Exp. Med., Feb. 1981.
25. Dy, M., Astoin, M., Rigaud, M., and Hamburger, J. Prostaglandin release in the mixed lymphocyte culture. Eur. J. Immunol., *10:*121, 1980.
26. Dy, M., Debray-Sachs, M., and Descamps, B. Role of macrophages in allograft rejection. Seventh International Congress of the Transplantation Society, Rome, 1978. Transplant. Proc., *11:*811, 1979.
27. Evans, R., and Alexander, P. Role of macrophage in tumour immunity. Immunology, *23:*615, 1972.
28. Feuillet, M. N., Descamps, B., Camus, A. M., N'Guyen, A. T., and Lacombe, M. Etude des macrophages dans les allogreffes cardiaques expérimentales. Ann. Biol. Clin., *37:* 275, 1979.
29. Fournier, C., and Charreire, J. Activation of a human T cell subpopulation bearing receptors for antologous erythrocytes by concanavalin A. J. Immunol., *12:*771, 1978.
30. French, M. E., and Batchelor, J. R. Immunological enhancement of rat kidney grafts. Lancet, *ii:*1103, 1969.
31. Guttmann, R. D., and Lindquist, R. R. Hematopoietic origin of immunological target in enhancement of renal allografts. Third International Congress of The Transplantation Society, The Hague, 1970. Transplant. Proc., *3:*717, 1971.
32. Hamburger, J. Un tournant de l'histoire des greffes. Bull. Acad. Natl. Med. (Paris), *154:* 606, 1970.
33. Hamburger, J. "Macrophage activation:" Imperfect terminology hiding imperfect knowledge. Ann. Immunol. Inst. Pasteur, *128C:*731, 1977.
34. Hamburger, J., Crosnier, J., and Dormont, J. Experience with 45 renal homotransplantations in man. Lancet, *i:*985, 1965.
35. Hamburger, J., Dimitriu, A., Bankir, L., Debray-Sachs, M., and Auvert, J. Collection of lymph from kidneys homotransplanted in man: cell transformation in vivo. Nature, 232: 633, 1971.
36. Hamburger, J., Dy, M., Debray-Sachs, M., and Descamps, B. Research on the role of macrophages in allograft immunity. In *10th International Course on Transplantation and Clinical Immunity*, vol. 10. Excerpta Medica, Amsterdam, 1974.
36a. Jaboulay, M. Greffe de reins au pli du coude par soudures arterielles et veineuses. Lyon Méd., *107:*575, 1906.

37. Keown, P., Stiller, C. R., Sinclair, N. R. StC., Fung, D. McGirr, D., Moseley, P., Howson, W., and Ulan, R. A. Recipient presensitization and renal allograft survival. First International Symposium on Immunologic Monitoring of the Transplant Patient, London, Ontario, 1977. *Transplant. Proc., 10:*459, 1978.
38. Kincaid-Smith, P. Histological diagnosis of rejection of renal homografts in man. Lancet, *ii:*849, 1967.
39. Lipinski, M., Tursz, T., Kreis, H., Finale, Y., and Amiel, J. L. Dissociation of natural killer (NK) cell activity and antibody-dependent cell-mediated cytotoxicity (ADCC) in kidney allograft recipients receiving high dose immunosuppressive therapy. Transplantation, *29:*214, 1980.
40. Marshall, W. H., Valentine, F. T., and Lawrence, H. S. Cellular immunity in vitro. Clonal proliferation of antigen stimulated lymphocytes. J. Exp. Med., *130:*327, 1969.
41. Myburgh, J. A., Cohen, I., Gecelter, L., Meyers, A. M., Abrahams, C., Furman, K. I., Goldberg, B., and Van Blerk, P. J. P. Hyperacute rejection in human-kidney allografts. Shwartzman or Arthus reaction? N. Engl. J. Med., *281:*131, 1969.
42. Nabarra, B., and Descamps, B. Ultrastructure of cells infiltrating human kidney allografts. Clin. Exp. Immunol., *24:*300, 1976.
43. Najarian, J. S., and Foker, J. E. Mechanisms of kidney allograft rejection. Transplant. Proc., *1:*184, 1969.
44. North, R. J. The concept of the activated macrophage. J. Immunol., *121:*806, 1978.
45. Oehler, J. R., Herbeman, R. B., Campbell, D. A., and Djeu, J. Y. Inhibition of rat mixed lymphocyte cultures by suppressor macrophages. Cell. Immunol., *29:*238, 1977.
46. Pedersen, N. C., and Morris, B. The role of the lymphatic system in the rejection of homografts: a study of lymph from renal transplants. J. Exp. Med., *131:*936, 1970.
47. Porter, K. A., Dossetor, J. B., Marchioro, T. L., Peart, W. S., Kendall, J. M., Starzl, T. E., and Terasaki, P. I. Human renal transplants. I. Glomerular changes. Lab. Invest., *16:*153, 1967.
48. Quadracci, L. J., Tremann, J. A., Marchiori, T. L., and Striker, G. E. Serum blocking factors in human recipients of renal allografts. Transplantation, *17:*361, 1974.
49. Rich, S. S., David, C. S., and Rich, R. R. Regulatory mechanisms in cell-mediated immune responses. VII. Presence of 1-C subregion determinants on mixed leukocyte reaction suppressor factor. J. Exp. Med., *149:*114, 1979.
50. Rinehart, J. J., Orser, M., and Kaplan, M. E. Human monocyte and macrophage modulation of lymphocyte proliferation. Cell. Immunol., *44:*131, 1979.
51. Rogentine, G. N., and Plocinik, B. A. Application of the ^{51}Cr cytotoxicity technique to the analysis of human lymphocyte isoantigens. Transplantation, *5:*1323, 1967.
52. Sasportes, M., Wollman, E., Cohen, D., Fradelizi, D., Carosella, E., Cathely, G., and Dausset, J. Mise en évidence d'un facteur soluble capable d'inhiber le prolifération lymphocytaire allogénique chez l'homme. C.R. Acad. Sci., Paris, *289 (Serie D):*41, 1979.
53. Starzl, T. E., Lerner, R. A., Dixon, F. J., Groth, C. G., Brettschneider, L., and Terasaki, P. I. Schwartzman reaction after human renal homotransplantation. N. Engl. J. Med., *278:*642, 1968.
54. Steinmuller, D., and Hart, E. A. Passenger leukocytes and induction of allograft immunity. Third International Congress of The Transplantation Society, The Hague, 1970. Transplant. Proc., *3:*673, 1971.
55. Stiller, C. R., Dossetor, J. B., and Sinclair, N. R. StC. (Eds). First International Symposium on Immunologic Monitoring of the Transplant Patient, London, Ontario, 1977. Transplant. Proc., *10:*301, 1978.
56. Strom, T. B., Tilney, N. L., Carpenter, C. B., and Busch, G. J. Identity and cytotoxic capacity of cells infiltrating renal allografts. N. Engl. J. Med., *292:*1257, 1975.
57. Stuart, F. P., Saitoh, F., and Fitch, F. W. Rejection of renal allografts: Specific immunologic suppression. Science, *160:*1463, 1968.
58. Thomas, F., Thomas, J., Mendez, G., and Lee, H. M. Pretransplant immune monitoring

of donor-recipient compatibility. First International Symposium on Immunologic Monitoring of the Transplant Patient, London, Ontario, 1977. Transplant. Proc., *10:*429, 1978.

59. Ting, A., and Terasaki, P. I. Influence of lymphocyte-dependent antibodies on human kidney transplants. Transplantation, *18:*371, 1974.
60. Togawa, A., Oppenheim, J. J., and Mizel, S. B. Characterisation of lymphocyte-activating factor (LAF) produced by human mononuclear cells: Biochemical relationship of high and low molecular weight forms of LAF. J. Immunol., *122:*2112, 1979.
61. Wagner, H., and Röllinghoff, M. T-T-cell interactions during in vitro cytotoxic allograft responses. J. Exp. Med., *148:*1523, 1978.
62. Waksman, B. H. Modulation of immunity by soluble mediators. Pharmacol. Ther. A., *2:*623, 1978.
63. Williams, G. M., Hume, D. M., Hudson, R. P., Jr., Morris, P. J., Kano, K., and Milgrom, F. "Hyperacute" renal-homograft rejection in man. N. Engl. J. Med., *279:*611, 1968.
64. Zimmerman, B., and Feldman, J. D. Enhancing antibody. I. Bioassay for normal skin grafts. J. Immunol., *102:*507, 1969.

CHAPTER TWO

The Graft Antigens

Jean Hamburger

Origin of the concept of histocompatibility—Major histocompatibility locus in mice, or H-2 locus—HLA system in man—Biochemistry of histocompatibility antigens—Significance of histocompatibility antigens—Are other types of antigens involved in graft rejection?

ORIGIN OF THE CONCEPT OF HISTOCOMPATIBILITY

Originally, there was no reason to think that the antigen system responsible for graft rejection was necessarily the same for all organs and all tissues. Only gradually did the idea develop that most of these antigens are characteristic of an individual and not of any particular tissue or organ. The simplest, and now traditional, demonstration of this concept is "second set" rejection. An animal which has rejected a first allograft is sensitized and rejects more rapidly a second graft from the same donor. This sensitization, following a skin graft for example, will cause accelerated rejection of any tissue from the same donor, whether spleen, liver, kidney or other. On the other hand, there is generally no acceleration of the rejection of a graft from another animal within the same species chosen at random. Thus, the tissues of a given individual have in common at least some antigens capable of provoking graft rejection. These antigens, which are specific for the individual and not for one or another organ or tissue, have been named histocompatibility antigens.

The systematic description of these antigens is a long story that begins in 1916 with the work of Little and Tyzzer,[15] who showed that mammary cancer of the Japanese waltzing mouse could be grafted to another mouse of the same race but not to the common laboratory mouse. The first generation hybrid (or F_1), obtained by crossing a waltzing mouse with a common mouse, would also accept the graft; but the F_2 generation, resulting from the union of F_1 with a common mouse, accepted the tumor in only 2% of the cases. This work was important in demonstrating the genetic determination of histocompatibility antigens; in addition, it set out for the first time the model of an experimental technique which was to form the basis of the genetic analysis of histocompatibility. By continuous inbreeding of the progeny of single pairs, "pure" strains were developed in which all the animals carried the same histocompatibility antigens. These animals, called syngenic or *syngeneic*, no longer rejected grafts taken from one another. The next stage was to develop strains which differed from one another only by a single histocompatibility locus—coisogenic strains*. This was achieved by careful crossing of various syngenic strains, followed by study of the rejection patterns of grafts among the progeny of these crosses. Step by step, it was finally possible to assemble the chromosome chart of the genes coding for histocompatibility antigens.

A first locus was isolated in mice by Gorer et al[9] and was named locus H-2. It is located on the mouse chromosome number 17. It carries strong histocompatibility factors which may provoke rejection of a skin graft in about 10 days. Ten other loci have been described in mice and 16 others are currently being studied. But none of these non-H-2 loci possesses the strength of the H-2 locus; grafts between mice sharing the same H-2 and differing in other histocompatibility loci will show only slow rejection, if any (for example after 20 days for a difference in H-4, 33 days for a difference in H-7 and more than 250 days for differences in H-1, H-9 or H-12).

Many other animal species have now been extensively studied. In all of them there is also a "major histocompatibility locus" similar to the H-2 system in mice. It has been named Rt-1 (or H-1 or Ag-B) in rats, DL-A in dogs, RL-A in rabbits, RhL-A in macacus rhesus monkeys, and so on. But none of these major histocompatibility systems is known as well as the mouse H-2. It is worth a brief description because it has remarkable similarities with the corresponding locus in man and has served as a model for human studies.

MAJOR HISTOCOMPATIBILITY COMPLEX IN MICE, OR H-2 LOCUS

The H-2 locus in mice is, in fact, a complex system including three categories of genes.

The *first category* consists mainly of two loci, H-2K and H-2D, responsible for the synthesis of histocompatibility antigens located on the surface of all cells of the animal. This category was the first to be thoroughly described because its study is facilitated by the easy produc-

* True coisogenicity is the result of punctual mutation in a pure strain. Partial coisogenicity may be obtained by serial cross breedings, during which the genetic makeup of a strain is maintained, except for a single gene taken from another strain. Partially coisogenic strains (i.e., those that differ not only at one locus but also probably with respect to a chromosomal segment of undetermined length adjacent to this locus) are called "congenic." Congenic mice that differ in a histocompatibility locus, and thus reject tissue grafts from the complementary strain, are said to be "congenic resistant."

tion of alloantibodies against these antigens coded by the K and D genes, hence the possibility of detecting these antigens with antisera, using classical serologic methods. The term "sero-defined," or SD antigens, has long been used for that reason.

H-2K and H-2D loci both have a large number of alleles (some 29 known for H-2K and 22 for H-2D). Since the presence of one given gene is always expressed by the corresponding antigen ("codominant" heredity), a large number of individual antigenic combinations are possible within only the K and D systems. In fact, the number of possible H-2 antigen patterns is even much greater because of the other categories of genes present within the H-2 complex.

The *second category* has long been termed LD (lymphocyte-defined) because it induces the cellular allogeneic response (detectable in vitro with the mixed lymphocyte reaction rather than with serologic methods). Hence, these LD antigens are opposed to the above described SD antigens. The genetic location of LD antigens differs from that of H-2K and H-2D antigens. Their main localization is in the region between the K and D loci, termed the I region. Hence, the LD genes located in the I region are now commonly termed Ia genes. The Ia antigens coded by Ia genes, contrary to K and D antigens, are not present on all cells. They are found mainly on B lymphocytes. More details about this type of histocompatibility antigen will be given below in the description of the human system. Studies in the mouse suggested the opposition between the first and the second categories of histocompatibility genes, but Ia alleles eventually proved more difficult to analyze in detail than the corresponding human genes.

The story of the I region is in fact related to the discovery of the genes termed Ir genes, which control the intensity of some immune responses. Some authors now believe that Ia antigens may be nothing other than products of the Ir genes.

Other genes in the H-2 region code for several components of serum complement and for various molecules which are not apparently involved in immune reactions. As we shall see now, these studies in the mouse have served as a remarkable introduction to the study of the major histocompatibility locus in man, termed the HLA system.

HLA SYSTEM IN MAN

The first human histocompatibility antigen was discovered by Jean Dausset in 1958.[5] He was studying leukocyte antigens in an effort to determine whether "groups" of individuals could be defined by applying serologic techniques to these cells, somewhat as red cell blood groups had been discovered at the beginning of the century. It so happened that Dausset was working in the hospital where we (J.H., J.C.) were studying allografts and searching for immunologic methods of donor selection. The hypothesis was raised that the series of leukocyte antigens studied by Jean Dausset were, in fact, histocompatibility antigens. This hypothesis was confirmed when skin grafts were found to be rejected earlier where antigenic differences between donor and recipient had been revealed by the battery of antisera detecting leukocyte groups. This discovery soon assumed considerable importance. It led the way to the serologic analysis of histocompatibility antigens in man.

From our early efforts at human kidney transplantation, the collaboration of Jean Dausset has enabled us to choose donors according to the results of leukocyte typing. This probably explains why, at that time, our results were slightly better than those in Boston, the only city other than Paris in which renal allografts were being essayed in man. In the case of the first successful transplant from a non-twin donor, the volunteer donor was chosen after serologic typing, admittedly very rudimentary at that time. Eighteen years later the grafted kidney is still functioning well.

The method was rapidly improved. After Dausset's 1958 publication announcing his discovery of the first human histocompatibility antigen, the antigen Mac ("Mac" was formed from the initials of the first three subjects in whom the antigen was identified),[5] we witnessed the development of an astonishing international effort. It has resulted in a detailed analysis of the major human histocompatibility system, the HLA (human leukocyte A) system.

General Description of the HLA Genetic Region

The HLA system is genetically located in the small arm of the sixth chromosome in man. It has remarkable similarities to the H-2 system in mice. Like H-2 genes, HLA genes are all polyallelic and codominant (if an allele is present in the chromosome it is always expressed on the cell surface). Like the H-2 system, the HLA region includes three categories of genes, those inducing SD antigens, serologically defined (HLA-A, B and C); those inducing LD antigens, defined by the lymphocyte reaction like mouse Ia antigens (HLA-D), although serologic methods may now also define D-related (DR) antigens, depending on a gene closely related (or identical) to the D gene; and finally a third category, including among others the gene responsible for C_2,C_4 and factor B of the complement system.

The First Category of HLA Antigens: HLA-A, B and C

HLA-A and HLA-B were the two histocompatibility loci first studied. The corresponding antigens easily induce specific antibodies in individuals who do not possess the antigen considered. Hence, batteries of antisera allow satisfactory typing of this series of antigens in any given individual. HLA-A has 20 well known alleles producing 20 different HLA-A antigens termed Al, A2, A3, A9, A10, A11, AW19, AW23, AW24, A25, A26, A28, A29, AW30, AW31, AW32, AW33, AW34, AW36 and AW43. HLA-B has 41 alleles and the 41 corresponding HLA-B antigens are called BW4, B5, BW6, B7, B8, B12, B13, B14, B15, BW16, B17, B18, BW21, BW22, B27, BW35, B37, BW38, BW39, B40, BW41, BW42, BW44, BW45, BW46, BW47, BW48, BW49, BW50, BW51, BW52, BW53, BW54, BW55, BW56, BW57, BW58, BW59, BW60, BW61 and BW63†. These antigens cover more than 95% of the human population. The "blank," corresponding to antigens not yet clearly defined, is now less than 5%, for HLA-A as well as for HLA-B.

The HLA-C gene, located between A and B, has been more recently described. Only eight alleles (and antigens) are known (CW1, CW2, CW3, CW4, CW5, CW7 and CW8), and the "blank" is still high, approximately 50% of genotypes.

Each individual has two HLA *haplotypes*,‡ one inherited from the father and the other from the mother. Since each haplotype induces three antigenic structures, A, B and C, the typing of one given individual will reveal 2 HLA-A antigens, 2 HLA-B antigens (and 2 HLA-C, but these are less routinely typed). For example, an individual will be HLA-A 2, 9 and HLA-B 8, 12. Figure 2.1 shows how these antigens are distributed within a family. A child always shares one HLA haplotype with his mother and one with his father: one parent and one child are said to be "semi-identical" (or haploidentical). Siblings may have 0 or 1 or 2 HLA haplotypes in common; they are termed HLA-different in the first case, HLA-semi-identical in the second and HLA-identical in the third.

The Second Category of HLA Antigens: HLA-D/DR

As already mentioned, the HLA system includes structures which, contrary to HLA-A, B and C, do not easily induce antibody formation in other individuals, but rather stimulate blast transformation of allogeneic

---

† The letter W in the name of an antigen indicates that the nomenclature is perhaps not final but is a provisional number proposed during an international workshop (histocompatibility testing workshops take place regularly). Another remark: The reader may have noticed that the above lists of specificities exceed the announced numbers of antigens. This is because some specificities have been shown to represent subsets of others. HLA-A9 includes AW23 and AW24; HLA-A10 includes A25 and A26; HLA-B5 includes BW51 and BW52; HLA-BW16 includes BW38 and BW39; and HLA-BW21 includes BW49 and BW50. More generally, the definition of histocompatibility antigens has been hindered by the phenomenon of *cross reactions*, i.e., antigenic determinants apparently common to different HLA specificities. The latter concept presently has important practical significance. However, it may be predicted that the use of "monoclonal antibodies" will progressively reduce this difficulty and clarify the distinction between the true HLA specificities.

‡ A haplotype is the set of genes present on a single chromosome.

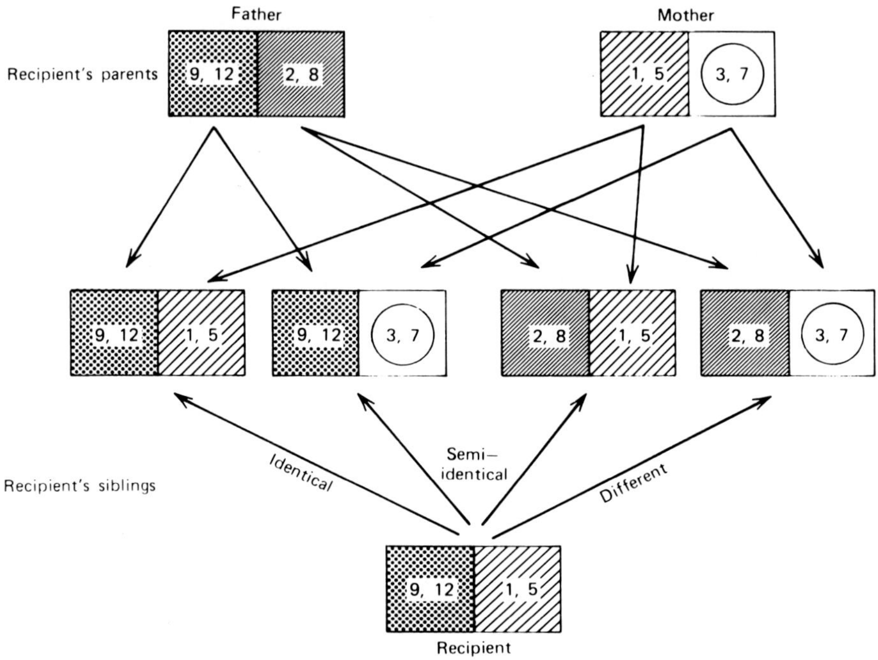

Fig. 2.1. HLA genotype. A parent (father or mother) donor always has one HLA haplotype in common with the child recipient. A sibling donor may have 0 (HLA-different donor), 1 (HLA semi-identical donor) or 2 (HLA-identical donor) HLA haplotypes in common with the recipient.

lymphocytes in MLC (mixed lymphocyte cultures). These LD antigens are similar to the LD antigens of mice and more precisely to the Ia antigen. In the human they have been termed HLA-D.

Contrary to the mouse LD genes, the HLA-D locus is not located between but outside the two main SD loci, between the HLA-B locus and the chromosome centromere (Fig. 2.2). The whole region is, of course, frequently transmitted as a whole in a family, so that HLA-D rarely differs between two members of the family when HLA-A and B are identical. In other words, the mixed lymphocyte reaction (MLR) is negative (little blast transformation and low thymidine incorporation) when HLA-A and B are identical, exception in only 7% of cases. Conversely, MLR is frequently positive between unrelated individuals in spite of identical HLA-A and B antigens. This was the first evidence that HLA-D is independent from HLA-A and B. This independence is, however, not complete, and the fact that MLR is negative in 10% of cases when the two unrelated individuals share identical A and B antigens is

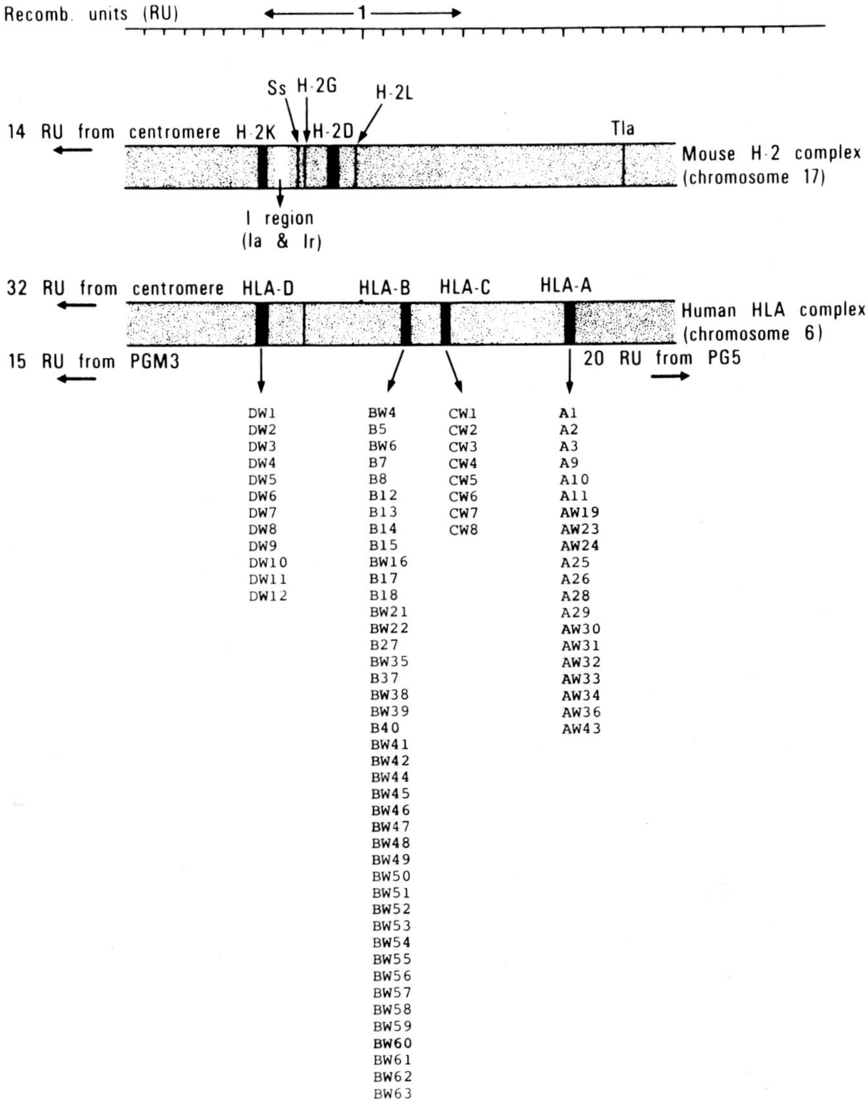

Fig. 2.2. The mouse H-2 complex and the human HLA complex in 1980.

interpreted as a "linkage disequilibrium"§ between the D locus and the A and B loci.

HLA-D typing requires special techniques. One of them uses cells

---

§ Preferential genetic association, the frequency of association of two genes in the population studied being greater than predicted based on the individual frequency of each of these genes.

homozygous with respect to the HLA-D locus as stimulatory cells in MLR; a negative MLR with such cells defines the D locus of the tested lymphocytes. Another method, termed PLT (primed LD typing), is based on MLR between the cells to be typed (previously mitomycin-treated) and stored cells specifically presensitized by cells of known HLA-D; the MLR is of the secondary response type (accelerated reaction) if the cells to be tested possess the same HLA-D. These techniques have led to the description of twelve D specificities, respectively termed HLA-DW1, DW2, DW3, DW4, DW5, D6, DW7, DW8, DW9, DW10, DW11 and DW12. It is likely that more D specificities will be found in the coming years. It is even possible that several D loci will eventually be described.

The DR (D-related) locus is detectable by serologic methods, exactly like A, B and C, although satisfactory anti-DR sera are not yet as readily available as are the anti A or B test sera. DR is probably very close to D since D or DR testing usually coincides. Some authors have even suggested that they corresponded to a single locus. Evidence against this suggestion has now been presented, but it does not diminish the value of DR typing, which is much easier than D typing for exploring the D region. Ten HLA-DR specificities have been described and termed DR1, DR2, DR3, DR4, DR5, DRW6, DR7, DRW8, DRW9 and DRW10. DR1 is usually associated with DW1, DR2 with DW2 and so on.

Contrary to HLA-A, B and C antigens, HLA-D structures are not equally found on the surface of all cells. They are mainly present on B lymphocytes, macrophages, skin Langerhans cells and spermatocytes. They are practically nonexistent on quiescent T lymphocytes and on platelets, which may thus be used to absorb anti-A, B and C antibodies from antisera without removing anti-HLA-DR antibodies. The amount of HLA-D antigens in the renal tissue has not been established, but it may be of interest that in pigs, analogues of I region antigen of the mouse have been detected on kidney parenchymal cells, while they are not detectable in other organs such as the liver.[7]

The respective significance of HLA-A, B and C antigens, on the one hand, and HLA-D, on the other, will be discussed in the following pages.

There is also a possibility that "immune response" genes (Ir), controlling the magnitude of antibody formation against one given antigen, exist in the same genetic region of man as they do in mice. But their study is just beginning and appears difficult in the human.[2]

Other Loci of the HLA Region

Histocompatibility antigens are not the only molecules coded for by the HLA region. Genes responsible for some important components of complement are probably located between HLA-B and HLA-D. They control C_2, C_4 and factor B (C_3-proactivator) of the complement system. They also control erythrocyte antigens Chido and Rodgers, which are now known to be fragments of C_4 secondarily fixed on red blood cells.

Finally, various enzymes are also coded in the HLA genetic region, particularly the erythrocyte glyoxalase (GLO) and the third enzyme of phosphoglucomutase (PGM3).

BIOCHEMISTRY OF HISTOCOMPATIBILITY ANTIGENS

Extensive biochemical research has permitted isolation and characterization of mouse and human histocompatibility antigens using treatment with proteolytic enzymes such as papain or detersive agents, like deoxycholate or triton, followed by chromatography, electrophoresis or sucrose gradient analysis.[18] The whole sequence of amino acids of several H-2 and HLA antigens such as HLA-A2, B7 and B12 has now been established.

Human HLA-A and B are glycoproteins whose molecular weights approximate 45,000 (like mouse H-2K and D antigens). These molecules are associated on the surface of the cell with a light chain common to all these antigens, $\beta 2$-microglobulin (molecular weight 11,600); this light chain is linked with the heavy HLA chain in a noncovalent way. Figure 2.3 shows that the overall structure is somewhat similar to that of immunoglobulins.

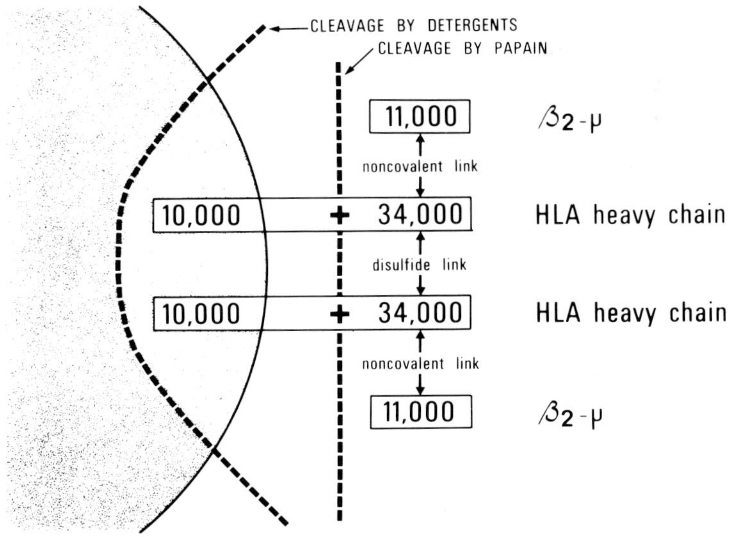

Fig. 2.3. Hypothetical arrangement of the HLA antigens on the cell surface. β_2-μ: β_2-microglobulin. (Inspired by Lars Rask et al. The subunit structure of transplantation antigens. Transplant. Rev., *21*:85, 1975.)

HLA-DR antigens are different. They are constituted of two chains of 28,000 and 33,000 daltons respectively. No β2-microglobulin is associated. Such a structure is identical to that of mouse Ia antigens.

SIGNIFICANCE OF HISTOCOMPATIBILITY ANTIGENS

Respective Significance of the First (HLA-A, B and C) and Second (HLA-D) Categories in Allograft Rejection

It is generally accepted that HLA-A, B and C structures present on the surface of all nucleated cells are the target molecules of the antiallograft immune reaction responsible for rejection.[18] This is clearly demonstrated with regard to the humoral contribution to rejection: recipient antibodies directed against donor A or B antigens usually induce hyperacute rejection when they are preformed prior to a renal transplantation, as already mentioned. Conversely, the presence of anti-HLA-DR antibodies before a renal transplantation does not prevent satisfactory graft tolerance;[19] it should, however, be mentioned that some consider preformed anti-DR antibodies as potentially harmful,[4] while, on the contrary, others believe that these antibodies may enhance tolerance.[12] The targets of cytotoxic lymphocytes are probably also antigens of the first category. This was at least demonstrated in vitro in the study of lymphocyte cytotoxicity produced in an MLC test. In summary, HLA-A, B and C antigens are the main target of the rejection reaction. This does not mean that they do not play important roles in the initial phase of the allogenic response, in addition to the early differentiation of cytotoxic T cell or B cell precursors, but this function is not as clear as for HLA-D antigens or for helper T cells.

D antigen stimulated T cells will proliferate (hence their major contribution to MLR) and produce various factors, particularly helper factors. HLA-D products probably also possess other functions, but this is suggested by research on mouse structures (Ia) homologous to HLA-D rather than actually demonstrated in man. In mice, the I genetic region, where Ia products are coded, has an overall regulatory function on immune responses.[13] It controls cell interactions among the different lymphocyte populations, between lymphocytes and macrophages and even, to a certain degree, between these cells and the antigen. Products of the I region play a role in the antigen "presentation" by macrophages, and this may be important in the mechanism by which Ir genes modulate the immune response, weak or strong, against various molecules. Ia specificities are found in soluble activating or suppressing factors, antigen specific or nonspecific, released by immunocompetent cells. Finally, I genes control the receptors binding these same soluble factors to the responding cell to which they communicate their message. In summary, Ia antigens may be considered as the tool allowing Ir genes to regulate the immune response by transmitting a sort of "password" among the various cells expressing these genes. Much work remains to be done before extending the same interpretation to the human.

General Significance of the HLA Region in Biology

The HLA genetic region has been revealed by research in transplantation, but clearly enough its initial function is not to prevent organ grafting. Its actual significance is far from being elucidated. But it is already certain that it is of the utmost importance in various fields of biology,[10] as the following examples will suffice to show.

The phenomenon of H-2 or HLA "restriction" was first described by Zinkernagel.[20] Lymphocytes infected by a virus may become cytotoxic against all cells infected by the same virus, provided that these cells are recognized as sharing the same H-2 histocompatibility antigens. A similar requirement has been found with human HLA.[16] This appears to be a general phenomenon, since H-2 or HLA identity is also a preliminary requirement for several other cellular interactions, such as lymphocyte homing into lymph nodes[8] or—and this is of interest for allograft immunology—recognition of minor non-HLA histocompatibility antigens, which paradoxically do not add their effect to that of HLA but rather appear effective only when HLA antigens of donor and recipient are identical.[3]

Other examples of the way in which the discovery of the HLA system has resulted in unexpected biologic and medical advances are: progress in the concept of genetic polymorphism (the HLA region is so polymorphic that the number of potential HLA combinations greatly exceeds the number of humans living on this earth); progress in human phylogeny and the study of movements of human populations; progress in the understanding of recognition and tolerance of the "self" and the genesis of autoimmune disease; progress in the understanding of host-parasite interactions, with the discovery that parasites may acquire the host's histocompatibility antigens and by this means escape the immune response;[17] and progress in the understanding of various diseases, whose incidence varies greatly, according to the HLA genotype of the subject.[6]

ARE OTHER TYPES OF ANTIGENS INVOLVED IN GRAFT REJECTION?

As mentioned at the beginning of this chapter, the term "histocompatibility antigens" usually refers to antigens characteristic of the individual as a whole and not of any particular organ or tissue. To say that graft rejection depends only on these antigens implies that all organs and tissues have an identical antigenic behavior in the natural history of allografting. In fact, nothing is less certain. There is evidence that specific tissue antigens are involved in the rejection of tissues such as skin[14] or thrombocytes.[11] More generally, it is clear that most tissues and organs may contain specific antigens, undetectable in other tissues or organs. In the human kidney, for example, at least 11 soluble antigens have been described, several of which appear to be totally kidney-specific.[1] The question is open as to whether or not some of these tissue antigens may present slight structural differences that would characterize various human groups, just as immunoglobulin allotypes may differentiate one group of subjects from another. If this is the case (and the phenomenon of "allotypic" determinants is so extensively found in biology that it may well be found in tissue-specific antigens), there is a possibility that some kidney antigens of the donor may become immunogenic when the kidney is transplanted if the corresponding antigens are not perfectly identical in the recipient.

REFERENCES

1. Bao-Linh Dinh, Brassard, A., Raghavan, S. R. V., Mardini, A., and Poirier, L. Immunochemical and enzymatic studies on the soluble antigens of normal human kidney. Nephron, *17:*104, 1976.
2. Benacerraf, B., and Germain, R. N. The immune response genes of the major histocompatibility complex. Immunol. Rev., *38:*70, 1978.
3. Bevan, M. J. The major histocompatibility complex determines susceptibility to cytotoxic T cells directed against minor histocompatibility antigens. J. Exp. Med., *142:*1349, 1975.
4. d'Apice, A. J. F., and Tait, B. D. The positive B-Cell cross-match: A marker of active enhancement? Transplant. Proc., *11:*954, 1979.
5. Dausset, J. Iso-leuco anticorps. Acta Haematol., *20:*156, 1958.
6. Dausset, J., and Svejgaard, A. (Eds). *HLA and Disease.* Munksgaard, Copenhagen, 1977.
7. Davies, H. S., Taylor, J. E., Daniel, M. R., and Wakerley, C. Differencs between pig tissues in the expression of major transplantation antigens: Possible relevance for organ allografts. J. Exp. Med., *143:*987, 1976.
8. Degos, L., Pla, M., and Colombani, J. M. H-2 restriction for lymphocyte homing into lymph nodes. Eur. J. Immunol., *9:*808, 1979.
9. Gorer, P. A., Lyman, S., and Snell, G. D. Studies of the genetic and antigenic basis of tumour transplantation. Linkage between a histocompatibility gene and "fused" in mice. Proc. R. Soc. B, *135:*499, 1948.
10. Hamburger, J. Some implications of transplantation research for biology and medicine. Transplant. Proc. , *9:*1313, 1977.
11. Hanna, N., and Nelken, D. Thrombocyte specific antigens. Detection of organ specific antigens by heterospecific antithrombocyte serum. Immunology, *16:*601, 1969.
12. Iwaki, Y., Terasaki, P. I., Park, M. S., and Billing, R. Enhancement of human kidney allografts by cold B lymphocyte cytotoxins. Lancet, *i:*1228, 1978.
13. Katz, D. H. *Lymphocyte Differentiation, Recognition and Regulation.* Academic Press, New York, 1977.
14. Lance, E. M., Bayse, E. A., Cooper, S., and Carswell, E. A. Rejection of skin allografts by irradiation chimeras: evidence for skin-specific transplantation barrier. Transplant. Proc., *3:*864, 1971.
15. Little, C. C., and Tyzzer, E. E. Further experimental studies on the inheritance of

susceptibility to a transplantable tumor carcinoma of the Japanese waltzing mouse. J. Med. Res., *33:*393, 1916.

16. McMichael, A. J., Ting, A., Zweerink, H. J., and Askonas, B. A. HLA restriction of cell-mediated lysis of influenza virus-infected human cells. Nature, *270:*524, 1977.
17. Sher, A., Hall, B. F., and Vadas, M. A. Acquisition of murine major histocompatibility complex gene products by schistosomula of Schistosoma mansoni. J. Exp. Med., *148:*46, 1978.
18. Snell, G. D., Dausset, J., and Nathenson, S. Histocompatibility. Academic Press, New York, 1976.
19. Ting, A., and Morris, P. J. Pre- and posttransplant B-cell antibodies in renal transplantation. Transplant. Proc., *11:*393, 1979.
20. Zinkernagel, R. M., and Klein, J. H-2 associated specificity of virus-immune cytotoxic T cells from H-2 mutant and wild mice. Immunogenetics, *4:*581, 1977.

CHAPTER THREE

Selection of a Donor

Henri Kreis

Immunologic selection of a donor—Selection using the HLA system—Other immunologic methods used in donor selection—Donor selection in everyday practice—Nonimmunologic factors in donor selection: living donors, cadaver donors.

IMMUNOLOGIC SELECTION OF A DONOR

The role of the human leukocyte A (HLA) antigens in the rejection of transplanted organs and tissues has received considerable interest in the past years. Although progress has been made in the definition of the HLA antigens, certain areas remain debated.

Selection Using the HLA System

Selection on the Basis of HLA-A, B and C Loci

Principles of the Techniques for Determining A, B and C Products. The story of typing for the products of HLA-A and B genes dates back to the early 1950s when it was demonstrated that blood transfusion and/or pregnancy could induce agglutinins against leukocyte antigens drawn from the blood of certain individuals.[20, 37, 115] Thus it became possible to produce large quantities of reliable typing antisera and consequently to define initially the four, then the six antigens controlled by the sero-defined (SD) region of the major histocompatibility complex (see p. 26).

In 1964, the introduction by Walford et al[121] of cytotoxic methods using rabbit complement for the serologic typing of human lymphocytes was a major improvement in the serologic definition of HLA antigens. Terasaki and McClelland's[98] subsequent description of a microdroplet assay provided the means enabling most centers to routinely type for HLA SD antigens. Today HLA typing is generally performed by microcytotoxicity techniques[19, 49] and in a few instances by the complement fixation test as defined by Colombani et al.[17] In both techniques, target lymphocytes are incubated with an antiserum and rabbit complement. Lymphocytes are lysed whenever they carry a membrane antigen recognized by antibodies in the serum.

In some cases, a serum might fail to react with all cells presenting a given specificity. This phenomenon has been termed "agglutination negative-adsorption positive" (ANAP) or "cytotoxicity negative-adsorption positive" (CYNAP) by van Rood.[113] Although not clearly understood, this phenomenon must be kept in mind when analyzing the results of HLA antigen typing.

Antisera used for typing can be obtained from various sources. Recipients of multiple blood transfusions frequently develop detectable antilymphocyte antibodies. A similar situation is observed in multiparous females who produce antibodies directed against fetal antigens inherited from the father but foreign to the mother. Multiparous sera are readily available in large amounts through plasmapheresis and are usually directed against a limited number of antigens.

More specific antisera can be produced by voluntary immunization with skin grafting.[105] For such purposes, donor-recipient combinations differing by only one HLA-A, B or C antigen are chosen.

Measuring the Degree of Histocompatibility. Using these methods and immune sera of increasing specificity, specialized laboratories can now determine the presence or absence of each HLA-A, B and C antigen from a study of the lymphocytes of a given subject.

Since nearly all the HLA-A and B antigens can be recognized, a phenotype of only two or three antigens is usually considered to correspond to a four-gene genotype, with two or one gene respectively homozygous. On the contrary, all HLA-C antigens cannot be determined at the present. In these conditions, the undetermined antigen(s) may be either identical with or different from the homologous antigen(s). In the former case, a blank in the phenotype does not modify the degree of histocompatibility between a prospective donor and recipient. In the latter case, however, a blank must be considered as "potential incompatibility."

In fact, matching for the C series of antigens does not seem to be important in kidney transplantation.[91] Although only a limited amount of data has so far been gathered on the subject, no evidence has emerged that C series antigens are particularly relevant to graft outcome.

Thus, at present the degree of histocompatibility refers only to the matching for A and B loci antigens.

Several methods have been used to measure the degree of compatibility between the four alleles of the A and B loci of two individuals.

1. *Determination of the number of incompatibilities,* i.e., the number of HLA antigens present in the donor which are not present in the recipient. This method has been used by Terasaki's group since 1971.[58] In

this sytem, Match Grade A represents identical antigen profiles, Grade B includes nonidentical donor-recipient pairs with no donor-to-recipient mismatched antigens, Grade C is one mismatched antigen and Grade D applies to mismatching of two or more antigens. This method underestimates the number of incompatibilities each time the donor possesses antigens which are still undefined by available sera. However, it can be used quite safely now to measure A and B loci compatibility since nearly all antigens governed by these loci have been accurately determined.

2. *Determination of the number of identical HLA antigens*, i.e., those present in both the donor and the recipient. This method assumes that all antigens not detected in the donor are incompatible with those present in the recipient. Because of the possibility of compatibility due to homozygosity in the donor, or that unknown antigens in the donor and the recipient are the same, this method underestimates the degree of compatibility between the donor and the recipient.

3. In an attempt to take all these possibilities into account, several formulas have been used to calculate the *degree of compatibility*. Rapaport and Dausset[82] suggested the use of a "net histocompatibility ratio" (NHR) calculated on the basis of incompatibilities. The NHR makes it possible to define 14 different classes of histocompatibility. It is infrequently used today.

In our own group we frequently use a formula developed by Hors et al[39] based on known gene frequencies to determine whether or not a blank allele could be due to homozygosity. This formula calculates compatibility in a fractional scale from 0 to 4, with 0 the most compatible and 4 the most incompatible.

In sum, the need to refine the method of determining compatibility and incompatibility reflects the relative difficulty of demonstrating an influence of the HLA-A and B antigens on transplantation.

Correlation of HLA-A, B and C Matching with Clinical Results. It is difficult at the present time to formulate a comprehensive view of the importance of HLA matching in kidney transplantation because much of the recent flood of data is conflicting. However, the importance of matching for the A and B series of antigens now appears quite well established. There has never been any question about the importance of HLA matching in the case of transplantation from a family donor,[20, 80, 100, 118] where HLA-identical sibling grafts do significantly better than haplo-identical (only one haplotype identical) grafts, which in turn do better than two-haplotype incompatible grafts (see below).

On the contrary, in cadaver donor transplantation, the question of matching has generated a great deal of controversy. The first reports in the late 1960s indicated a more successful graft outcome in well matched donor-recipient combinations.[9, 63, 77, 119] A few years later these preliminary reports were questioned by Terasaki's group,[96] which found no direct correlation between the number of HLA compatibilities and graft outcome. However, despite the large number of patients included in this pooled study (over 1,000), its results can be debated. In such studies it is impossible to control multiple variables, which are probably more important than tissue typing in determining the success or failure of a graft. Among these factors are a wide variety of insults in terms of trauma and ischemia that a kidney may be subject to between the accident which led to the donor's death and the actual connection of the recipient artery supply to the kidney. This bias can be minimized only by analyzing a very large number of cases originating from the fewest possible centers. Moreover, at the time of Terasaki's and other early reports, HLA specificities were not as well defined as they are now. The report of a recent study in which 11 of the principal European tissue typing laboratories collaborated concludes: "Although HLA antigen recognition is generally a reproducible procedure in Europe, the lesson to be learned is that, even with highly selected sera tested in experienced laboratories with the same technique, discordant results can be obtained."[114] If this was still true in 1976, it is probable that greater discordance was present a few years earlier.

Nevertheless, following the early reports, several studies[10, 58, 81] appearing in the early 1970s failed to show a correlation between HLA matching and graft survival. Such scepticism was common, especially in American centers. Various attempts have been made to explain this transatlantic discordance. It is generally thought[6, 108] to be due to heterogeneity in the genetic background of the American and European populations, which can account for a linkage disequilibrium between the genes of the loci controlling the A-B and the DR (D-related) antigens. Because so many different racial groups migrated to America only recently, it is less likely that identity for HLA-A and HLA-B locus antigens will be associated with HLA-D/DR identity in this population than in a comparable group of Europeans living in Europe.

Another reason for this apparent discordance is that transplant groups in the United States have not considered tissue matching to be a prime determinant in selecting donor-recipient pairs. Consequently, they have performed relatively small numbers of well matched cadaver grafts. This fact, in association with differences in the management of transplant patients in transfusion policy or in the quality of cadaver kidneys among the many cooperating centers, leads to stratification of the analyzed material at the extreme of that allowed by statistical principles.

Whatever the real explanation, within the last few years nearly all groups with sufficient experience in cadaver kidney transplantation have shown significantly better outcome in well matched than in poorly matched grafts. In Europe recent results obtained with the expanded patient population have confirmed previous results. Studying graft outcome within France Transplant, Dausset[13] found that 65% of the most compatible grafts (less than two incompatibilities)but only 47% of the most incompatible (more than two incompatibilities) survive at 5 years. In a joint London-France study including 918 first cadaver kidney grafts,[25] it was observed that 70% of zero mismatched kidneys and only 34% of three or four mismatched kidneys survived 2 years. Similar results were reported by Scandinavian transplanters[48] in their last joint analysis[88] comprising 540 transplants performed between "full house" donors and recipients. Although the difference observed between the best and the very poor matches was not very impressive (less than 20% after 2 years), the kidney survival curves paralleled the degree of HLA-A and B matching ($P = 0.02$). In fact, the number of very poor matches (three or four incompatibilities) was very low ($n = 16$). In a recent analysis of 259 first cadaver grafts reported by the Norwegian group alone, it was concluded that graft survival decreases with increasing HLA-A and B disparity.[91] The difference between compatible combinations and one or two antigen incompatible combinations reaches statistical significance at 2 years. Matching for C antigens does not seem to improve graft survival.

For the London Transplant Group[34] the rank order of survival of 769 cadaver renal grafts also corresponds to the number of matched HLA-A and B antigens between donor and recipient. The difference between the percentage of 1 year surviving kidneys in the "full house" matched grafts (63%) and in the zero identical matched grafts (25%) is among the highest reported.

The opinion of the Eurotransplant group is more equivocal. In analyzing their material they demonstrated that in recipients without leukocyte antibodies between HLA-A and B the overall correlation between matching and graft survival is not significant.[108] On the contrary, matching for the B locus only is of importance in patients with leukocyte antibodies. We shall refer again to this issue elsewhere.

In our own material (Fig. 3.1), the influence of matching on transplant outcome was not clear-cut for our overall results. In a 1976 study of 252 cadaver renal grafts, compatible recipients ($n = 135$), i.e., those with zero or one mismatched HLA-A or B antigens, had a 2-year survival of 66%, while that of 117 incompatible recipients (two, three or four mismatched antigens) was 53%. Even though the P value of this difference is 0.05, it is hardly possible to conclude that the difference between the two groups is highly significant. On the contrary, HLA matching appears to be of great importance in various subgroups of patients, as will be discussed below.

European transplant groups have thus confirmed that, at least in their

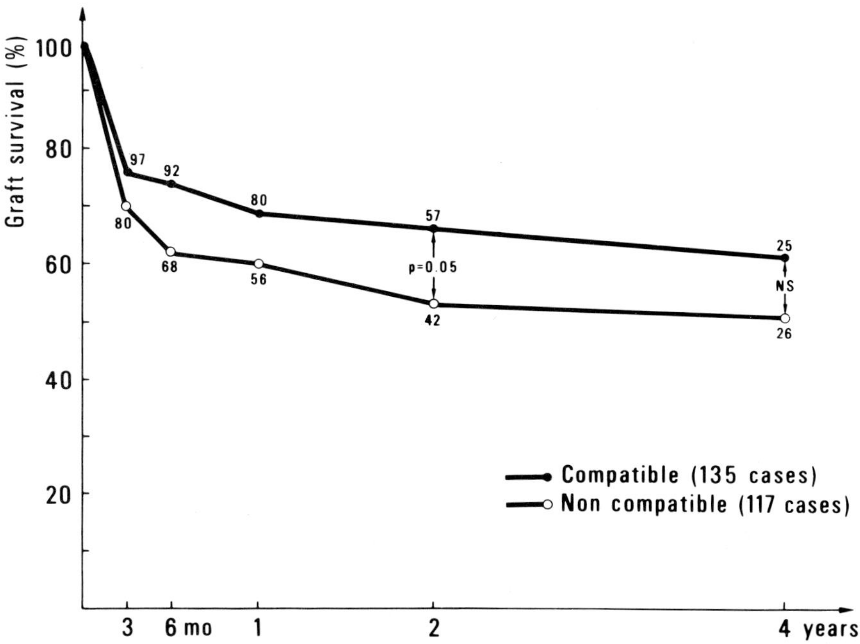

Fig. 3.1. Renal transplant survival according to donor-recipient HLA compatibility in 252 cadaver grafts performed at Necker Hospital.

population, there is a direct relationship between donor-recipient HLA matching and the results of cadaver kidney transplantation. Numerous reports published by the four major organ sharing organizations in Europe fully support this statement.

It also appears now that more and more United States transplant centers are accepting the idea that matching could improve graft prognosis. In 1975, for the first time, the 12th Renal Transplant Registry[2] indicated that prospective HLA serotyping is valuable in cadaver kidney transplantation. Opelz and Terasaki[71] have provided evidence that matching for the HLA-A and B loci is highly important, but only in certain subsets of patients. Data from a single large center such as the Minneapolis Transplantation Center[90] have recently demonstrated an overall clear superiority in patient survival and transplant function with the better matched kidneys. For example, individuals who were matched for only zero or one antigen had 61.9% kidney function survival, compared with 81.4% survival when two to four antigens were matched. Tissue matching failed to improve survival and function only in diabetic patients, who frequently die of problems unrelated to rejection.

For the Nashville group,[122] donor-recipient tissue matching affects both the rate of graft loss and the percentage of patients surviving with a functioning transplant. At 5 years, kidney survival among first cadaver grafts were 83%, 48% and 36% for, respectively, four, three and two HLA-A and B matches.

Nevertheless, the San Francisco group[87] still cannot demonstrate any influence of HLA match grade on renal allograft survival. It must be pointed out, however, that only three of their patients were four-antigen matched and 36 were three-antigen matched. These 39 compatible donor-recipient pairs were compared to 424 incompatible transplants, a method which is certainly open to criticism.

In sum, nearly all transplant reports published today are in agreement with the concept that matching for HLA antigens has a beneficial effect on the outcome of cadaver kidney transplantation. The chances of successful grafting are increased by 10 to 15% in well matched kidney recipients over those who are poorly matched. This difference might appear not sufficiently significant to merit all the effort required for exchanging compatible organs. However, it should be pointed out that, although the major histocompatibility complex is known today to have at least four loci (A, B, C and D; see p. 26), all the data analyzed above have dealt only with the A and B loci. It is also clear that certain HLA-A and B antigens or antigen combinations are probably of more importance than others.

Other immunologic factors, in addition to the immunologic status of the recipient, may also intervene to bias the results obtained in small or pooled series. It is not surprising that the controversy about HLA-A and B matching has been so long-lasting. As shown above, however, the current tendency appears to be toward closer agreement on the question. In any case, even if the benefit of A and B matching on graft survival is not patent, it has been shown that when histocompatibility is lacking, rejections are more likely to occur. The resulting need for increased immunosuppression entails severe side effects and an increased mortality rate. This has recently been re-emphasized by Van Rood et al,[117] who demonstrated that in the absence of mismatched A and B antigens, the 5-year survival of 150 patients studied was over 85%. In contrast, with three or four mismatches only 57% of patients survived after 5 years. This is certainly a much more important argument in favor of matching than a 15% increase in graft survival.

Relative Importance of Certain Antigens or Antigen Combinations. It is clear from currently available data that matching for the A and B loci is not sufficient to improve significantly the outcome of kidney transplantation. Various authors have suggested that certain antigens or antigen combinations might play a more important role than others.[25, 86, 108, 110]

Oliver et al[68] were the first to show directly that the antigens of the second locus are more important in graft rejection than are those of the first locus. These findings have been substantiated by other reports. In the study reported by Dausset et al,[25] the long-term survival of 62 "full house" grafts with one A locus incompatibility (63% at 2 years) was compared with that of 100 "full house" grafts with one B locus incompatibility (44% at 2 years). Although the difference between the two groups of recipients was not significant, the authors concluded that they found a clear trend indicating a more detrimental influence of B locus incompatibility. A similar trend was found by Sachs et al[86] and Festenstein et al.[34] The Leiden group[110] reported a highly significant ($P < 0.001$) difference between the greater influence of matching for the HLA-B as compared to the HLA-A antigens, but only for patients having circulating cytotoxic HLA antibodies.

In our own series the graft survival rates up to 10 years after transplantation are exactly the same, whether recipients are compatible or incompatible for B locus antigens (see Fig. 9.10, p. 277). This remains true whatever the status of the donor-recipient pair with regard to the A locus. Other authors[103] have also been unable to confirm reports correlating serologic HLA-B matching and improved graft survival.

The explanation that is generally given for a greater influence of the B locus antigens is based on the existence of a linkage between the B locus and the D locus, the latter being more important for graft survival.[7, 104, 110] For example, there is a linkage disequilibrium between BW35 and DW1, B7 and DW2, B8 and DW3, BW15 and DW4 and BW16 and DW5. Thus, identity for one of these B locus antigens is likely to mean an identity for the D locus antigen as well.

It has also been shown that some HLA-A and B phenotype combinations are more frequent than expected on the basis of frequencies of the individual genes.[56] That is the case, for example, for HLA-A1 and HLA-B8 or HLA-A3 and HLA-B7. Thus it has become clear that there exists a linkage disequilibrium not only between the A and B locus products but also between the latter and the products of the lymphocyte-defined (LD) locus.[3, 47] Here again, donor-recipient combinations sharing one such haplotype (1–8, 3–7 or 2–12) are more likely than other donor-recipient combinations to share an LD determinant.[21] Supporting this hypothesis are some reports demonstrating a better graft survival when the recipient of an unrelated cadaver kidney shares at least what has been called a haplophenotype with the donor.[108]

Such observations suggest that loci other than A and B are also important in determining graft survival. Among these may well be the LD loci, but other as yet undefined loci might also play a role. It is undeniable that matching for the HLA-A and B loci improves graft survival, but this is clearly not the only factor determining transplant prognosis.

Selection on the Basis of HLA-D or DR antigens

If the favorable influence of some haplotypes on the outcome of cadaver kidney grafts is the consequence of a linkage disequilibrium between HLA-A and B antigens and the mixed lymphocyte culture (MLC) or D locus, this might imply that matching for HLA-D antigens would be more effective than matching for HLA-A and B antigens.

Matching for HLA Antigens of the D Locus. The observation that the reaction in the MLC is the weakest when the tested cells come from closely related individuals[6, 22] was discussed in Chapter Two. In addition, there is increasing evidence that a weaker negative response in MLC between donor and recipient lymphocytes, probably indicating identity for the HLA-D locus (see p. 7), is extremely important in determining the outcome of the allograft.

The mixed lymphocyte reaction (MLR) can provide indirect assessment of donor-recipient matching for HLA-D antigens. A remarkable correlation between the results of MLR and the clinical outcome of kidney transplantation from living related donors has been reported by several authors,[44, 89] as well as by our group.[8, 38] In our series, a significant difference was observed between the clinical results obtained at 2 years in 23 cases having positive MLR and 27 having negative MLR (33% versus 74% graft success, $P < 0.01$). Since graft results obtained with positive MLR living donor-recipient combinations are not better than with cadaver kidneys, our group considers that living related donor transplantation is contraindicated in the presence of MLR incompatibility.

In cadaver kidney transplantation, Cochrum et al[15, 16] have shown a striking correlation between graft survival and the degree of responsiveness in bidirectional MLR. Opelz and Terasaki,[72] in a recent series of 131 cadaver donor transplants, observed a correlation between both unidirectional and bidirectional MLR cultures which, although not as strong as that reported by Cochrum et al, was statistically highly significant. Such a correlation was not found by Sachs et al[86] using one-way MLR, but they did observe a tendency toward a better 1-year graft survival in the D-compatible than in the D-incompatible group (74% versus 63%). However, all patients in this study were well matched for A and B antigens and already had a good survival. On the other hand, two recent reports failed to show any correlation between the outcome of cadaver kidney transplants and lymphocyte stimulation in MLR.[18, 45]

Thus, indirect matching for the D locus antigens appears to greatly improve the outcome of living related grafts when the donor and recipient are not genetically identical. Its interest in cadaver organ transplantation is more debated. It is possible that varying technical conditions may explain the discrepancy observed in the literature. Highly significant experimental data reported by van Es et al[107] showed that SD-identical, MLR-positive kidney allografts in unrelated rhesus monkeys had a mean survival time of 12.4 days, while that of SD-identical, MLR-negative allografts was 24.4 days. This supports the trend noted in some human studies that a low degree of MLR stimulation between donor and recipient may improve the outcome of unrelated kidney grafts and may even outweigh HLA-A and B matching.

Matching human related donors on the basis of HLA-D locus determination is possible because there is time to wait for the MLR results. However, in the case of cadaver kidney grafting, the technical time requirements make it still impossible to match prospectively for the HLA-D alleles. Considerable effort is being made at the present to perfect the techniques available for defining HLA-D alleles. Three techniques are in current use:

1. Cells from individuals who are homozygous[46, 47] for the HLA-D locus can be used as stimulators, because when a responder has the antigen for which the stimulating cell is homozygous, no response will be detectable. Using this type of cell, 11 specificities (DW1 to DW11) have been defined. At present, this test takes up to 6 days to perform. A recent variation, however, gives results in 24 to 48 hours; it is based on using homozygous cells prestimulated by phytohemagglutinin as MLR responders.[13]

2. PLT, or the primed lymphocyte test, defines determinants very similar to those detectable using homozygous typing cells.[6] The primed cells are prepared by a specific primary MLR response and, when subsequently set up in secondary response, show the strongest response toward those cells carrying the same determinant as was used for priming. This test has an advantage over the standard MLR in that results are available within 36 to 48 hours.

3. van Leeuwen et al[111, 112] have introduced a serologic approach to the definition of the LD alleles, based on the finding that certain antisera block the lymphocyte response in MLR (see p. 30). These blocking antisera probably react solely with B lymphocytes and not with the platelets which carry SD but not Ia antigens. The latter antigens were defined by the 1977 International Histocompatibility Workshop as D-related (DR) antigens. Thus, a complement-dependent type of reaction permitting recognition of the anti-Ia antibodies can be perfected. It would seem that the anti-Ia antibodies recognize the LD determinants, or at least determinants of a locus very closely linked to LD, thus permitting serologic definition of the D locus products. Serological definition of D

locus antigens will have an extremely important practical application because the complement-dependent antibody technique for DR antigens can be performed in 3 hours.

Matching for HLA Antigens of the DR Locus. Matching for HLA-DR antigens increases the possibility of a negative MLR test between responder and stimulator. If such a close relationship between D and DR locus determinants does exist, it can be assumed that matching for HLA-DR will be as useful as matching in MLR for predicting the outcome of kidney graft survival. At the present, the literature does not contain sufficient data to assess the value of DR matching. Nevertheless, various studies,[4, 34, 55, 82, 92, 106, 116] most of them retrospective, contain evidence favoring an important role for DR antigens in allotransplantation. The Leiden group[82] found that matching for both HLA-DR antigens improves kidney graft prognosis up to 18 months post-transplantation in unrelated donor-recipient combinations and appears to do so more effectively than HLA-A or HLA-B matching. This appears to be true as early as 6 months after grafting; when donor and recipient share both DR antigens,[4, 117] the 6-month actuarial graft survival is over 90%.[2, 106]

In the few prospective studies concerning the effectiveness of HLA-DR matching reported so far, similar results were observed, confirming the retrospective data. Albrechtsen et al[4] in a prospective study reported that in transplantation involving no detectable HLA-DR incompatibility, results after 1, 3, 6 and 12 months were significantly better (75%) than in those involving one or two HLA-DR incompatibilities (38 and 31% respectively) ($P < 0.05$). All of these preliminary data strongly suggest that matching for HLA-DR may influence graft survival. It is still too early, however, to draw any definite conclusion. The influence of matching for only one HLA-DR antigen is still debated. Persijn et al,[82] as well as Ting et al[106] and Martins da Silva and associates,[55] reported that matching for only one HLA-DR determinant drastically improves graft survival. Their data suggest that the prognosis of kidney grafting is just as good with matching for one DR antigen as for four HLA-A and B antigens.

On the other hand, other groups have found no improved graft survival with matching for only one HLA-DR antigen over those with no DR antigen in common.[4, 34] This is in agreement with the observation that combinations sharing only one HLA-DR determinant are always MLR positive. Our group has already shown that, for up to 2 years, no difference in graft survival can be demonstrated between HLA semi-identical pairs (parent-child or siblings sharing only one haplotype) who share only one HLA-DR determinant and HLA-different pairs (unrelated or genotypically HLA-different siblings).[29, 38] This is indirect evidence that matching for one HLA-DR antigen probably has little influence. Why is it, then, that grafts mismatched for one HLA-DR antigen do so well in certain groups? One answer might be that HLA-DR alone is not sufficient to attain the highest survival rate and that the HLA-A and B matches should also be taken into account. Compatibility for A and B loci seems to reinforce the effect of one DR match.[82] Another answer, suggested by Van Rood,[117] is that matching for only one HLA-DR is effective only when the recipient has been transfused before transplantation.

At the present, eight HLA-DR specificities can be typed for. The sum of the gene frequencies of these eight DR specificities approximates 0.85[55] to 0.76,[4] suggesting that 15 to 24% of the alleles belonging to this locus remain to be identified. When HLA-DR antigens cannot be detected in a prospective organ donor, graft prognosis appears to be favorable.[4] This indicates that a blank phenotype of the HLA-DR locus may be poorly immunogenic.

From all the above, it can be concluded that further data must be collected on HLA-A, B, C and D/DR donor-recipient matching before definite conclusions can be drawn on the value of HLA-D/DR matching in kidney graft survival. But there is no doubt that this new SD locus creates hope for a much improved practical solution over the matching for HLA-A, B and C loci. This is especially true in the light of the fact that without any attempt at prospective matching for DR specificities, about 50% of transplanted patients received a graft identical for one DR antigen.

Phenotypic and Genotypic Compatibility

Within the members of a family the HLA genetic map can be reconstructed from HLA-A and B phenotypes. The inheritance of four parental haplotypes belonging to chromosome No. 6 can be accurately determined if a sufficient number of the members of the family, especially parents and siblings, is typed. Thus, the actual HLA genotype of one particular individual may be confirmed and completed (see p. 27). In practice, this reconstruction of the probable haplotype structure of donor and recipient has been possible in nearly all of the transplantations which we have carried out between related donors.

Living related donors may then be classified into three categories: (Fig. 2.1)

1. *HLA-identical* donors, when both donor and recipient have the same two HLA haplotypes in common. This situation is found only in siblings who have inherited the same paternal and maternal haplotypes. The probability of two siblings being HLA-identical is 25%.

2. *HLA-semi-identical* donors, when only one of the two HLA haplotypes is the same in the donor and the recipient. This situation is found in all parent-child pairs and with a probability of 50% in siblings.

3. *HLA-different* donors, when both paternal and maternal haplotypes are different in the recipient and the donor; its probability is 25% in siblings and almost 100% in unrelated individuals. It is, however, occasionally possible to find a haplotype match between a cadaver donor and a potential recipient.[103] In fact, in such cases only the HLA-A and B genotype is determined and no evidence indicates whether other histocompatibility systems may be identical.

Using this system, it is possible to locate living related couples who are genotypically identical for all histocompatibility systems controlled by genes on the sixth chromosome pair. In these circumstances, the antigens of the HLA-A and B loci are, in fact, only acting as markers of a chromosome whose role in the outcome of transplantation is undisputed. It is thus clear that genotypic HLA identity between related donor-recipient pairs and phenotypic HLA identity between unrelated individuals each has its own significance in predicting graft outcome. In the former case, where haplotypes are identical, all the corresponding antigens are identical; however, when antigenic identities are compared one by one as in the latter case, some antigens, such as the D/DR antigens or others still unknown, are probably overlooked. We have already shown that haplotyping is much more reliable in predicting graft survival than is simple phenotyping.[51] On the other hand, results obtained in HLA-identical siblings are much better than those in other transplantation from living related donors: 96% of allografts functioning at 4 years in our own series[29] and 85% at 2 years in other series.[14] The differences are statistically significant when compared with HLA-semi-identical pairs, as well as with HLA-different pairs ($P < 0.01$), while no significant difference is found between these two groups in spite of the fact that semi-identical pairs are related and the majority of different pairs in this study involved unrelated cadaver kidneys.[29]

Since the results with kidneys taken from HLA compatible cadaver donors are as good as those obtained from HLA-semi-identical related donors and much better than those obtained with HLA-different related donors, transplantation from living related donors should be restricted to those cases in which genotypic compatibility is perfect (HLA-identical siblings or HLA-semi-identical siblings sharing the same D/DR locus).

Donor Selection for the Immunized Recipient

In addition to matching for major histocompatibility complex (MHC) products, we are now faced with the controversial and somewhat confusing problems of presensitization.

Recipient Presensitization to Donor Antigens. *Presensitization to HLA-A, B and C Antigens.* First, Terasaki et al[97] and Kissmeyer-Nielsen and associates[50] clearly showed that the presence of preformed circulating antibodies to donor antigens in the serum of an allograft recipient, demonstrated by a positive cross-match, inevitably results in an immediate and irreversible rejection of the graft. For example, Patel and Terasaki[78] reported a series of 24 hyperacute rejections in 30 subjects who were presensitized to their donors. This remains an important fact in transplantation today, and a negative cross-match, generally based on the microcytotoxicity technique,[59] now is an important prerequisite for organ transplantation.

However, it is interesting to note that in the above series, six grafts (20%) did not undergo hyperacute rejection. In these cases, the validity of the cross-match can be questioned. In fact, very little is known today about the specificities of these antibodies. They are usually thought to have anti-HLA-A, B and C specificity, but it is almost certain that other systems, whether a part of the HLA or not, are also involved. In 1976 and 1978, Ettenger et al[31, 32] demonstrated that it was possible to find patients with preformed antibodies against donor B lymphocytes and not against T lymphocytes. When a graft was performed in such cases, no hyperacute rejection was observed and the incidence of graft failure was not higher than in cross-match negative donor-recipient pairs. Similar findings by other groups[53, 62, 76] could suggest that when a positive cross-match is found to be positive against donor B lymphocytes and not T lymphocytes, a renal allograft might be safely carried out in most instances. The present situation, however, is more complex: 1) because the above hypothesis is far from being confirmed or universally accepted, and many authors[4, 28, 95] have reported either acute rejection or poorer graft survival in B cell cross-match positive transplants, while the lack of such presensitization is associated with stable graft function; and 2) because B cell antibodies are certainly not of a unique type. Terasaki's group[42, 43] was the first to show that sera of prospective kidney transplant recipients[41] contain not only antibody to HLA antigens but also antibody to non-HLA antigens. Thus, patients who have antibodies reactive to B lymphocytes in the cold have a higher graft survival rate than patients with either no preformed antibody or with B or T warm antibodies. The graft survival rate in the latter case is lower than that of patients with no cytotoxins. The opinion of these authors is that warm B cell cytotoxins are probably not only directed against HLA-DR but in many instances against HLA-A, B and C specificities. In fact, HLA-A, B and C antibodies that are too weak to react against T lymphocytes can react against B lymphocytes only.[43] Simple sera dilution can discriminate between these two types of antibodies. It also appears that antibodies which react against B lymphocytes in the cold do not have HLA specificities and are not demonstrated after dilution of the HLA antibodies. Cold antibodies reacting against B lymphocytes are probably autoreactive antibodies.

Thus, antibodies responsible for a positive cross-match can be characterized as being: T (or T + B) cell reactive, and thus directed against allogeneic HLA-A, B and C specificities, although T cell autoreactive antibody can be found; or B cell reactive, which can then be directed at HLA-DR antigens or at HLA-A, B and C antigens when they are weak, because of the greater density of the HLA-A, B and C antigens on B cells than on T cells; they can as well be present in the cold and can be directed at non-HLA antigens found specifically on B cells.

From all these rather confusing data two facts emerge: 1) that warm antibodies directed at donor T lymphocytes are associated with rapid rejection of the graft, and 2) that a positive cross-match reaction due to autoreactive or cold anti-B cell antibodies is likely not to affect graft outcome. The influence of other varieties of preformed anti-donor antibodies on graft survival, especially warm anti-B cell antibody, is still a matter of debate.

For practical purposes, it should be remembered that a strongly positive cross-match reaction, even with 50 or 60% cell death, does not always indicate the presence of anti-HLA-A, B or C antibody, particularly when spleen cells are tested. Because of the present policy of transfusing patients awaiting kidney transplantation, more and more potential recipients have high concentrations of preformed anti-B cell antibody only. In these cases, a positive cross-match reaction probably is not a definite contraindication to grafting. In any case, the need to identify the precise type of anti-donor antibodies in the sera of a potential recipient requires that cross-match reaction be performed at least on T cells and B cells, both at 37°C and in the cold.

Other Donor-Specific Assays. 1. Antibody Directed at Nonlymphocyte Targets. The sera of potential recipients may contain IgG antibodies directed against antigens on the endothelium of donor kidney arteries. Cerilli et al[12a] reported a three-fold increase in the number of accelerated rejections in such cases over that in recipients without endothelial antibodies. On a panel of endothelial cells isolated from umbilical veins they showed that the presence of pre-existing endothelial antibodies prior to grafting correlates more closely to the occurrence of accelerated transplant rejection than does the presence of antilymphocyte antibodies. Although several histocompatibility antigens, such as HLA-SD, HLA-DR and ABO, are known to be present on endothelial cells, an antigen system expressed both in endothelial cells and monocytes was recently described by Moraes and Stastny.[61] Such antigens are not present in T and B lymphocytes. They were demonstrated to bind to antigens on the endothelial cells of the peritubular capillaries and on monocytes.[79] Blood transfusion can induce endothelial antibodies in the serum of potential recipients. They are associated with accelerated acute rejection only when they are directed against the donor kidney.[79] These endothelial antibodies, also present in monocytes, are possibly involved in the vascular lesions which are known to play the major role in kidney allograft failure. Thus, cross-matching recipient serum with donor monocytes may become a necessity.

2. Antibody-Dependent Cell-Mediated Cytotoxicity (ADCC). ADCC positive cross-matches against a potential donor are frequent. Whether it is a contraindication to transplantation is still debated. In fact, the main question involved has to do with the specificity of the ADCC. ADCC can be directed at HLA-A, B and C antigens or at B cell antigens. Adsorption of the serum with platelets from the donor thus appears to be an essential step for precisely determining the specificity against HLA-A, B and C antigens or against anti-Ia antigens. This may partly explain the great discrepancy in results reported by various groups. The Richmond group[101] reported a statistically significant association between a positive pretransplant ADCC and chronic rejection or early severe acute rejection. On the other hand, the Johannesburg group[66] found no correlation between the ADCC cross-match and graft rejection, and in Dossetor's experience, platelet nonadsorbable ADCC was not detrimental to graft survival.[94] It thus appears that present data on ADCC are so conflicting that the ADCC cross-match should not be taken into account in donor selection.

3. Lymphocyte-Mediated Cytotoxicity (LMC). The pretransplant detection of LMC and its correlation with kidney transplant survival has been studied by many groups. Almost all studies report a significant correlation between a positive LMC cross-match and kidney graft loss from rejection.[66, 94] Results obtained by the various groups with this assay were so similar that the conclusion of a session especially devoted to this matter at the Sixth Congress of The Transplantation Society was to recommend that the LMC cross-match be included as a part of routine cross-matching.[94] As this will make the cross-match procedure much more complicated, further data are still required before including this test in everyday practice.

Recipient Presensitization to Nondonor Specific HLA Antigens. The question of whether a previous immunization of the recipient against nondonor specific HLA antigens has any influence on graft survival is still without a clear answer. Terasaki et al[94] were the first to show an unfavorable influence of recipient presensitization to HLA antigens. In their large series of more than 1,000 cases, the authors showed that the incidence of early rejection during the first 6 months after transplantation was significantly greater in recipients who had preformed anti-HLA antibodies. A similar poor graft prognosis in recipients with preformed antibodies was not observed by other groups except when additional factors were considered. Dausset et al[24] did not find any harmful effect of preformed antibodies unless their reactivity spectrum was above 50% of the panel cells. Van Hoof et al[110] found this effect only among HLA incompatible recipients; Thomas et al[101] found no correlation between pretransplant humoral antibody levels and graft survival. A retrospective analysis of 191 cadaveric renal transplantations performed in our group[30] shows virtually no difference in the 2-year graft survival rate between 121 patients without pre-existing anti-HLA-A and B antibodies (58%) and 70 preimmunized recipients (60%) (Fig. 3.2*A*). However, when compatible and incompatible recipients are distinguished in each group, a striking difference appears between the two groups (Fig. 3.2*B*); i.e., presensitized patients have a significantly lower graft survival rate when they receive kidneys from incompatible donors (42% at 2 years) than from compatible donors (79% at 2 years). This difference is not seen among nonsensitized patients, where graft survival at 2 years is similar in compatible (56%) and incompatible (61%) pairs. Similar results observed by other authors[25, 47, 68, 70, 110] clearly indicate that close HLA compatibility is of great importance in patients having anti-HLA preformed antibodies but appears to be unnecessary in nonpresensitized patients.

However, in retrospective studies the terms "presensitized recipient" (or responder) and "nonpresensitized recipient" (or nonresponder) are based on the demonstration of the absence of cytotoxic antibodies at any moment prior to transplantation. It is well known today, however, that antibodies may develop after antigenic stimulation, such as blood transfusion, and then disappear, giving a false negative result. Sera must thus be screened for antibodies at frequent intervals and after every blood transfusion. On the other hand, in a retrospective study, potential responders may be classed as "nonresponders" if they have not received antigenic stimulation. A "nonsensitized" recipient must not be confused with a "nonresponder," for the latter implies that adequate antigenic stimulation has been provided. Thus, the "antibody negative" group of patients reported in retrospective studies includes both nonsensitized and true nonresponder patients. In order to clarify this situation, we have undertaken a prospective study (still in progress) in which all potential allograft recipients receive up to 10 units of blood, unless they develop antibodies with less. Only those who do not produce antibody after 10 units of blood are labeled "nonresponders." Our preliminary results are in complete agreement with those of the retrospective study. They reemphasize the fact that matching for HLA-A and B antigens does not influence post-transplantation outcome, and they confirm that HLA compatible "responder" recipients have a much better outcome than "nonresponder" recipients, whatever the degree of compatibility. This latter fact is somewhat troublesome since a better graft survival rate was expected among transfused "nonresponder" recipients. This observation

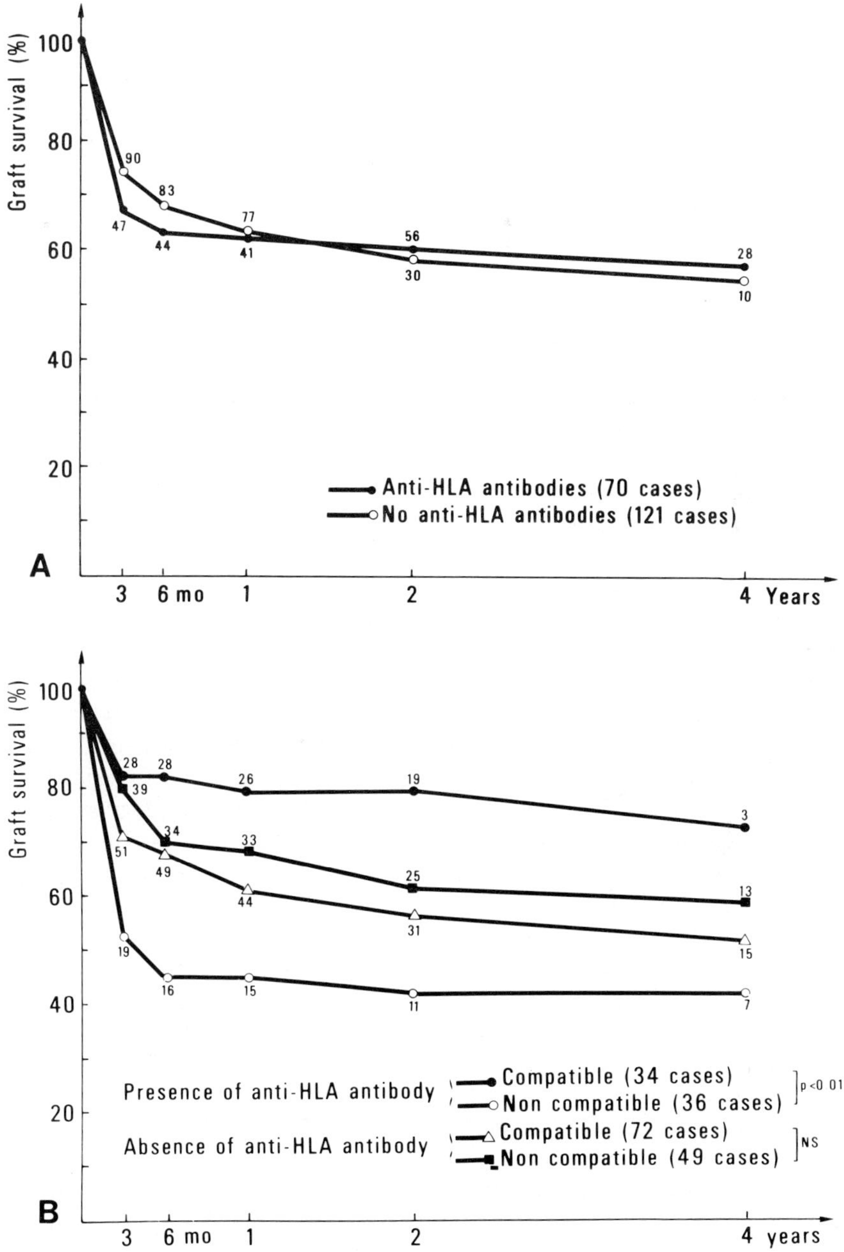

Fig. 3.2. Effect of recipient anti-HLA preimmunization on renal transplant survival in 191 cadaver grafts. *A*, overall results; *B*, results in HLA compatible and noncompatible recipients.

probably means that "responders" produce not only cytotoxic antibodies after blood transfusions but also other factor(s) beneficial to graft tolerance. HLA compatibility would prevent the harmful effect of cytotoxic antibodies, revealing the favorable effect of blood transfusion. On the contrary, "nonresponder" recipients are unable to develop either a cytotoxic or a beneficial response after stimulation by blood transfusion. This explains the lesser influence of HLA compatibility in such recipients, as well as the inferior graft survival rate observed in nonresponders even when HLA antigens are well matched.

Other Immunologic Methods Used in Donor Selection

Although it is undeniable that HLA-A, B, C and D/DR matching improves graft survival, these are certainly not the only factors determining transplant prognosis.

Red Blood Cell Groups

ABO Groups. Since the early 1960s, compatibility between the ABO blood groups of donor and recipient has been considered an absolute requirement for transplantation.[26, 40, 64, 93] Almost all transplantations made across this barrier have ended in more or less rapid destruction of the graft. This rejection is probably due to the fact that A and B antigens are present in the vascular endothelium of the kidney and blood group antibodies directed against the incompatible ABO antigens are presumed to be responsible for graft rejection.[123] However, binding of these antibodies has never been demonstrated in vascular sections of the rejected kidney.

Nearly all reported cases of ABO incompatible kidneys were observed during the early years of human transplantation when the overall kidney graft survival rate was still poor. It is interesting to note that in some reports A to O or B to A grafts were successful.[93] In our own series an O recipient received an A cadaver kidney, which has not been rejected. Nevertheless, the lack of more reliable data makes it reasonable to accept only the relatively safe pattern already defined for blood transfusions.

The observation first reported by Oliver et al[67] that kidneys from blood group A donors transplanted into A recipients have a lower 1-year survival rate than do O kidneys transplanted into O recipients has not been confirmed by others.[69] This might result from a greater immune response of group A individuals, possibly due to an immune response gene in linkage disequilibrium with genes controlling the ABO antigens.

Rhesus Antigens (Rh). Since the work of Boorman and Dodd,[12] it appears that, in addition to A and B antigens, Rh antigens are present in the homogenates of kidneys from Rh positive individuals. However, the possible role of Rh antigen in kidney transplantation is still debated. Although no difference in graft survival rate could be demonstrated between patients who had received an Rh incompatible kidney and those who had received an Rh compatible kidney by some groups,[109] on the contrary Murray et al[65] and Opelz and Terasaki[73] found a better graft outcome for Rh-positive recipients than for Rh-negative recipients. Rh antigens are probably poor immunogens in allotransplantation and are probably not really harmful to the graft.

Lewis Antigens. Oriol et al[74] have recently shown that the Lewis system may play a role in renal transplantation. Lewis-negative recipients had significantly lower graft survival rates than did Lewis-positive recipients. It seems that the effects of Lewis and HLA incompatibilities are additive[75] and that the effects of the Lewis system alone are more evident in A, B and AB recipients than in O recipients. This observation requires confirmation. If so, it will be of great practical importance, especially for Black recipients who are Lewis-negative in nearly 50% of cases.

Other Blood Group Antigens. The possible role of P antigen, initially discussed in the Kidney Registry,[36] has not been clearly confirmed in kidney transplantation. MN antigens are not considered important as far as transplantation is concerned.[109]

Donor Selection in Everyday Practice

Because of the extreme complexity of the HLA system, it is not always possible to make the very best HLA match in practice.

Donor for "HLA-Responder" Recipients

For recipients who have been shown to be antibody producers, it is very important to make every effort for the best match possible. At the present, there is still no evidence that HLA-DR matching alone can abrogate the deleterious influence of HLA-A and B mismatching in responders. Therefore, a B locus identity probably represents the minimal requirement for successful graft outcome. Under these conditions, as we have seen in our own series,[30] more than 70% of recipients have normal graft function at 4 years.

Donor for "HLA-Nonresponder" Recipients

When dealing with patients in whom it has never been possible to detect any anti-HLA antibody, despite numerous well controlled transfusions prior to grafting, it is possible to be less strict with regard to the degree of HLA compatibility necessary for considering a particular donor. Whatever the compatibility for HLA-A and B antigens between donor and recipient, graft outcome appears to be similar. It is probable that matching for DR antigens will be important in "nonresponders," but the possibility should be regarded with caution at this time.

Donor for Recipient not Tested for HLA Response

When the search for anti-HLA antibodies has not been properly performed after blood transfusions, it is not possible to determine the capacity of the potential recipient to produce antibodies if this search was negative in the pretransplantation period. In this case, the patient must be considered as if he were a responder and close matching is the only means of ensuring a successful outcome.

NONIMMUNOLOGIC FACTORS IN DONOR SELECTION

The conditions required for regarding a donor as acceptable are different with volunteer living donors and in transplantation of a cadaver kidney.

Living Donors

For reasons which will be discussed in more detail in Chapter 11, the decision to accept a kidney from a volunteer living donor is always a very serious matter and requires detailed consideration. Naturally, immunologic factors are paramount, but they are by no means the only factors involved.

Age Limits for Living Donors

A child is never an acceptable donor. Only an individual who has reached full maturity can arrive at a valid decision to donate a kidney. We have settled on 18 years as the minimum age. Although the removal of organs from minors is authorized by French law "if he or she is a brother or sister of the recipient,"[54] we feel that a minor must never be considered as a donor. Treatment by chronic hemodialysis will allow the patient to wait until his potential donor reaches the age of 18. Exceptions to this rule can be considered only in very rare cases, such as with identical twins, when it appears better for the recipient to receive an early transplantation and avoid chronic hemodialysis.

The upper age limit is more difficult to fix. Most transplant groups prefer not to use elderly donors because of the distinct possibility of nephrosclerosis, the increased surgical risk of nephrectomy in the donor and the failure of compensatory hypertrophy beyond a certain age. It seems, however, that the increase in size of the donor's remaining kidney is not related to his age. Although the most pronounced loss of function observed in living kidney donors usually occurs in those over 50 years of age,[85] there appears to be no correlation between the age of the donor and the function of the graft.[84] Thus, setting an upper age limit for volunteer living donors is clearly an arbitrary matter. It is our practice not to consider donors over the age of 50 years whenever cadaver kidney transplantation can be reasonably anticipated.

Assessment of the Donor's General Health

Careful general examination is obviously necessary in order to ascertain that the donor is in perfect health and that there is no reason to suspect an increased operative risk.

Renal Studies in the Donor

Careful nephrologic study, including urography, is obviously essential. We perform renal arteriography in every case to make sure that the arrangement of the renal arteries is suitable for transplantation. When there are two or even three renal arteries transplantation is often, but not always, possible (see Appendix I, p. 326). It is up to the surgeon in charge of the transplantation to decide on the technical feasibility.

In general, the left kidney is preferred because of the greater length of the renal vein. It has been suggested, however, that when the donor is a young woman, the right kidney should be used because of the greater risk of right-sided hydronephrosis or pyelonephritis during subsequent pregnancy.

Psychological Assessment of the Donor

It is not sufficient to ascertain that the potential donor is in full possession of his faculties and has no psychiatric disease. He must be entirely free in his decision and must retain a genuine, reasoned and disinterested wish to donate a kidney after being made fully aware of the risks involved and of the fact that there is no guarantee that the transplantation will be successful (for more details see p. 294). So that the donor will be perfectly free in his ultimate decision, we tell him that his family will not be told should he decide against donation and that technical reasons will be given for abandoning the project.

Special Considerations

Identical Twins. No immunologic risk of rejection exists in kidney transplantation between identical twins. The circumstances are particularly favorable, and this is why we have broken our own rules on age limits on two occasions in this situation. One case was a young girl, aged 14, and the other was a man aged 61, who unfortunately died of stomach carcinoma 21 months after transplantation.

Related Donors (Excluding Identical Twins). It should be recalled that from the immunologic viewpoint HLA-identical siblings are by far the best allograft donors and that, of genetically HLA semi-identical donors, siblings are slightly better than parents. Actually the outcome of semi-identical kidney transplantation is not that much better than that of cadaver kidney transplantation. It is therefore our opinion that living donor transplantation should be restricted to those cases in which 1) compatibility is perfect and 2) it is certain that there is no hidden family pressure interfering with the freedom of decision of the proposed donor.

Unrelated Living Donors. The results with unrelated living donors are now no better than with cadaver kidneys. There thus seems to be no justification for putting a living donor to any risk, and in our view unrelated living donor transplantation should not be considered.

Cadaver Donors

As a result of improved preservation techniques and better understanding of histocompatibility systems, the success obtained with cadaver grafts is increasing and attaining that of semi-identical living donors. Thus, the proportion of grafts performed with cadaver donors, which was only 26% in France in 1964, reached 71% in 1970 and was as high as 98% in 1978 (Fig. 3.3).

Age Limits of the Donor

Although transplantation has been performed with a kidney taken from a cadaver aged 84 years,[1] it is generally advised that the donor should not be more than 50 years old. The 11th Report of the Human Renal Transplant Registry shows that the rate of graft loss is higher during the first 6 months in transplantation from donors of more than 51 years but subsequently the rate of graft loss per year is similar to that of donors in their middle years.[1]

Theoretically there is no lower age limit, and neonatal kidneys taken from anencephalic donors have been transplanted into infants and children. In fact it is not known whether such kidneys could be used in adult

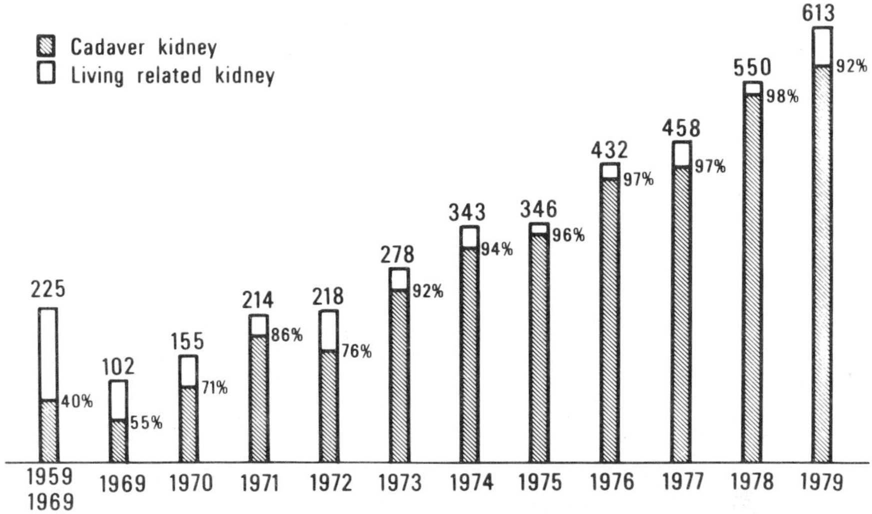

Fig. 3.3. Yearly kidney transplantations in France. Hatched columns represent the percentage of cadaver kidney grafts.

recipients. It seems that kidneys from donors under 5 years of age have a success rate inferior to those from older donors.[1] Nevertheless, many authors have reported adequate graft function of pediatric cadaver kidneys transplanted into adult recipients.[5, 11, 35, 57]

In our opinion, therefore, except in cases of extreme urgency, it appears unreasonable to use kidneys from donors of more than 50 years of age. It is more difficult to fix a lower age limit, but in practice the use of kidneys from children of less than 10 years of age should be restricted to transplantation into children.

Nature of the Disease Causing Death

Any cadaver in which vascular or hypertensive disease is suspected should be eliminated. Equally unacceptable are cadavers with a general infection, whether bacterial or viral, or hepatitis.

Kidneys from cancerous cadavers should not be used for transplantation because after a few months the recipient may develop metastases, perhaps fostered by treatment with immunosuppressive drugs.

Renal status can be evaluated by the volume of urine output, the absence of proteinuria, the results of urine cultures and serum creatinine levels. Nevertheless, it is preferable not to use kidneys from women who died after abortion or in the immediate postpartum period because of the risk of cortical necrosis. It should also be remembered that kidneys from individuals with cirrhosis of the liver are frequently affected by glomerulonephritis with immunoglobulin A deposits.

Different Types of Cadaver Donors

The conditions of death have a marked influence on the post-transplantation function of cadaver grafts, as clearly seen when comparing the function of kidneys from the two types of cadaver donors currently employed.

Beating Heart Donor. The ideal potential donor is an individual who has entered the state of cerebral death,[60] i.e., where the nervous system has been irreversibly destroyed but the heart continues to beat regularly, maintaining normal systemic vascular circulation. This state can generally be prolonged for several hours or even days by the use of artificial ventilation. The diagnosis of cerebral death can easily be made on the basis of certain strict criteria, the most important of which is the absence of all electrical activity in the cerebral cortex. However, it is also extremely important to consider the circumstances of the accident that produced the cerebral condition. The above criteria are valid only if the individual has received no barbiturate and is not in a hypothermic state. Under these circumstances, all the organs other than the brain continue to function normally, and the quality of the kidneys equals that of kidneys from a living donor. The reasons for this are: 1) there is no agonal phase of insufficient renal blood flow and no prolonged period of ischemia prior to cooling of the kidney; 2) the time of removal can be set in advance, providing time for determining tissue groups and locating the most compatible recipient; and 3) once cerebral death has been diagnosed by two physicians outside the transplantation team, it is possible to undertake treatments that will actually improve the quality of the transplant, e.g. renal vasodilators (phenoxybenzamine, dopamine or regitine) which prevent the appearance of arterial vasoconstriction during surgical removal of the kidney.

Unfortunately, a number of difficulties limit the retrieval of kidneys from beating heart donors. Only a small number of organs actually becomes available for transplantation because: 1) although statistics show that the number of cerebral deaths each year far surpasses that which would be required for transplantation, the need to obtain the active cooperation of intensive care and/or neurosurgical units which handle these cases is an important limiting factor; and 2) harvesting techniques require a rather complicated organization.

Cardiac Arrest Donor. It is possible to remove kidneys from individuals who have just died under circumstances other than cerebral death. After cardiac arrest, irreversible ischemic damage of the kidneys occurs within approximately 60 to 120 min (See p. 71). Thus, it is rare to obtain good quality kidneys from individuals who have had cardiac arrest, since the time required to assemble the surgical team and to undertake transplant nephrectomy is usually at least 1 hour. This explains why the same transplant group obtained much poorer results with this type of donor than with beating heart donors.[33] As a consequence, most groups throughout the world have given up using these donors, except under exceptional circumstances when there is an urgent need for the donor kidney.

Organization of Cadaver Kidney Transplantation

The organization of cadaver kidney transplantation must take into account both the immunologic requirements and the limited length of time for which the kidney can be preserved after death.

To obtain an adequate number of kidneys suitable for transplantation under the best circumstances and at the lowest possible cost, a relatively complex and wide ranging organization is required. In Europe, at present four separate organizations cover Western Europe: France Transplant (France, Switzerland, Spain), Eurotransplant (Benelux, Germany, Austria, Switzerland, Italy), U.K. Transplant (England, Ireland) and Scandiatransplant (Sweden, Norway, Denmark, Finland). These four organizations function with almost identical structures. In France (Fig. 3.4), each transplantation unit has three principal roles: 1) to assume responsibility for the care of patients awaiting transplantation in its region; 2) to organize and promote the collection of organs on a regional basis; and 3) to make every effort to increase the number of HLA compatible transplantations performed.

This necessitates educating the public as well as the physicians and surgeons in every general hospital to the problems and possibilities of organ transplantation. Whenever a local hospital signals the presence of a potential donor, the regional transplant team should have personnel on call to take immediate charge of all problems related to the particular donor. HLA typing should be organized through the regional histocompatibility laboratory, and the most compatible recipients should be identified by a central computer. Priority should be given, among the more compatible recipients, to those available at the transplantation center nearest the donor. If the kidneys have to be sent a long distance, it is advisable to eliminate any center having only one potential recipient if he has a large number of HLA antibodies in his serum. Using the Collins washout technique and preservation on ice, it is possible to transport the kidney in a relatively small insulated box by regular commercial transportation (air, rail, taxi, etc.), keeping the cost to a minimum.

Today, short-term preservation using the washout technique provides

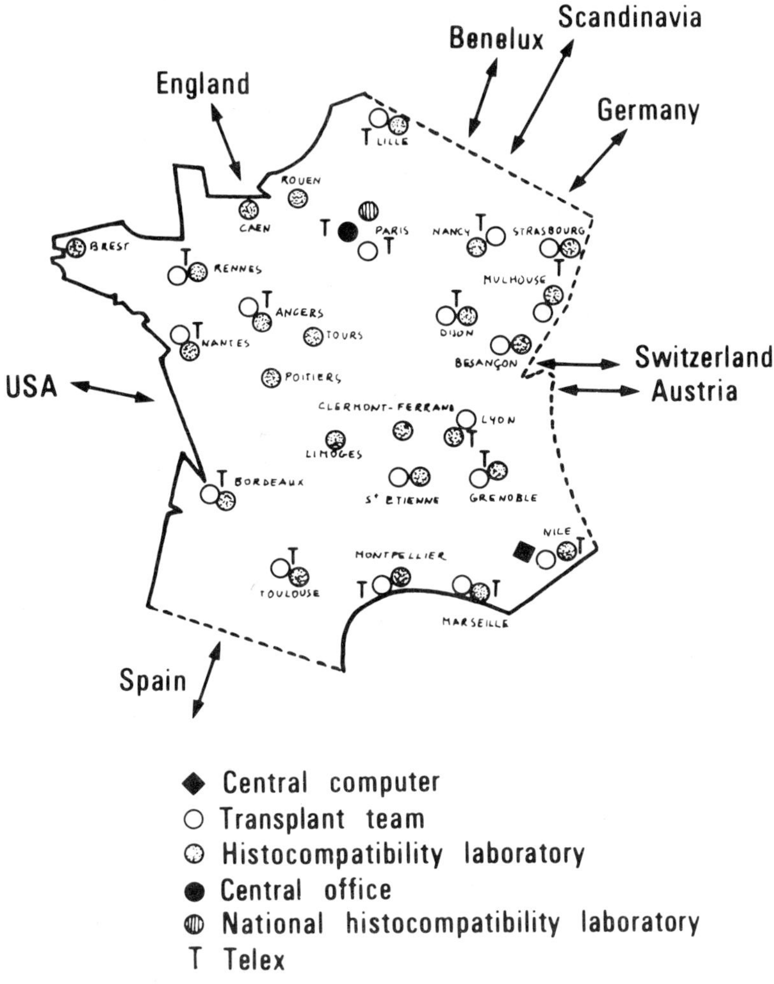

Fig. 3.4. Organization of France Transplant, 1979.

sufficient time for exchange with all countries in Europe. Thus, if no compatible recipient can be found in the three countries which are part of the France Transplant organization, the kidney will be offered to the other three European organizations. This enlarged pool includes a population of 10,000 potential recipients, and there is, thus, a very good chance of finding a recipient that will be compatible for every kidney.

It has been clearly established that this type of exchange has no detrimental effect on the quality of the graft after transplantation.[52, 120] Similar exchanges of kidneys are now being developed in the United States, and more recently transatlantic exchanges have been undertaken. This demonstrates that in the future it may well be possible to seek a recipient for any potential kidney within a worldwide pool.

REFERENCES

1. ACS/NIH Organ Transplant Registry. The 11th Report of the Human Renal Transplant Registry. J. Am. Med. Assoc., *226:*1197, 1973.
2. ACS/NIH Organ Transplant Registry. The 12th Report of the Human Renal Transplant Registry. J. Am. Med. Assoc., *233:*787, 1975.
3. Albert, E. D., Mempel, W. Q., and Grosse-Wilde, H. Linkage disequilibrium between HL-A 7 and the MLC specificity Pi. Transplant. Proc., *5:*1551, 1973.
4. Albrechtsen, D., Arnesen, E., Solheim, B. G., and Thorsby, E. Significance of HLA-DR matching and of B cell cross-match tests in vitro and in cadaver renal transplantation. Transplant. Proc., *9:*743, 1979.
5. Andersen, O. S., Jonasson, O., and Merkel, P. K. En bloc transplantation of pediatric kidneys into adult patients. Arch. Surg., *108:*35, 1974.
6. Bach, F. H., and van Rood, J. J. The major histocompatibility complex. Genetics and biology (second of three parts). N. Engl. J. Med., *295:*872, 1976.
7. Bach, F. H., and van Rood, J. J. The major histocompatibility complex. Genetics and biology (third of three parts). N. Engl. J. Med., *295:*927, 1976.
8. Bach, J. F., Debray-Sachs, M., Crosnier, J., Kreis, H., and Dormont, J. Correlation between mixed lymphocyte culture performed before renal transplantation and kidney function. J. Clin. Exp. Immunol., *6:*821, 1970.
9. Batchelor, J. R., and Joysey, V. C. Influence of HL-A compatibility on cadaveric renal transplantation. Lancet, *1:*790, 1969.
10. Belzer, F. O., Perkins, H. A., Fortmann, J. L., Kountz, S. L., Salvatierra, O., Cochrum, K. C., and Payne, R. Is HL-A typing of clinical significance in cadaver renal transplantation? Lancet, *1:*774, 1974.
11. Bolkzo, S., Tellis, V., and Veith, F. J. Transplantation of children's kidneys into adult recipients. Surg. Gynecol. Obstet., *146:*387, 1978.
12. Boorman, K. E., and Dodd, B. E. The group specific substances, A, B, M, N, and Rh: Their occurrence in tissues and body fluids. J. Pathol., *55:*329, 1944.

12a. Cerilli, J., Holliday, J. E., and Fesperman, D. P. Role of antivascular endothelial antibody in predicting renal allograft rejection. Transplant. Proc., *9:*771, 1977.

13. Charmot, J. S., Comoy, A., Mawas, C., and Sasportes M. Rapid HLA-D matching method using PHA blasts as responding cells. Transplant. Proc., *9:*410, 1977.
14. Cheig, J. S., Chami, J., Stenzel, K. H., Riggio, R. R., Saal, S., Mouradian, J. A., Fotino, M., Stubenbord, W. T., and Rubin, A. L. Renal transplantation between HLA identical siblings. Comparison with transplants from HLA semi-identical related donors. N. Engl. J. Med., *296:*1030, 1977.
15. Cochrum, K. C., Perkins, H. A., Payne, R. O., Kountz, S. L., Belzer, F. O. The correlation of MLC with graft survival. Transplant. Proc., *5:*391, 1973.
16. Cochrum, K. C., Salvatierra, O., Perkins, H. A., and Belzer, F. O. MLC testing in renal transplantation. Transplant. Proc., *7:*659, 1975.
17. Colombani, J., D'Amaro, J., Gabb, B., Smith, G., and Svejgaard, A. International agreement on a microtechnique of platelet complement fixation. Transplant. Proc., *3:* 121, 1971.
18. Cullen, P. R., Lester, S., Rouch, J., and Morris, P. J. Mixed lymphocyte reaction (MLR) and graft survival in 40 cadaveric renal transplants. Clin. Exp. Immunol., *28:* 218, 1977.
19. D'Amaro, J. The micro-complement fixation test. I. A solution of the technical problems of HL-A typing? Vox Sang., *18:*334, 1970.

20. Dausset, J. Leuco-agglutinins. IV. Leuco-agglutinins and blood transfusion. Vox Sang., *6:*190, 1954.
21. Dausset, J. Le complexe HLA. I. Immunogénétique du système HLA. Les séries alléliques HLA-A, -B et -C. Nouv. Presse Med., *5:*1301, 1976.
22. Dausset, J. Le complexe HLA. II. Immunogénétique du système HLA. La série allélique HLA-D et les spécificités des sous-populations lymphocytaires. Nouv. Presse Med., *5:*1353, 1976.
23. Dausset, J. International Forum. Fifteen years of HL-A: What is the importance of HL-A compatibility for clinical outcome of renal transplantations? Vox Sang., *34:*171, 1978.
24. Dausset, J., Hors, J., and Busson, M. Histocompatibilité et transplantation rénale. In *Proceedings of the Sixth International Congress on Nephrology, Florence, 1975*, p. 728. Karger, Basel, 1976.
25. Dausset, J., Hors, J., Busson, M., Festenstein, H., Oliver, R. T. D., Paris, A. M. I., and Sachs, J. A. Serologically defined HL-A antigens and long-term survival of cadaver kidney transplants. N. Engl. J. Med., *18:*979, 1974.
26. Dausset, J., and Rapaport, F. T. The role of blood group antigens in human histocompatibility. Ann. NY Acad. Sci., *129:*408, 1966.
27. Dausset, J., Rapaport, F. T., and Legrand, L. *Advance in Transplantation*, p. 750. Munksgaard, Copenhagen, 1968.
28. Dejelo, C. L., and Williams, T. C. B. Cell cross-match in renal transplantation. Lancet, *2:*241, 1977.
29. Descamps, B., Hinglais, N., and Crosnier, J. Renal transplantation between 33 HL-A identical siblings. Transplant Proc., *5:*231, 1973.
30. Descamps, B., N'Guyen, A. T., and Kreis, H. New insights into immunologic selection of human cadaver renal allograft recipients based on immune response capacity criteria. Transplant. Proc., *10:*497, 1978.
31. Ettenger, R. B., Opelz, G., Walker, J., Terasaki, P. I., Uittenbogaart, C., Pennisi, A. J., Malekzadeh, M. H., and Fine, R. N. Antibodies to donor B. lymphocytes and mixed lymphocyte culture blocking in cadaveric renal transplantation. Transplantation, *25:* 169, 1978.
32. Ettenger, R. B., Terasaki, P. I., Opelz, G., Malekzadeh, M., Pennisi, A. J., Uittenbogaart, C., and Fine R. Successful renal allografts across a positive cross-match for donor B-lymphocyte alloantigens. Lancet, *2:*56, 1976.
33. Festenstein, H., Oliver, R. T. D., Sachs, J. A., Burke, J. M., Adams, E., Divver, W., Hyams, A., Pegrum, G. D., Balfour, I. C., and Moorhead, J. F. Multicentre collaboration in 162 time-typed renal transplants. Lancet, *2:*225, 1971.
34. Festenstein, H., Pachoula-Papasteriadis, C., Sachs, J. A., Jaraquemada, D., and Burke, J. M. Collaborative scheme for tissue typing and matching in renal transplantation. X effect of HLA-A, B, D and DR matching and pretransplant blood transfusion on 769 cadaver renal grafts. Transplant. Proc., *11:*752, 1979.
35. Fine, R. N. Renal transplantation in children. In *Advances in Nephrology*, edited by J. Hamburger, J. Crosnier, and M. H. Maxwell, vol. 5, p. 201. Year Book Medical Publishers, Chicago, 1975.
36. Gleeson, R. E., and Murray, J. E. Report from kidney transplant registry: Analysis of variables in the function of human kidney transplants. Transplantation, *5:*343, 1967.
37. Goudsmit, R., and van Loghem, J. J. Studies on the occurrence of leukocyte antibodies. Vox Sang., *3:*58, 1953.
38. Hamburger, J., Crosnier, J., Descamps, B., and Rowinska, D. The value of present methods used for the selection of organ donors. Transplant. Proc., *3:*260, 1971.
39. Hors, J., Feingold, N., Fradelizi, D., and Dausset, J. Critical evaluation of histocompatibility in 179 renal transplants. Lancet, *1:*609, 1971.

40. Hume, D. M. *Transplantation of Tissues*, edited by L. Peer, p. 534. Williams & Wilkins, Baltimore, 1959.
41. Iwaki, Y., Terasaki, P. I., Park, M. S., and Billing, R. Enhancement of human kidney allograft by cold B-lymphocyte cytotoxins. Lancet, *1:*1228, 1978.
42. Iwaki, Y., Terasaki, P. I., Park, M. S., Hientz, R., Silberman, H., and Berne, T. Dilutions and specificity analysis of pretransplant sera. Transplant. Proc., *11:*944, 1979.
43. Iwaki, Y., Terasaki, P. I., Weil, R., Koep, L., and Starzl, T. Retrospective tests of B-cold lymphocytotoxins and transplant survival at a single center. Transplant. Proc., *11:*941, 1979.
44. Jeannet, M. Histocompatibility testing using leukocyte typing and mixed lymphocyte culture in kidney transplants. Helv. Med. Acta., *35:*168, 1970.
45. Jones, A. R., Vaughan, R. W., Beswick, M., and Batchelor, J. R. Transformation of lymphocytes from patients awaiting cadaver renal transplants. Lancet, *2:*529, 1976.
46. Jorgensen, F., Lamm, L. U., and Kissmeyer-Nielsen, F. Mixed lymphocyte cultures with inbred individuals. An approach to MLC typing. Tissue Antigens, *3:*323, 1973.
47. Keuning, J. J., Termijtelen, A., Blusse van Oud Alblas, A., Gabb, B. W., D'Amaro, J., and van Rood, J. J. LD (MLC) population and family studies in a Dutch population. In *Histocompatibility Testing, 1975*, edited by F. Kissmeyer-Nielsen, p. 533. Munksgaard, Copenhagen, 1975.
48. Kissmeyer-Nielsen, F. International Forum. Fifteen years of HL-A: What is the importance of HL-A compatibility for clinical outcome of renal transplantations? Vox Sang., *34:*171, 1978.
49. Kissmeyer-Nielsen, F., and Kjerbye, K. E. Lymphocytotoxin micro-technique: Purification of lymphocytes by flottation. In *Histocompatibility Testing 1967*, edited by E. S. Curtoni, P. L. Mattius, and R. M. Tosi, p. 381. Williams & Wilkins, Baltimore, 1967.
50. Kissmeyer-Nielsen, F., Olsen, S., Petersen, V. P., and Fjeldborg, O. Hyperacute rejection of kidney allografts associated with pre-existing humoral antibodies against donor cells. Lancet, *2:*662, 1966.
51. Kreis, H., Leski, M., Crosnier, J., and Hamburger, J. The value of a genetic expression of leucocyte typing in renal transplantation. Clin. Exp. Immunol., *6:*815, 1970.
52. Kreis, H., Noel, L. H., Moreau, J. F., Barbanel, C., and Crosnier, J., Devenir des transplants rénaux conservés par la méthode de Collins. Nouv. Presse Med., *7:*429, 1978.
53. Lobo, P. I., Westervelt, F. B., and Rudolf, L. E. Kidney transplantability across a positive cross-match. Cross match assays and distribution of B lymphocyte in donor tissues. Lancet, *1:*925, 1977.
54. Loi N°76-1181 du 22 Décembre 1976 relative aux prélèvements d'organes ("Journal Officiel" de la République Française du 23 Décembre 1976).
55. Martins da Silva, B., Jeannet, M., Vassali, P., Harder, F., Largiader, F., and Montandon, A. Influence of HLA-DR matching in cadaver kidney transplantation in Swisstransplant. Transplant. Proc., *11:*760, 1979.
56. Mattiuz, P. L., Ihde, D., Piazza, A., Ceppellini, R., and Bodmer, W. F. New approaches to the population genetic and segregation analysis of the HL-A system. In *Histocompatibility Testing 1970*, edited by P. I. Terasaki, p. 193. Williams & Wilkins, Baltimore, 1970.
57. Merkel, F. K., Ing, T. S., Ahmadian, Y., Lewy, P., Ambruster, J. O., Sulieman, J. S., Belman, A. B., and King, L. R. Transplantation in and of the young. J. Urol., *3:*679, 1974.
58. Mickey, M. R., Kreisler, M., Albert, E. D., Tanaka, N., and Terasaki, P. I. Analysis of HL-A incompatibility in human renal transplants. Tissue Antigens, *1:*57, 1971.
59. Mittal, K. K., Mickey, M. R., Singal, D. P., and Terasaki, P. I. Refinement of microdroplet lymphocyte cytotoxicity test. Transplantation, *6:*913, 1968.

60. Mollaret, P., and Goulon, M. Le coma dépassé (mémoire préliminaire). Rev. Neurol., *101:*3, 1959.
61. Moraes, J. R., and Stastny, P. A new antigen system expressed in human endothelial cells. J. Clin. Invest., *60:*449, 1977.
62. Morris, J. P. Histocompatibility antigens in human organ transplantation. Surg. Clin. North Am., *58:*233, 1978.
63. Morris, J. P., Kincaid-Smith, P., Ting, A., Stocker, J. W., Marshall, V. C. Prospective leucocyte typing in cadaver transplantation. Lancet, *2:*803, 1968.
64. Murray, J. E., and Harrison, J. H. Surgical management of fifty patients with kidney transplants including eighteen pairs of twins. Am. J. Surg., *105:*205, 1963.
65. Murray, S., Dewar, P. J., Uldall, P. R., Wilkinson, R., Kerr, D. N. S., Taylor, R. M. R., and Swinney, J. Some important factors in cadaver-donor kidney transplantation. Tissue Antigens, *4:*458, 1974.
66. Myburgh, J. A., and Smit, J. A. Pre-transplant lymphocyte mediated cytotoxicity (LMC) and antibody dependent cell-mediated cytotoxicity (ADCC) in kidney transplantation. Transplant. Proc., *10:*425, 1978.
67. Oliver, R. T. D. An assessement of the role of HL-A antigens and the other factors which influence cadaver renal graft survival. Thesis, Cambridge, 1974.
68. Oliver, R. T. D., Sachs, J. A., Festenstein, H., Pegrum, G., and Moorhead, J. F. The influence of HL-A matching, antigenic strength and immune responsiveness on the outcome of 349 cadaver renal grafts. Lancet, *2:*1381, 1972.
69. Opelz, G., and Terasaki, P. I. Effect of blood-groups on relation between HLA match and outcome of cadaver kidney transplants. Lancet, *1:*220, 1977.
70. Opelz, G., Mickey, M. R., and Terasaki, P. I. HLA matching and cadaver kidney transplant survival in North America. Influence of center variation and presensitisation. Transplantation, *23:*490, 1977.
71. Opelz, G., and Terasaki, P. I. Factors influencing effect of HLA matching on cadaver kidney transplants. Transplant. Proc., *9:*1795, 1977.
72. Opelz, G., and Terasaki, P. I. Significance of mixed leukocyte culture testing in cadaver kidney transplantation. Transplantation, *23:*375, 1977.
73. Opelz, G., and Terasaki, P. I. Cadaver kidney transplants in North America, Analysis 1978. Dial. Transplant, *8:*167, 1979.
74. Oriol, R., Cartron, J., Yvart, J., Bedrossian, J., Duboust, A., Bariety, J., Gluckman, J. C., and Gagnadoux, M. F. Rôle des systèmes Lewis (Le-le) et sécréteur (Se-se) dans le rejet des greffes rénales, C. R. Acad. Sci., Paris, *285:*1083, 1977.
75. Oriol, R., Cartron, J., Yvart, J., Bedrossian, J., Duboust, A., Bariety, J., Gluckman, J. C., and Gagnadoux, M. F. The Lewis system: New histocompatibility antigens in renal transplantation. Lancet, *1:*574, 1978.
76. Parks, M. S., Terasaki, P. I., and Bernoco, D. Autoantibody against B lymphocytes. Lancet, *2:*465, 1977.
77. Patel, R., Mickey, M. R., and Terasaki, P. I. Serotyping for homotransplantation. XVI. Analysis of kidney transplants from unrelated donors. N. Engl. J. Med., *279:*501, 1968.
78. Patel, L., and Terasaki, P. I. Significance of the positive cross-match test in kidney transplantation. N. Engl. J. Med., *280:*735, 1969.
79. Paul, L. Antibodies directed against donor antigens in human renal allograft. Thesis, p. 140. Drukkerij J. H. Pasmans, Gravenhage, 1979.
80. Payne, R., Perkins, H. A., and Najarian, J. S. *Advance in Transplantation*, p. 221. Munksgaard, Copenhagen, 1968.
81. Perkins, H. A., Kountz, S. L., Payne, R., and Belzer, F. O. Achievements and limitations of histocompatibility testing for ten HL-A factors in kidney transplantation. Transplant. Proc., *3:*130, 1971.

82. Persijn, G. G., Gabb, B. W., van Leeuwen, A., Nagtegaal, A., Hoogeboom, J., and van Rood, J. J. Matching for HLA antigens of A, B and DR loci in renal transplantation by Eurotransplant. Lancet, *1:*1278, 1978.
83. Rapaport, F. T., and Dausset, J. Ranks of donor recipient histocompatibility for human transplantation. Science, *167:*1260, 1970.
84. Reeve, C. E., Martin, D. C., Gonick, H. C., Kaufman, J. J., Rubini, M. E., Mims, M. M., Goodwin, W. E., Koppel, M. H., Kopple, J. D., and Goldman, R. Kidney Transplantation. A comparison of results using cadaver and related living donors. Am. J. Med., *47:*410, 1969.
85. Ringden, O., Friman, L., Londgren, G., and Magnusson, G. Living related kidney donors: Complications and long-term renal function. Transplantation, *25:*221, 1978.
86. Sachs, J. A., Festenstein, H., Tuffnell, V. A., and Paris, A. M. I. Collaborative scheme for tissue typing and matching in renal transplantation. XI. Effects of HLA-A, -B and -D locus matching, pretransplant transfusion, and other factors on 612 cadaver renal grafts. Transplant. Proc., *9:*383, 1977.
87. Salvatierra, O., Perkins, H. A., Cochrum, K. C., Duca, R. M., Potter, D. E., Amend, W. J., and Feduska, N. J. HLA typing and primary cadaver graft survival. Transplant. Proc., *9:*495, 1977.
88. Scandiatransplant Reports. HL-A matching and kidney graft survival. Lancet, *1:*240, 1975.
89. Segall, M., Bach, F. H., Bach, M. L., Hussey, J. L., and Vehling, D. T. Correlation of MLC stimulation and clinical course in kidney transplants. Transplant. Proc., *8:*41, 1975.
90. Simmons, R. L., Yunis, E. J., Noreen, H., Thompson, E. J., Fryd, D. S., and Najarian, J. S. Effects of HLA matching on cadaver kidney function: experience at a single large center. Transplant. Proc., *9:*941, 1977.
91. Solheim, B. G., Flatmark, A., Halvorsen, S., Jervell, J., and Thorsby, E. Influence of HLA-A, -B, -C and -D matching on the outcome of clinical kidney transplantation. Transplant. Proc., *9:*445, 1977.
92. Solheim, B. G., Flatmark, A., Halvorsen, S., Jervell, J., and Thorsby, E. Influence of HLA-A, -B, -C, and D matching and pretransplant blood transfusions on kidney graft survival. Transplant. Proc., *11:*748, 1979.
93. Starzl, T. E., Marchioro, T. L., Holmes, J. H., Hermann, G., Brittain, R. S., Stonington, O. H., Talmage, D. W., and Waddel, W. R. Renal homografts in patients with major donor-recipients blood group incompatibilities. Surgery, *55:*195, 1964.
94. Stiller, C. R., Dossetor, J. B., Carpenter, C. B., and Myburgh, J. A. Immunologic monitoring of the transplant recipient. Transplant. Proc., *9:*1245, 1977.
95. Suthanthiran, M., Gailiunas, P., St Louis, G., Fagan, G., Carpenter, C. B., and Garovoy, M. R. Presensitization to donor B-cell ("Ia") antigens associated with early allograft failure. Transplant. Proc., *9:*1807, 1977.
96. Terasaki, P. I., Kreisler, M., Mickey, M. R., and Sengar, D. P. S. Analysis of histocompatibility data from 1000 kidney transplants. In *Third International Congress of the Transplantation Society*. The Hague, 1970.
97. Terasaki, P. I., Marchioro, T. L., and Starzl, T. E. First finding of preformed cytotoxic antibodies against donor cells. In *Histocompatibility Testing 1965*, p. 83. National Academy of Sciences, Washington, D.C., 1965.
98. Terasaki, P. I., and McClelland, J. D. Microdoplet assay of human serum cytotoxins. Nature *204:*998, 1964.
99. Terasaki, P. I., Mickey, M. R., and Kreisler, M. Presensitization and kidney transplant failures. Postgrad. Med. J., *47:*89; 1971.
100. Terasaki, P. I., Vredevoe, D. L., and Mickey, M. R. Serotyping for homotransplanta-

tion. X. Survival of 196 grafted kidneys subsequent to typing. Transplantation, *5:*1057, 1967.

101. Thomas, F., Thomas, J., Mendez, G., and Lee, H. M. Pretransplant immune monitoring of donor-recipient compatibility. Transplant. Proc., *10:*429, 1978.
102. Thompson, J. S., Bonney, W. W., Lawton, R. L., Flink, R. J., and Corry, J. R. Effect of HL-A haplotype matching on renal transplantation. Transplantation, *17:*438, 1974.
103. Thompson, J. S., Corry, R. J., Lawton, R. L., Bonney, W. W., and Kaloyanides, G. J. Effect of prospective HLA-haplotype matching on renal transplantation. Transplant. Proc., *9:*205, 1977.
104. Thorsby, E., Helgesen, A., Rankin, B., Möller, E., and Kaakinen, A. Identification of five lymphocyte activating determinants in man. Tissue Antigens, *6:*147, 1975.
105. Thorsby, E., and Kissmeyer-Nielsen, F. Lymphocytotoxin antisera of limited isospecificity after skin grafting in man. Vox Sang., *14:*417, 1968.
106. Ting, A., and Morris, P. J. The influence on renal transplantation of a positive crossmatch due to autoantibodies and alloantibodies against B lymphocytes. Lancet, *2:* 1095, 1977.
107. van Es, A., Marquet, R. L., van Vreeswijk, W., Tank, B., and Balner, H. The influence of matching for RhL-A (SD) antigens and of mixed lymphocyte reactivity on allograft survival in unrelated rhesus monkeys. Transplant. Proc., *9:*257, 1977.
108. van Hoof, J. P., Hendriks, G. F. J., Schippers, H. M. A., and van Rood, J. J. Influence of possible HL-A haploidentity on renal graft survival in Eurotransplant. Lancet, *1:* 1130, 1974.
109. van Hoof, J. P., Hendriks, G. F. J., and van Rood, J. J. The influence of a number of immunogenetic and non immunogenetic factors on the graft prognosis. The relative importance of HL-A matching in kidney transplantation, p. 69. Academic Thesis, University of Leiden, 1976.
110. van Hoof, J. P., Schippers, H. M. A., van der Steen, G. J., and van Rood, J. J. Efficacy of HL-A matching in Eurotransplant. Lancet, *2:*1385, 1972.
111. van Leeuwen, A., Schuit, H. R. E., and van Rood, J. J. Typing for MLC (LD). II. The selection of nonstimulator cells by MLC inhibition tests using SD-identical stimulator cells (MISIS) and fluorescence antibody studies. Transplant. Proc., *5:*1539, 1973.
112. van Leeuwen, A., Winchester, R., and van Rood, J. J. Serotyping for MLC. II. Technical aspects. Ann. NY Acad. Sci., *254:*289, 1975.
113. van Rood, J. J. Leukocyte grouping: A method and its application. Thesis, University of Leiden, 1962.
114. van Rood, J. J. The search for standard HLA reagents. Vox Sang., *31:*380, 1976.
115. van Rood, J. J., Eernisse, J. G., and van Leeuwen, A. Leucocyte antibodies in sera from pregnant women. Nature, *181:*1735, 1958.
116. van Rood, J. J., Persijn, G. G., Lansbergen, Q., Cohen, B., van Leeuwen, A., and Bradley, B. A. How can HLA matching improve kidney graft survival? Proc. Eur. Dial. Transplant. Assoc., *16:*297, 1979.
117. van Rood, J. J., Persijn, G. G., van Leeuwen, A., Goulmy, E., and Gabb, B. W. A new strategy to improve kidney graft survival: The induction of CML non responsiveness. Transplant. Proc., *11:*736, 1979.
118. van Rood, J. J., van Leeuwen, A., and Bruning, J. W. The redevance of leucocyte antigens for allogeneic renal transplantation. J. Clin. Pathol. (Suppl.), *20:*504, 1967.
119. van Rood, J. J., van Leeuwen, A., Pearce, R., and Does, J. Leucocyte typing and kidney transplantation in unrelated donor recipient pairs. Transplant. Proc., *1:*372, 1969.
120. van Rood, J. J., van Leeuwen, A., Persijn, G. G., Lansbergen, Q., Goulmy, E., Termijtelen, A., and Bradley, A. HLA compatibility in clinical transplantation. Transplant. Proc., *9:*459, 1977.

121. Walford, R. L., Gallagher, R., and Sjaarda, J. R. Serologic typing of human lymphocytes with immune serum obtained after homografting. Science, *144:*868, 1964.
122. Walker, W. E., Niblack, G. W., Johnson, H. K., and Richie, R. E. Relationship of cadaveric renal transplant results to HLA tissue matching. Transplant. Proc., *9:*487, 1977.
123. Wilbrandt, R., Tung, K. S. H., Deodhar, S. D., Nakamoto, S., and Kolff, W. J. ABO blood group incompatibility in human renal homotransplantation. Am. J. Clin. Pathol., *51:*15, 1969.

CHAPTER FOUR

Renal Preservation

Henri Kreis

Basic principles—Simple hypothermic storage—Hypothermic perfusion by machine—Deepfreezing for long-term storage—Assessment of viability—Practical application.

A few years after the first successful attempts to transplant human kidneys, it became apparent that living donors were not the clue to the treatment of end-stage renal diseases by transplantation. It therefore became necessary to seek more fruitful sources of organs, and cases where brain death has been declared fulfill all the requirements. These cases, however, are not necessarily located near the best suitable recipient, and after removal the kidney usually has to be transported from the harvesting hospital to the transplant center. In addition, when human leukocyte A (HLA) compatibility is desired, typing and cross-match procedures are time consuming. Preservation of the isolated kidney for many hours is thus inevitable, both for transplantation and for immunologic assays between donor and recipient.

For these reasons, the past decade has witnessed a renewed interest in organ preservation. Isolated kidney preservation, which is possible for only a few minutes without special care, is now practicable for 2 to 3 days with relatively simple methods. This amount of time is sufficient to allow long distance transportation, HLA-A, B and DR (D-related) typing and all types of cross-match procedures. However, induction of specific immunologic tolerance could be attempted were a longer period of time available before transplantation between specific donors and recipients. On the other hand, the present shortage of kidneys and the resultant long waiting lists for transplantation provide a wide range of recipient choice and the possibility of good HLA compatibility. Without this large recipient pool it would be quite impossible to make such highly compatible pairings. Another means of providing a wide choice of pairings is long-term kidney preservation by deepfreezing whole kidneys. These methods, however, are still at an early stage and are not available for practical use. In sum, at the present, short-term storage for about 2 days is readily achieved, long-term storage is in an embryonic stage and intermediate storage for a week or so will probably be as difficult to attain as long-term storage and will be of little profit. The assessment of the quality of a preserved kidney also remains a fundamental, but unachieved, task.

BASIC PRINCIPLES AND REQUIREMENTS FOR KIDNEY PRESERVATION

If the kidneys removed from living donors were to be preserved for many hours, many fewer problems would have to be solved. The preservation status of these kidneys is excellent; they had normal function, their diuresis was maintained until vascular clamping and they suffered only a few minutes' warm ischemia before cooling began. In this situation one can hope to attain the longest possible cold ischemia time with the method used and immediate recovery of normal function after transplantation. Unfortunately, kidneys harvested from cadavers are seldom in such good condition. Agonal damage to the kidney is almost always present and is of varying and unforseeable intensity. Cardiac arrest or severe vascular collapse is frequent and aggravates previous damage. Furthermore, harvesting of cadaver kidneys is not always performed by fully experimented teams, resulting in various traumas which are almost impossible to assess. This creates a background which is undoubtedly detrimental to long-term cold storage, and whatever the preservation method used, it will certainly not improve previous damage.

It is our feeling that factors such as agonal injury before harvesting or surgical mishaps are more important to subsequent renal function than is the method of preservation itself. Unfortunately, none of these factors is easy to evaluate, with the exception of warm ischemia time before cooling. However, the consequences of warm ischemia differ according to whether it is due to prolonged cardiac arrest or just to clamping of renal vessels on a perfectly well hydrated young donor.

It is now well known that resistance to ischemia varies considerably among organs. The brain will suffer irreversible damage after a circulatory collapse of a few minutes, while the skin is far more resistant, being able to tolerate several hours of ischemia. Resistance of the kidney appears intermediate.

In experimental autotransplantation in pigs[52] I demonstrated that 45 min of warm ischemia followed by 2 days of cold storage resulted in an increased duration of postoperative renal failure but did not prevent complete recovery (Fig. 4.1). When the human kidney is submitted to ischemia of 60 to 120 min, progressive irreversible damage is usually observed even when functional recovery occurs.[63] With more than 2 hours, kidneys are unlikely to recover normal function, and most of them will never function again. Their cellular ultrastructure undergoes irreversible destruction: vacuolization, distension of the endoplastic reticulum and mitochondrial lesions.[61] Metabolism continues, but the supply of

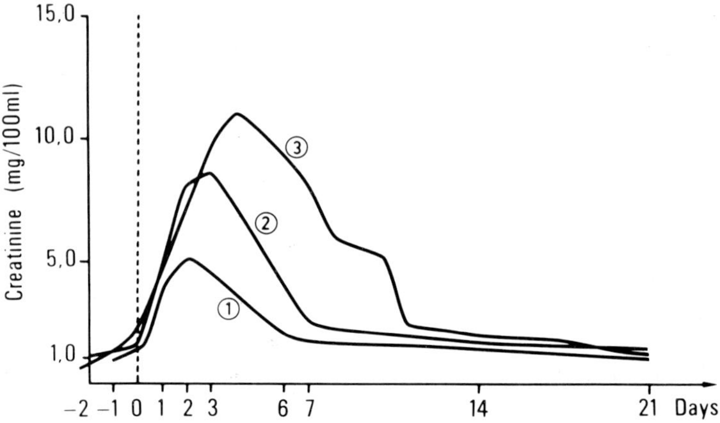

Fig. 4.1 Serum creatinine level after autotransplantation of pig kidneys preserved with Collins C_3 solution for: 1) 24 hours, 2) 48 hours and 3) 48 hours after a 45 min warm ischemia (6 animals in each series).

nutrients essential for this metabolism has been cut off. Early tissue death is thus inevitable.

To keep an isolated organ alive, or at least to avoid irreversible damage, it might seem reasonable to mimic physiologic conditions, that is, to supply essential nutrients artificially by perfusing the organ at normal body temperature. This approach, however, has failed in practice, primarily because of the early appearance of progressively increasing vascular resistance, resulting in a decreased perfusion flow rate. Even if this problem were overcome, the technique itself would be much too complex to be practical.

Many authors[58, 80] showed that hypothermia reduces renal oxygenation to a considerable degree (less than 5% of normal at 5°C) and switches off enzyme systems controlling the sodium pump.[5] The obvious corollary, that hypothermia alone would improve renal tolerance to ischemia, was soon confirmed, and preservation from 8 hours[78] to 12 hours[10, 17, 32] was obtained either by simple in situ cooling or by plunging the kidney into a cold solution after removal.

To the effects of ischemia, however, are added those of hypothermia, a more or less complete inactivation of the cellular, energy-requiring sodium pump. Thus, the potassium, phosphate and magnesium ions which are the normal constituents of renal cells are released into the extracellular medium, and sodium ions and water are free to break into the cells,[57] resulting in cell swelling. The obvious prerequisite for successful organ preservation was thus to maintain membrane potential despite the absence of an active mechanism. The solution was found in 1966 by

Keeler et al:[49] the use of a potassium and magnesium rich solution preventing ionic loss from cold ischemic cells.

Today, hypothermia, as a means of reducing metabolic demand during ischemia, is an essential part of all methods of kidney preservation.

SIMPLE HYPOTHERMIC STORAGE

The first approach to kidney preservation was simple cooling by placement in a cold medium. Among the first reports were those of Calne et al[10] and Dormont et al[27] in our group, who succeeded in storing dog kidneys by simple surface cooling in a cold medium for up to 12 hours. Better results were obtained when kidneys were initially flushed with autologous cold blood, but after 12 hours irreversible damage was observed, and after 24 hours kidneys were not life-sustaining. Based on the suggestion of Pegg et al,[71] that sufficiently fast cooling could not be achieved by surface transmission, attempts were made to increase the cooling rate by perfusion with cooled solutions. Heparinized antologous cold blood was first used, and we[47] and others[71] successfully reached a storage period of 24 hours. But in general, readily available commercial electrolyte solutions were used for rapid cooling, to remove the blood from the vascular bed of the graft and to wash out potentially harmful particulate elements such as platelet aggregates,[38] cells and fibrinoid thrombi.[44] The first solutions used were composed of extracellular electrolytes, and, in fact, little or no benefit could be demonstrated when these results were compared with simple surface cooling.[6, 16, 21, 24, 50] We then achieved satisfactory preservation up to 12 hours using low molecular weight dextran, or serum albumin, containing extracellular-like solutions, but after 17 to 27 hours of ischemia there was incomplete recovery of function.[27] Similar results were reported by many other workers.[56] Up to 1969 most cadaver kidneys were preserved using solutions such as Rheomacrodex, Ringer's, plasma, medium 199, Perfudex or dextran-bicarbonate. But 50% of the kidneys were stored for less than 120 min, and only 10% had an ischemic time of 240 min or longer[67] (Fig. 4.2).

The next step in the development of this technique stemmed from the work of Keeler et al[49] mentioned above. It was Collins and associates[18] who tested in a dog model an electrolyte solution formulated to resemble intracellular fluid. They achieved a 100% success rate in autotransplantation after 24-hour storage, and even after 30 hours when using their C_4 solution containing both procaine and phenoxybenzamine. Using this solution in pigs, we[54] (Fig. 4.1), and others using it in dogs,[59] obtained satisfactory 48-hour preservation. It was also demonstrated by our group that a 48-hour storage period was not detrimental even when kidneys had been subjected to 45 min of warm ischemia prior to removal.[52] After

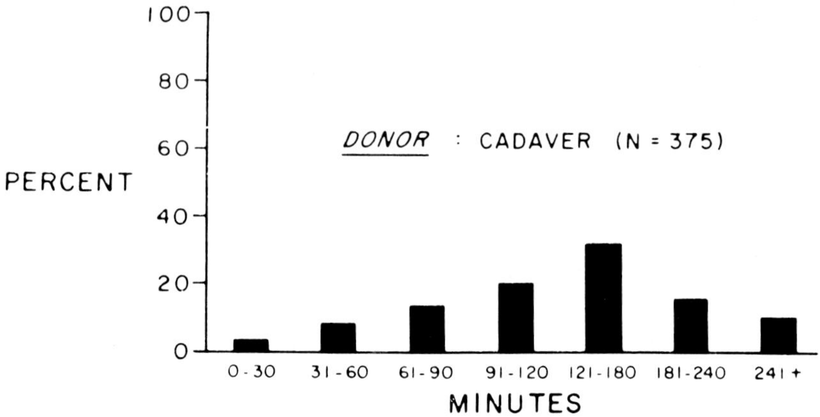

Fig. 4.2 Frequency distribution of total ischemic period. (Reprinted by permission from: J. E. Murray, B. A. Barnes and J. C. Atkinson. Transplantation, *5*:752, 1967.)

72-hour preservation using this method, we found that 50% of pigs which had undergone autotransplantation and immediate contralateral nephrectomy recovered completely normal function of the preserved kidney.[1]

Further research demonstrated that the various components of this solution were not equally important.[22, 45] Watkins et al[84] noted that the magnesium present in C_3 solution was probably not necessary, and in 1973 we confirmed this by obtaining identical results with C_3 solution whether or not magnesium was present.[52] Watkins also questioned the necessity of procaine hydrochloride, which is now considered more toxic than useful.[19] Heparin also appears unnecessary, probably because of the calcium chelating phosphate ions which are present in very high concentration and because there is hardly an opportunity for thrombi to develop as the washing fluid rapidly becomes clear.[19, 84] Regarding the use of phenoxybenzamine, it was clearly shown that it forms a precipitate in the solution and consequently loses its activity.[19]

In 1973 Sacks et al[77] reported success after transplantation of dog kidneys preserved 48 to 72 hours using a solution very close to that described by Collins but in which the osmolarity had been increased to 410 mmol by the use of mannitol. Hypertonic solutions containing mannitol glucose or sucrose were proposed[28, 39] to minimize cellular swelling during the storage period. However, although these substances are poorly diffusable, they will in time diffuse into the cell, increasing cellular osmolarity and resulting in disastrous cell swelling after reimplantation and revascularization.[5] In fact, according to Collins and Halasz,[20] hyperkalemic solutions lacking indiffusible anions may actually cause cell swelling and be harmful. On the other hand, hyperosmolar sodium-based flush solutions can give relatively good preservation results for periods of up to 48 hours.[19, 28] Most hyperosmolar solutions, however, are basically of the intracellular type. The most recent formula is that proposed by Ross et al,[75] which differs from Collins and Sacks solutions principally in that it contains citrate as the major anion. It was considered by Collins and Halasz[20] to provide better results than either of the former for 72-hour kidney storage because it avoided the risk of insoluble magnesium precipitation. This is no longer a valid argument since magnesium is not now considered to be necessary in preservation solutions.

For all the above reasons, the Collins C_2 solution,[18] depleted of magnesium sulfate and heparin but with osmolarity increased to 355 mmol/liter by raising glucose content to 35 g/liter, is now used by most European groups for cadaver kidney preservation (trade name, EuroCollins; see formula, Table 4.1). At present there is no evidence that results obtained with this solution are fundamentally different from those using the Sacks or Ross solutions.

Thus, experimental kidney conservation for up to 72 hours can be achieved with a very simple method. In man, preservation for as long as 48 hours has been followed by immediate function after transplantation (G. Alexandre, personal communication). In a previous work, we reviewed our own series of 225 kidneys preserved by simple cooling after an initial washout perfusion with Collins C_3 solution.[55] The duration of cold ischemia has progressively increased since 1969 from 80 min to 30 hours, with a mean of approximately 20 hours (Fig. 4.3). This is enough time to direct the kidney toward the best possible recipient and to undertake the transplant at a time convenient to the medicosurgical team rather than as an emergency procedure in the middle of the night. Retrospectively, this policy appears to have no deleterious effect on the immediate function of kidney grafts. Less than 20% of recipients in our series have

TABLE 4.1
EuroCollins solution

Components	G/liter	Components	mEq/liter
KH_2PO_4	2.05	K^+	115
K_2HPO_4	7.4	Na^+	10
KCl	1.12	Cl^-	15
$NaHCO_3$	0.84	HCO_3^-	10
		HPO_4^{--}	85
Glucose	35	$H_2PO_4^-$	15

Osmolarity: 355 mosm/liter
pH
20°C:7.33
4°C:7.20

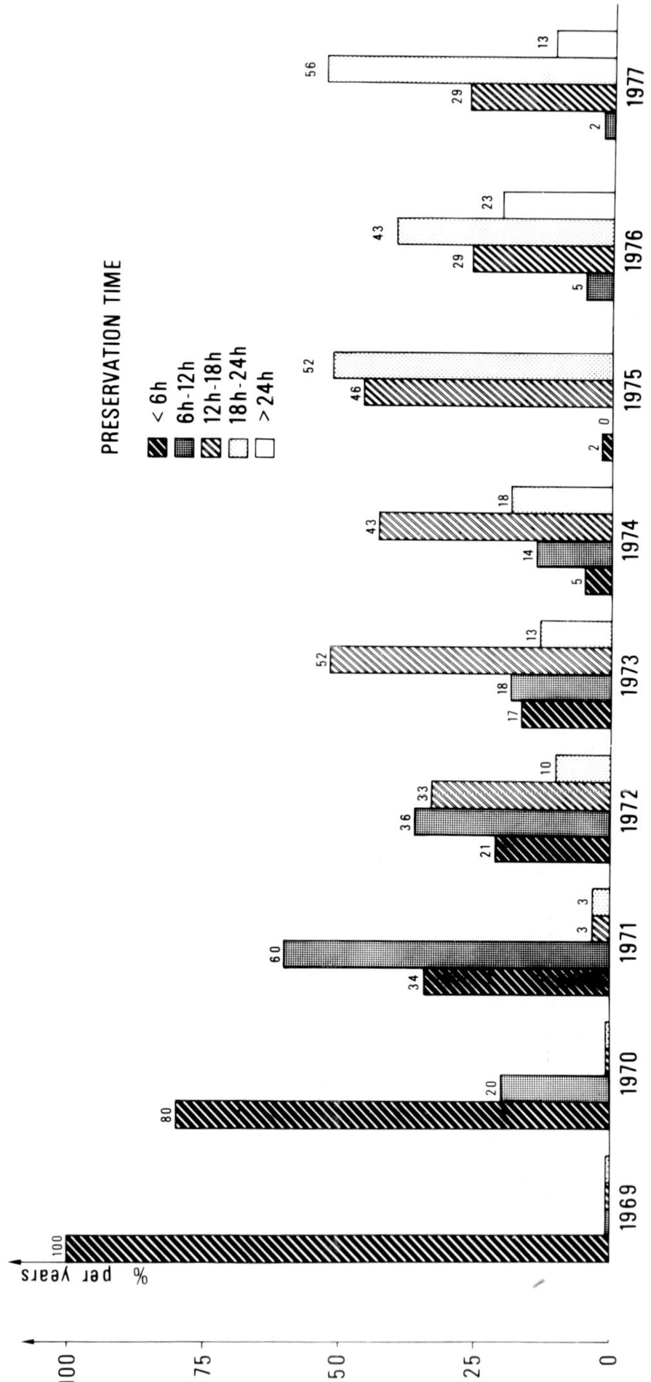

Fig. 4.3. Duration of storage period of cadaver kidneys transplanted at Necker Hospital from 1969 to 1977.

required hemodialysis in the postoperative period, and this incidence was the same whether grafts had more or less than 12 hours of total ischemia. It is also probable that even the few cases of renal insufficiency that we observed were not due to the preservation technique but instead were the result of trauma during the prepreservation period. In our experience,[51] this technique can even be applied to kidneys that have been subjected to warm ischemia of from 10 to 60 min.

An increasing number of reports from other groups[5, 15, 19, 25, 60] indicates that this method of preservation gives satisfactory functional results, as assessed by the recovery of graft function during the first days. We have recently shown[55] for the first time that this type of cadaver kidney preservation does not adversely affect the long-term prognosis of the graft, which is in fact the goal of kidney preservation. Kidneys preserved up to 30 hours in Collins solution have a 2-year survival rate of 65%, which is as good as that of kidneys preserved less than 12 hours (59%) (Fig. 4.4). It is worth noting, however, that the percentage of transplanted kidneys exhibiting tubular or interstitial changes on 2-year routine biopsy was higher, although not significantly, when the storage period was between 12 and 30 hours than when it was less than 12 hours. The incidence of vascular lesions, however, was very similar (Table 4.2).

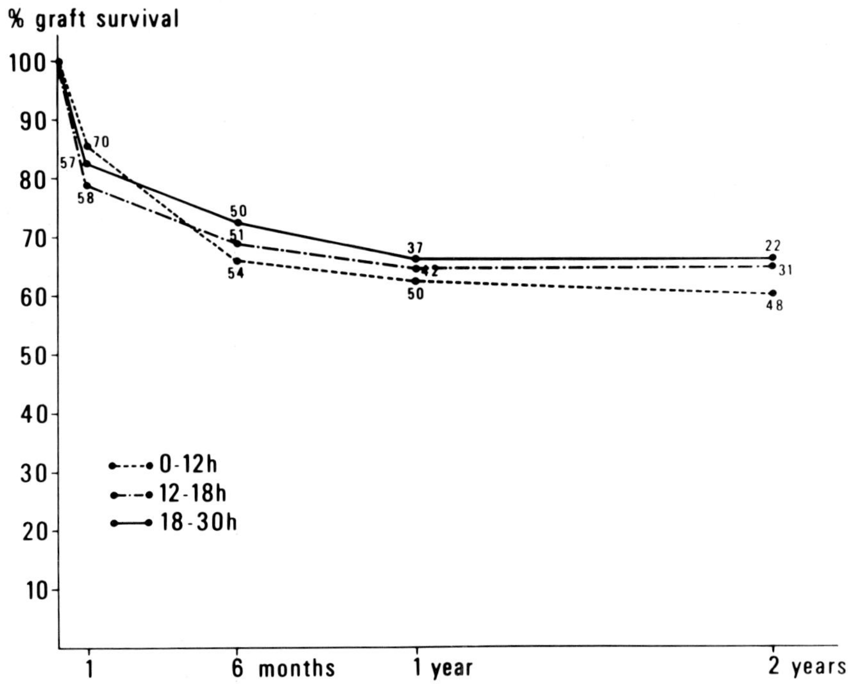

Fig. 4.4. Influence of preservation time on the long-term outcome of cadaver kidney grafts preserved with Collins C_2 solution.

TABLE 4.2
Type and frequency of pathologic changes in 2-year routine cadaver transplant biopsies[a]

Location of Changes	0–12 Hours		12–30 Hours	
	No. of Biopsies Available	Percentage With Changes	No. of Biopsies Available	Percentage With Changes
Tubules	45	56	44	59
Interstitium				
Cells	45	38	44	48
Fibrosis	45	56	44	70.5
Loose fibrosis	45	7	44	20.5
Arteries				
arcuate	12	100	9	89
interlobular	44	59	43	47
arterioles	45	45	44	39

[a] Kidneys which were preserved for less than 12 hours before transplantation are compared with those which were preserved between 12 and 30 hours.

Finally, our results, as well as those of a number of other groups, show that the simple hypothermic storage of kidneys which have been washed through with an intracellular-like solution, whether hyperosmolar or not, provides cadaver kidney preservation for at least 30 hours and probably for 48 hours when kidneys are correctly removed from a well treated brain-dead donor, without detrimental effects either on the immediate functional recovery of the graft or on its long-term prognosis. On the other hand, no poor quality kidney can be improved by any kind of preservation method, and as metabolic activity is not entirely abolished at 0°C, there is necessarily a finite limit on the duration of storage attainable by this method.[20]

HYPOTHERMIC PERFUSION BY MACHINE

At present, the only real alternative to the simple washout technique is continuous hypothermic perfusion. After the preliminary works by Carrel and Lindbergh[11] in 1938, the first important reports were those of Humphries et al in 1963,[43] 1964[42] and 1968.[44] Using blood, serum or plasma diluted with a balanced salt solution, they succeeded in perfusing dog kidneys for 1, 2 and 3 days at 10°C in a perfusion circuit that included a pulsatile pump, a membrane oxygenator and a filter. The method was further developed by Belzer et al,[3] who obtained more reproducible results. In fact, their perfusion circuit (Fig. 4.5) was similar to that of Humphries, but they showed that detrimental increasing vascular resistances usually observed in previous perfusion studies employing plasma could be prevented with the use of cryoprecipitated plasma. A highly sophisticated pulsatile perfusion machine including a membrane oxygenator was later devised, and cadaver kidneys were thus preserved for 17

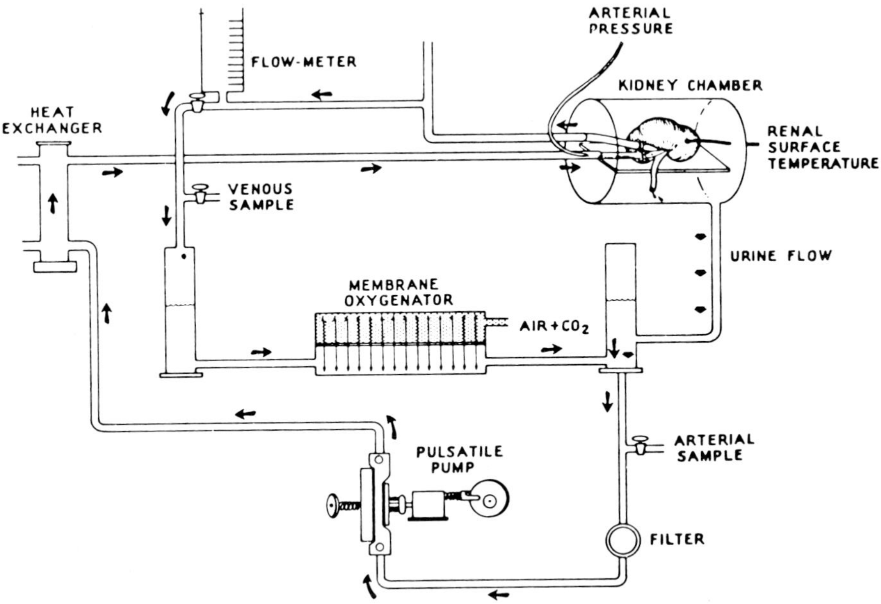

Fig. 4.5. Belzer kidney perfusion circuit.

hours for the first time.[4] Further research concentrated primarily on two objectives: 1) determining an optimum perfusate and 2) simplification of the initial Belzer machine without loss of efficiency.

A large number of experimental *perfusates* have been used in place of the probably harmful cryoprecipitated plasma first proposed by Belzer.[3] This perfusate is generally not used at the present, at least in Europe, not only because its preparation is complex and expensive, but also because it is probably toxic for the perfused kidney.[40, 76, 8] The presence of cytotoxic antibodies has been demonstrated in the plasma after cryoprecipitation.[31] Rents have also been demonstrated in the endothelium.[40] They were presumed to originate from mechanical damage to the kidney by the perfusion apparatus. In both cases, nonspecific thrombosis secondary to endothelial damage may develop after reimplantation of the perfused kidney.[76] Among other solutions which have been assayed, two were extensively studied: purified protein fractions[46, 64] and albumin.[13, 23, 34, 36] Claes and Blohme,[13] using a perfusate containing 45 g/liter of purified human albumin, were able to store dog kidneys up to 96 hours. The extreme variability of results observed with this method appears to be due to high variations in the composition of various commercial solutions.[14] In particular, osmolarity can vary from 164 to 310 mmol/liter. The most hyperosmolar solutions have given the best results, better than those obtained with cryoprecipitated plasma.[34] Free fatty acid content also varies markedly from one manufacturer to another.[41] In addition, highly or partially purified albumin solutions, which at present seem to be considered the best,[70] are very costly.

Several types of *perfusion machines* are commercially available today. All consist of a pump producing a pulsatile perfusate flow, a membrane oxygenator, a heat exchanger controlling the degree of hypothermia and a chamber for attaching one or several kidneys. In most, the perfusion pressure of the kidney can be measured.

The equipment required for permanent hypothermic perfusion of human kidneys is complex, expensive, bulky and difficult to integrate into a routine and active kidney exchange program. As recently pointed out by Pegg,[70] the Belzer approach was entirely empirical and there is no evidence of the necessity for each of the components in his machine. For example, the pulsatile pump and high perfusate flow rate can probably be replaced by constant pressure perfusion;[72] the membrane oxygenator has been omitted from new small machines without any harmful effect for the perfused kidney, whose oxygenation is provided by the small gas-liquid interface which exists in the preservation chamber. Finally, the necessity of permanent perfusion itself can be questioned.

Although successful kidney preservation of up to 7 days has been reported in rare animal experiments with this method,[85] the results of cadaver kidney transplantation after continuous flow preservation have not proven to be better than those obtained after much simpler methods of washout and surface cooling. It is generally agreed that despite careful donor selection and elimination of 6 to 10% of cadaver kidneys because of poor perfusion characteristics on the machine, postoperative renal failure still requires dialysis in approximately 20% of cases. Some groups, notably that in Los Angeles,[15] have even found a significantly high incidence of late failure in kidneys preserved on continuous flow machines. Enthusiasm for this method survives, particularly in North America[7, 12, 29, 65, 79] and Sweden.[14] However, the costly capital outlay for equipment and training of personnel, the expense of the perfusate and the difficulty involved in transporting the kidney attached to the machine, have led most European and many American transplant teams to abandon the technique.

DEEPFREEZING FOR LONG-TERM STORAGE

Since metabolic activity is not entirely abolished at 0°C, it is unlikely that washout techniques will ever provide long-term storage of kidneys. With continuous perfusion, even if technically possible, long-term preservation would be of such a complexity and cost as to make it unrealistic. Thus, deepfreezing at very low temperatures seems to be the only technique which could conceivably allow long-term preservation of organs. Unfortunately, although indefinite storage of cells and simple tissues[69] is already routine with this technique, the problems posed by freezing a large organ such as the kidney to −80°C or less are still far from solved.[30]

The first problem is the choice of an effective and nontoxic cryoprotective agent. Dimethyl sulfoxide (DMSO) has been the most commonly used,[28, 48, 66] but it was responsible for increased vascular resistance and endothelial damage.[68] Glycerol presently appears to be the best known cryoprotectant,[73] providing osmolality of the perfusate is close to 400 mmol/kg. But the next steps, i.e., cooling, storage, thawing and assessment of viability before transplantation, are still subjects of conjecture. It is very difficult to control the freezing rate so as to avoid a temperature gradient between the cortex and the medulla. The optimum cooling rate is still unknown, although fast cooling (−1°C/min) seems to be superior to slow cooling. Storage temperature must be at −80°C or below if storage periods are to exceed 1 year. For rewarming, the temperature must rise more than 100°C/min without creating any temperature gradient and without allowing the external temperature to rise above 40°C. Microwave heating, which was thought to bring a solution,[35] seems in fact to create many problems. None of these problems may be entirely insoluble, but the first question is whether their solution is necessary, or whether a simpler approach might be possible.[74] So far only Dietzman et al[26] and Guttman et al[35] have successfully frozen, then thawed and retransplanted dog kidneys, but they did not lower the temperature below −22°C. After transplantation, the function of the kidneys was really only mediocre.

When an efficient process for deepfreezing has been developed, interest in other preservation methods will be considerably less, and donor kidney banks could be established. This would considerably modify the general concept of transplantation and its results.

ASSESSMENT OF VIABILITY

There is an urgent need for a reliable method of predicting the viability of a preserved organ because much of the potential damage which could affect the kidney before transplantation is clinically undetectable. Several criteria have been proposed,[8, 9, 33, 62] ranging from simple evaluation of physiologic parameters of the whole organ to the study of intracellular biochemistry.

Most of these approaches are designed to detect the secondary effects of cellular anoxia:[83] inhibition of oxidative phosphorylation, reduction in the total adenine nucleotides, alteration of membrane potential and modification in intracellular as well as surface pH, reduction of oxygen consumption and release of lysosomal enzymes. Despite all these approaches for measuring cellular viability, it is still not possible to predict the long-term outcome for a preserved kidney. The well known reversible tubular cell damage is sufficient to render most of the tests positive in a significantly viable organ. They may, nevertheless, be of value for predicting acute postoperative tubular necrosis.

In everyday practice, the viability test most frequently used is the study of renal perfusion flow during the preservation period, when a perfusion machine is employed. Flow less than 100 ml/min has been assumed to indicate very poor prognosis.[2] However, numerous reports have emphasized the fact that perfusion parameters are far from being consistently predictive.[33, 82]

Although these tests can give indications of cellular damage in a preserved organ, none can predict whether these lesions are reversible. In our experience with hypothermic storage and washout perfusion, the percentage of immediate and irreversible failures is less than 10%[53] and it is difficult and even impossible to know whether these failures result from poor preservation or reflect hyperacute rejection (see p. 201). The same problem exists in kidneys that develop chronic rejection lesions, since there is no clear distinction between lesions due to aggressive immunologic reaction and those due to ischemia. Nevertheless, it is certain that lesions caused by poor preservation can slowly lead to progressive destruction of the kidney. Thus, tests which reflect only the presence of tubular cell damage rather than predicting long-term viability, are not really helpful. On the other hand, as suggested by Collins,[20] some of the injury sustained by the organ is not measurable before vascular reflow because it is not present before implantation (i.e., cortical ischemia secondary to altered cortical revascularization). Such changes are probably very important for the long-term prognosis of the transplanted kidney but are not predictable during preservation.

PRACTICAL APPLICATION TO HUMAN KIDNEY PRESERVATION

In transplantation from living donors, only simple cooling is required because ischemia time is no longer than a few minutes or hours. We perfuse the kidney as soon as it is removed with 500 ml of EuroCollins solution, previously stored at 0 to 4°C. The kidney is then kept immersed in this solution and maintained at 0°C. Diuresis always appears immediately after transplantation, and renal function is usually close to normal in less than 48 hours.

With cadaver kidneys, we are faced with a different and more complicated situation. It is necessary to prevent kidneys from sustaining damage while still in the dead donor and then to preserve them using the most efficient techniques.

Prevention of Damage to the Kidney before its Removal

There are several ways of decreasing the risk of cadaveric changes in the kidneys during the interval from death to removal of the kidney.

When the donor is not on a respirator, kidneys are likely to suffer ischemia before preservation and to exhibit acute tubular necrosis after revascularization. Such kidneys should not be preserved for a long time, even on a perfusion machine. If they are to be used, it should be locally. It is always possible to try to avoid ischemia by external cardiac massage from the moment of death.

If the donor is on a respirator and declared dead from irreversible brain damage, the respirator should not be switched off until after the kidney has been removed. It is important that kidneys be harvested in the best possible conditions; when this is done by a well experienced surgeon, they can be stored or perfused for at least 2 days and will recover their function immediately after transplantation.

It is also important that the kidney not suffer poor blood perfusion during the period between death to surgical removal of the kidney, in order to ensure that it will be able to endure a cold ischemia period of up to 24 or 48 hours without vascular supply.

Beating Heart Donor

It is vital that the donor be in good cardiovascular state with a normal heart rate and normal venous and arterial pressure. In addition, there must be normal electrolyte balance and urinary output, and hematocrit should not be less than 20%. To ensure this, care of a potential donor should be by physicians with experience in intensive care, with careful monitoring of arterial and venous blood pressure, urinary volume, heart and respiratory rates, ECG and serum electrolytes. Fluid balance should be maintained by replacement with plasma or a substitute such as low molecular weight dextran, blood or physiologic saline or glucose solution. If vasopressive drugs are necessary, it is important to use only those which do not cause renal vasoconstriction, such as dopamine or isoprenaline chlorhydrate or dobutamine. Phenoxybenzamine administered intravenously or phentolamine injected directly into the renal artery before nephrectomy can reverse to a certain extent the renal vasoconstriction that occurs during surgical manipulations. Despite these precautionary measures, dissection of the vascular pedicle and of the kidneys must be performed as atraumatically as possible.

Induction of Cardiac Arrest

Despite the use of vasodilatators, vasoconstriction of renal vessels frequently occurs when perfoming nephrectomy in a beating heart donor. It can be avoided by inducing cardiac arrest before removing the kidneys. The best technique is to introduce a catheter into the aorta, which is ligatured above and below the renal arteries (or by using a double balloon catheter), while perfusing the kidneys with an intracellular-like electrolyte solution at 0°C. This technique permits subsequent rapid perfusion and cooling of the kidneys.

Choice of Preservation Techniques

It is now established from experimental studies and human experience that kidneys preserved between 0°C and 4°C after simple washout by either EuroCollins solution or other hyperosmolar intracellular-like solutions can recover normal function after preservation for between 30 and 48 hours. Since this method is less complicated and substantially less expensive than continuous perfusion, since neither technique provides preservation long enough to perform donor-recipient HLA-D matching with the standard mixed lymphocyte reaction (MLR) technique or to try to induce specific tolerance in the recipient, and since results after simple washout as mentioned above are as good as if not better than those after machine perfusion, there is still considerable doubt about the necessity of continuous perfusion.[70] Logistic considerations clearly favor ice storage techniques, which allow intercity (or even international) kidney exchange.[20]

There is little evidence in the human to support the hypothesis that kidneys preserved by machine do better than those on ice if they are previously submitted to a warm ischemia period.[37] Whatever the answer, it is certainly easier to avoid warm ischemia than to develop preservation and exchange programs using perfusion machines. Thus, there seems little justification for their use at the present time, except on an experimental basis.

REFERENCES

1. Barbanel, C., and Kreis, H. Further evaluation of kidney preservation with Collins' solution. Annual Report of the Eurotransplant Meeting, Leiden, 1973.
2. Belzer, F. O. Renal preservation. N. Engl. J. Med., *1*:774, 1974.
3. Belzer, F. O., Ashby, B. S., and Dunphy, J. E. 24-hour and 72-hour preservation of canine kidney. Lancet, *2*:536, 1967.

4. Belzer, F. O., Ashby, B. S., Gulyassy, P. F., and Powell, M. Successful seventeen-hour preservation and transplantation of human-cadaver kidney. N. Engl. J. Med., *278:*608, 1968.
5. Belzer, F. O., Hoffman, R. M., and Southard, J. H. Kidney preservation. Surg. Clin. North Am., *58:*261, 1978.
6. Brunius, U., Fritjofsson, A., and Gelin, L. E. Organ and tissue transplantation: Microcirculatory aspects on the preservation of kidneys for transplantation. Bibl. Anat., *9:* 374, 1967.
7. Burleson, R. L., Jones, D. B., Yenikomshian, A. M., Cornwall, C., Devoe, C., Derito, J., and Schiff, M. Clinical renal preservation by cryoperfusion with an albumin perfusate. Renal perfusion with albumin. Arch. Surg., *113:*688, 1978.
8. Calman, K. C. The prediction of organ viability. I. An hypothesis. Cryobiology, *11:*1, 1974.
9. Calman, K. C. The prediction of an organ viability. II. Testing and hypothesis. Cryobiology, *11:*7, 1974.
10. Calne, R. Y., Pegg, D. E., Pryse-Davies, J., and Leigh-Brown, F. Renal preservation by ice cooling. An experimental study relating to kidney transplantation from cadavers. Br. Med. J., *2:*651, 1963.
11. Carrel, A., and Lindbergh, C. A. *The Culture of Organs.* Hamish Hamilton Medical Books, London, 1938.
12. Cho, S. I., Der Hagopian, R. P., Krane, R. Z., and Nabseth, D. O. Regional organ preservation program in the New England area. Surgery, *75:*528, 1974.
13. Claes, G., and Blohme, I. Experimental and clinical results of continuous albumin perfusion of kidneys. In *Organ Preservation,* edited by D. E. Pegg, p. 51. Churchill Livingstone, London, 1973.
14. Claes, G., Blohme, I., Gelin, L. E., and Heideman, M. Organ preservation. Renal transplantation as the treatment of choice for terminal renal failure. Scand. J. Urol. Nephrol. (Suppl.), *38:*29, 1976.
15. Clark, E. A., Opelz, G., Mickey, M. R., and Terasaki, P. I. Evaluation of Belzer and Collins kidney preservation methods. Lancet, *7766:*361, 1973.
16. Cleveland, R. J., Lee, H. M., Prout, G. R., and Hume, D. M. Preservation of the cadaver kidney for renal homotransplantation in man. Surg. Gynecol. Obstet., *119:*991, 1964.
17. Collins, G. M., Bravo-Shugarman, M., Novom, S., and Terasaki, P. I. Kidney preservation for transplantation. I. Twelve hour storage in rabbits. Transplant. Proc., *1:*801, 1969.
18. Collins, G. M., Bravo-Shugarman, M., and Terasaki, P. I. Kidney preservation for transportation. Initial perfusion and 30 hours ice storage. Lancet, *2:*1219, 1969.
19. Collins, G. M., and Halasz, N. A. Forty-eight hour ice storage of kidneys: Importance of cation content. Surgery, *79:*432, 1976.
20. Collins, G. M., and Halasz, N. A. Current aspects of renal preservation. Urology, *10:*22, 1977.
21. Collins, G. M., Hartley, L. C. J., and Clunie, G. J. A. Kidney preservation for transportation. 5. Comparison of perfusates for hypothermic storage. Med. J. Aust., *1:*1171, 1971.
22. Collins, G. M., Hartley, L. J. C., and Clunie, G. J. A. Kidney preservation for transplantation. Experimental analysis of optimal perfusate composition. Br. J. Surg., *59:*187, 1972.
23. Collste, H. Perservation of kidneys for transplantation. Experimental studies. Acta Chir. Scand. (Suppl.), *425:*1, 1972.
24. Dempster, W. J., Kountz, S. L., and Jovanovic, M. Simple kidney storage technique. Br. Med. J., *1:*407, 1964.
25. Diethelm, A. G., Sterling, W. A., Balch, C. M., and Clark, E. C. Preservation of cadaver

kidneys using hypothermic, hyperosmolar, intracellular washout solution. Transplantation, *21:*417, 1976.

26. Dietzman, R. H., Eira Rebelo, A., Graham, E. F., Crabo, B. G., and Lillehei, R. C. Long-term functional success following freezing of canine kidneys. Surgery, *74:*181, 1973.
27. Dormont, J., Auvert, J., Cukier, J., and Zmerli, S. Auto-transplantation rénale chez le chien après conservation prolongée à basse température. Rev. Fr., Etud. Clin. Biol., *9:* 1043, 1964.
28. Downes, G., Hoffman, R., Huang, J., and Belzer, F. O. Mechanism of action of washout solutions for kidney preservation. Transplantation, *16:*46, 1973.
29. Feduska, N. J., Belzer, F. O., Stieper, K. W., Duca, R. M., Mitchell, J. W., Vincenti, F., Cochrum, K. C., and Salvatierra, O. A ten year experience with cadaver kidney preservation using cryoprecipitated plasma. Am. J. Surg., *135:*356, 1978.
30. Filo, R. S., Bell, R. T., Small, A., and Sell, K. W. Current status of kidney freeze preservation. Transplant. Proc. (Suppl. 1), *8:*215, 1976.
31. Filo, R. S., Dickson, L. G., Suba, E. A., and Sell, K. W. Immunologic injury induced by in-vivo perfusion of canine renal autografts. Surgery, *76:*88, 1974.
32. Fisher, E. F., Copeland, C. H., and Fisher, B. Correlation of ultrastructure and function following hypothermic preservation of canine kidneys. Lab. Invest., *17:*99, 1967.
33. Foreman, J. Prediction of viability of rabbit kidneys preserved by hypothermic perfusion. Cryobiology, *12:*231, 1975.
34. Grundmann, R., Berr, F., Pitschi, H., Kirchhoff, R., and Pichlmaier, H. Ninety-six hour preservation of canine kidneys. Transplantation, *17:*299, 1974.
35. Guttman, F. M., Robitaille, P., Lizin, P., and Blanchard, H. Physiologic investigation of frozen-thawed canine kidneys. Transplant. Proc., *9:*255, 1977.
36. Halasz, N. A., and Collins, G. M. Simplification of perfusion preservation methods. Transplantation, *17:*534, 1974.
37. Halasz, N. A., and Collins, G. M. Forty-eight hour kidney preservation. A comparison of flushing and ice storage with perfusion. Arch. Surg., *3:*175, 1976.
38. Hansson, L. O. The influences of thrombocyte aggregation on renal circulation. Acta Chir. Scand. (Suppl.), *345:*1, 1965.
39. Hardie, I. R., Balderson, G., Hamlyn, L., Mackay, D., and Clunie, G. Extended ice storage of canine kidneys using hyperosmolar Collins solution. Transplantation, *23:*282, 1977.
40. Hill, G. S., Light, J. A., and Perloff, L. J. Perfusion-related injury in renal transplantation. Surgery, *79:*440, 1976.
41. Horsburgh, T. Possible role of free fatty acids in kidney preservation media. Nature (New Biology), *242:*122, 1973.
42. Humphries, A. L., Russel, R., Gregory, J., Carter, R. H., and Moretz, W. H. Hypothermic perfusion of the canine kidney for 48 hours followed by reimplantation. Am. Surg., *30:* 748, 1964.
43. Humphries, A. L., Russel, R., Ostafin, J., Goodrich, S. M., and Moretz, W. H. Successful reimplantation of canine kidney after 24 hour storage. Surgery, *54:*136, 1963.
44. Humphries, A. L., Russel, R., Stoddard, L. D., and Moretz, W. H. Three-day kidney preservation: Perfusion of kidneys with hypothermic, diluted blood or plasma. Surgery, *63:*646, 1968.
45. Jensen, E. H., and Kemp, E. Kidney preservation. III. The importance of the composition of perfusion fluids in the transplantation of rabbit kidneys. Scand. J. Urol. Nephrol., *6:*284, 1972.
46. Johnson, R. W. G., Anderson, M., Flear, C. T. G., Murray, S. G. H., Taylor, R. M. R., and Swinney, J., Evaluation of a new perfusion solution for kidney preservation. Transplantation, *13:*270, 1972.

47. Karlson, K. E., Dormont, J., and Hamburger, J. Twenty-four hours kidney storage at 4°C with the vascular bed filled with arterial blood. In *Organ Perfusion and Preservation*, edited by J. C. Norman, p. 687. Appleton-Century-Crofts, New York, 1968.
48. Karow, A. M., Webb, W. R., and Stapp, J. E. Preservation of hearts by freezing. Arch. Surg., *91:*572, 1965.
49. Keeler, R., Swinney, D. J., Taylor, M. R., and Uldall, P. R. The problem of renal preservation. Br. J. Urol., *38:*653, 1966.
50. Knight, P. R., Tonkiewicz, Z. M., and Couch, N. P. Evaluation of functioning canine renal allografts after six hours storage. Surg. Forum, *14:*171, 1963.
51. Kreis, H. Influence of ischaemia on post-transplant function of 188 cadaver renal grafts. A collaborative study from four Paris hospitals. Lancet, *2:*887, 1972.
52. Kreis, H. Organ procurement. Proc. Eur. Dial. Transplant. Assoc., *10:*31, 1973.
53. Kreis, H., Finch, T. W., Moreau, J. F., Noel, L. H., Lacombe, M., and Crosnier, J. Early renal failure after cadaver kidney transplantation. In *Advances in Nephrology*, vol. 8, p. 209, edited by J. Hamburger, J. Crosnier and M. H. Maxwell. Year Book Medical Publishers, Chicago, 1979.
54. Kreis, H., Lacombe, M., Ciancioni, C., and Marinov, V. 48-hour kidney preservation (initial perfusion with potassium and magnesium rich solution). Rev. Eur. Etud. Clin. Biol., *17:*192, 1972.
55. Kreis, H., Noel, L. H., Moreau, J. F., Barbanel, C., and Crosnier, J. Biologic, pathologic and radiologic studies of cadaver kidneys preserved in Collins' solution. Transplant. Proc., *9:*1611, 1977.
56. Ladaga, L. G., Nabseth, D. C., and Deterling, R. A., Jr. Kidney preservation by means of hypothermia and hyperbaric oxygen without perfusion. In *Organ Perfusion and Preservation*, edited by J. C. Norman, p. 677. Appleton-Century-Crofts, New York, 1968.
57. Leaf, A. Maintenance of concentration gradients and regulation of cell volume. Ann. NY Acad. Sci., *72:*398, 1959.
58. Levy, M. N. Oxygen consumption and blood flow in the hypothermic, perfused kidney. Am. J. Physiol., *194:*1111, 1959.
59. Liu, W. P., Humphries, A. L., Stoddard, L. D., and Moretz, W. H. 48-hour kidney storage, Lancet, *2:*423, 1970.
60. Lokkegaard, H. Experimental and clinical experiences with long term kidney preservation by use of simple hypothermia. Scand. J. Urol. Nephrol. (Suppl.), *42:*207, 1977.
61. Mackay, B., Moloney, P. J., and Rix, D. B. The use of electron microscopy in renal preservation and perfusion. In *Organ Perfusion and Preservation*, edited by J. C. Norman, p. 697. Appleton-Century-Crofts, New York, 1968.
62. Malinin, T. I., and Perry, V. P. A review of tissue and organ viability assay. Cryobiology, *4:*104, 1967.
63. Marshall, V. Renal preservation. In *Kidney Transplantation, Principles and Practice*, edited by P. J. Morris, p. 89. Academic Press, London, 1979.
64. Mendezpicon, G., Belle, C., Pierce, J. C., Thomas, F., Murai, M., Wolf, J., and Lee, H. M. Use of plasma protein fraction in preservation of cadaveric kidneys. Surgery, *79:*364, 1976.
65. Moore, T. C., Berne, T. V., and English, T. S. Use of a mobile transplant kidney preservation unit in a large metropolitan area. Am. J. Surg., *124:*229, 1972.
66. Mundth, E. D., De Falco, A. J., and Jacobson, Y. G. Functional survival of kidneys subjected to extracorporeal freezing and reimplantation. Cryobiology, *2:*62, 1965.
67. Murray, J. E., Barnes, B. A., and Atkinson, J. C. Fifth report of the human kidney transplant registry. Transplantation, *5:*752, 1967.
68. Pegg, D. E. Perfusion of rabbit kidneys with cryoprotective agents. Cryobiology, *9:*411, 1972.

69. Pegg, D. E. Long term preservation of cells and tissues: A review. J. Clin. Pathol., *29:* 271, 1976.
70. Pegg, D. E. An approach to hypothermic renal preservation. Cryobiology, *15:*1, 1978.
71. Pegg, D. E., Calne, R. Y., Pryse-Davies, J., and Leigh-Brown, F., Canine renal preservation using surface and perfusion cooling techniques. Ann. NY Acad. Sci., *120:*506, 1964.
72. Pegg, D. E., and Green, C. J. Renal preservation by hypothermic perfusion. III. The lack of influence of pulsatile flow. Cryobiology, *13:*161, 1976.
73. Pegg, D. E., and Wusteman, M. C. Perfusion of rabbit kidneys with glycerol solutions at 5°C. Cryobiology, *14:*168, 1977.
74. Rapatz, G., Luyet, B., and McKenzie, A. Effect of cooling and rewarming rates on glycerolated human erythrocytes. Cryobiology, *12:*293, 1975.
75. Ross, H., Marshall, V. C., and Escott, M. L. Seventy-two hours canine kidney preservation without continuous perfusion. Transplantation, *21:*498, 1976.
76. Rowlands, D. T., Hill, G. S., and Zmijewski, C. M. The pathology of renal homograft rejection. Am. J. Pathol., *85:*774, 1976.
77. Sacks, S. A., Petritsch, P. H., and Kaufman, J. J. Canine kidney preservation using a new perfusate. Lancet, *1:*1024, 1973.
78. Schloerb, P. R., Waldorf, R. D., and Welsh, J. S. The protective effect of kidney hypothermia on total renal ischemia. Surg. Gynecol. Obstet., *109:*561, 1959.
79. Schweizer, R. T., Stuphin, B. A., and Bartus, S. A. Fibrin formation in plasma perfusates during kidney preservation. Surg. Res., *24:*57, 1978.
80. Semb, G., Krog, J., and Johansen, J. Renal metabolism and blood flow during hypothermia. Study by means of renal perfusion in situ. Acta Chir. Scand. (Suppl.), *253:*196, 1960.
81. Spector, D., Limas, C., Frost, J. S., Zachary, J. B., Sterioff, S., Williams, G. M., Rolley, R. T., and Sadler, J. H. Perfusion nephropathy in human transplants. N. Engl. J. Med., *295:*1217, 1976.
82. Vehling, D. T., and Cossman, F. P. Renal preservation with a synthetic perfusion fluid. Invest. Urol., *10:*63, 1972.
83. Vogt, M. T., and Farber, E. On the molecular pathology of cell death. Am. J. Pathol., *53:*1, 1968.
84. Watkins, G. M., Prentiss, N. A., and Couch, N. P. Successful 24-hour kidney preservation with simplified hyperosmolar hyperkaliemic perfusate. Transplant. Proc., *3:*612, 1971.
85. Woods, J. E. Successful three-to-seven-day preservation of canine kidneys. Immediate life-sustaining function. Arch. Surg., *102:*614, 1971.

CHAPTER FIVE

Immunosuppression

Jean-François Bach

Introduction—Chemical immunosuppression: Azathioprine, corticosteroids, other drugs—Antilymphocyte sera—Other methods of nonspecific immunosuppression—Induction of specific unresponsiveness—Conclusions.

The normal fate of a renal allograft is inevitable rejection. Two approaches have been used to avoid this unfavorable outcome and permit clinical transplantation: selection of the most histocompatible donor and suppression of the recipient immune response (eventually specifically to the donor antigens).

The first approach is the more satisfactory since it does not involve manipulation of the recipient's immune system. It is difficult, however, and even if significant progress in clinical results has derived from our knowledge of the HLA (human leucocyte A) antigens [A, B and D-related (DR)],[235] it must be recognized that donor selection does not permit allograft survival without immunosuppression.

The suppression of immune responses has been successfully achieved by several methods using various chemical, biologic or physical treatments, which are discussed in the following pages. The problems encountered when using these treatments (toxicity, side effects due to non-graft-specific immunosuppression) will be emphasized and the present state of the search for new methods allowing the induction of specific allograft tolerance will be presented.

CHEMICAL IMMUNOSUPPRESSION

The chemical immunosuppressive agents are synthetic products which can suppress or depress immune responses. In 1958 Schwartz and Dameshek[237a] demonstrated that 6-mercaptopurine (6-MP) could prevent production of antibodies against bovine serum albumin. Since then, many other agents have been shown to have immunosuppressive properties, but it is remarkable that 6-MP (Purinethol) and its imidazole derivative, azathioprine (Imuran) are still the most used of these agents in human transplantation.

Prolongation of allograft survival is not, in fact, a general property of all immunosuppressive drugs. For example, cytosine arabinoside[121] gives complete inhibition of the humoral response of dogs to sheep red cells, but it has no effect on the survival of kidney grafts in dogs. Conversely, azathioprine produces remarkable prolongation of graft survival but has little or no ability to prevent the appearance of antibody after stimulation by flagellin.[234] The only drugs which will be considered here are those that have a high therapeutic index in the prolongation of graft survival, that is, those that combine the greatest degree of inhibition of graft rejection with the least possible toxicity for the recipient.

The problem is complicated by the fact that some *anti-inflammatory* drugs can prolong graft survival without having any true immunosuppressive effect. This is the case with indomethacin,[71] which acts in guinea pigs by specifically preventing cell infiltration of the graft. It is debatable if this can be regarded as immunosuppressive activity, but nonetheless such drugs have been used in the management of kidney grafts in man and so must be considered here. Even more important in this connection are the corticosteroids. Although steroids alone are probably incapable of preventing renal allograft rejection, they are widely used today in the conditioning of graft recipients. They are virtually specific in the treatment of "crises" and for this reason must be considered in detail.

Knowledge of chemical immunosuppression is developing rapidly. Various new and original immunosuppressive agents, such as asparaginase, or more important, cyclosporin A, have been discovered in recent years. Even more important is the considerable progress in understanding the metabolism and mode of action of the various drugs. Knowledge of these recent advances in pharmacology is essential if the drugs are to be used to best advantage in the treatment of transplant recipients. The reader can consult many general reviews of the subject for a more detailed account of the work done in the past decade.[14, 40, 111, 236]

Azathioprine

Chemical Structure

Azathioprine (Imuran, Burroughs Wellcome) was synthesized in 1961 by Elion et al,[96] 11 years after the same group had synthesized another thiopurine, 6-MP[95] (Purinethol, Burroughs Wellcome). Azathioprine is the imidazole derivative of 6-MP (see Fig. 5.1), which in turn is the analogue of a purine base, hypoxanthine (Fig. 5.1). Azathioprine has a molecular weight of 286 and is given in double the dose of 6-MP, which has a molecular weight of 170.

Immunosuppressive Action of Azathioprine

In animals, azathioprine and 6-MP depress antibody production against serum albumin in rabbits and against heterologous red cells in mice. The

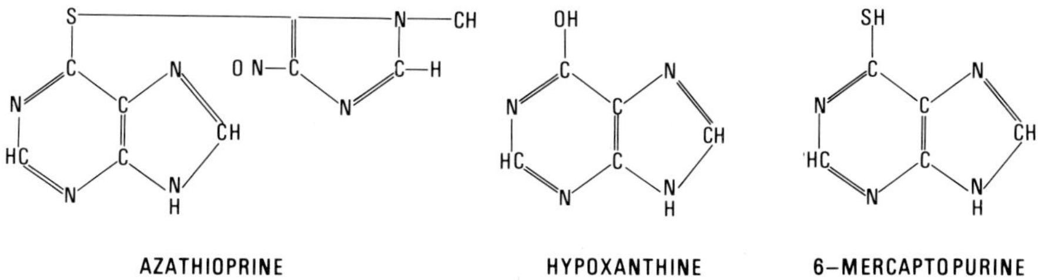

Fig. 5.1. Chemical formulae of azathioprine, hypoxanthine and 6-mercaptopurine.

immunosuppression is optimal when the drug is given in a single dose 2 days after the antigenic stimulation.[38] If the drug is given first and treatment is stopped more than 5 days before the antigenic stimulation, there may be an increase in the immune response,[67] which could be due to selective inhibition of certain categories of suppressor cells. Azathioprine is also active on cell-mediated immunity. It depresses delayed type hypersensitivity reactions and retards skin allograft rejection.[14]

In vitro, azathioprine alters most T cell markers and functions. In particular, it inhibits the mixed lymphocyte reaction[26] and the subsequent generation of cytotoxic T cells. Azathioprine is also active on B cells, but less intensely than on T cells. For example, mouse T cell rosettes are inhibited by low concentrations of the drug, whereas high concentrations are required for B cell rosette inhibition.[19]

In man, at the usual dose of 3 mg/kg, azathioprine does not alter antibody production after an injection of flagellin[234] or hemocyanin;[263] the secondary response after a further injection, however, is inhibited.[234] If 6-MP is given to man at the relatively higher dose of 2.5 mg/kg/day,[136] it inhibits the primary response to the Vi antigen and to the tularemia antigen and inhibits the onset of delayed hypersensitivity to *Pasteurella tularensis.* At the same dosage, 6-MP does not suppress delayed hypersensitivity established before treatment and does not affect the level of natural antibody.

In vitro, azathioprine inhibits most activities of human lymphocytes: mixed lymphocyte reaction (MLR), cell-mediated lympholysis (CML), antibody synthesis.[14, 19, 21, 112] It is particularly active on suppressor T cells,[79] an effect also found in vivo in renal transplant patients.[89] Lastly, it should be noted that azathioprine inhibits Natural Killer (NK) cell activity;[184] its effect on K (killer) cells is the subject of controversial reports.

Azathioprine and 6-MP also have an *anti-inflammatory* action under certain conditions.[145] This anti-inflammatory activity makes it difficult to interpret some of the immunosuppressive effects, especially in the field of delayed hypersensitivity and transplantation. Borel and Schwartz[49] have shown that the inhibition of delayed hypersensitivity may be due to a true immunosuppressive effect, to an anti-inflammatory effect or to a combination of the two, depending upon the experimental protocol.

Action of Azathioprine in Kidney Grafts

It has been verified in man that azathioprine and 6-MP, in sufficient dose, prolong skin graft survival.[136] But their action on kidney grafts is even more marked, both in animals and in man. This effect made it possible to produce a new situation, long-term graft survival; a great deal of information has been gathered from its study. Calne proved the efficacy of 6-MP (in 1960)[56] and of azathioprine (in 1961)[57] for the prevention of kidney allograft rejection in dogs. Many authors have confirmed that azathioprine prolongs the survival of the transplanted kidney and other organs.[3, 298] In some cases, survival was prolonged for many months, notably by Murray's group in dogs.[209, 241] These long survivals made it possible to analyze the situation in animals carrying a renal allograft, both *during* treatment with azathioprine and *after* treatment had been stopped.

During the period of azathioprine administration, a skin graft from the donor of the kidney graft may be rejected (the rejection is delayed but irreversible), and the rejection of the skin graft is accompanied by a reversible rejection crisis in the transplanted kidney. A skin graft from a dog unrelated to the kidney donor is also rejected, more rapidly than is the skin from the kidney donor; but this skin graft from a third dog produces a less severe rejection reaction in the transplanted kidney.

After the immunosuppressive treatment is discontinued, the kidney may be rejected spontaneously, but in some cases it continues to function normally. In the latter case, a skin graft from the kidney donor is rejected in an accelerated fashion (second set rejection), while a skin graft from a dog unrelated to the kidney donor is rejected in the normal way. As before, the rejection of these skin grafts is accompanied by rejection of the transplanted kidney. This rejection may be reversible (rejection crisis) or irreversible. A graft of the second kidney from the donor of the original graft is rejected like the skin grafts.

Mode of Action of Azathioprine

The biochemical impact of azathioprine is not univocal. Azathioprine inhibits DNA and RNA synthesis. Several possibilities can be considered with regard to its mode of action at the molecular level: interference with coenzymes, incorporation in nucleic acids, inhibition of enzymes, alteration of purine interconversions and inhibition of the de novo purine synthesis and binding to amino acids.[14] These actions explain the inhibition of nucleic acid synthesis but there are probably also many other subcellular actions which could be the basis of the immunosuppressive activity. This could explain why azathioprine inhibits rosette formation by quiescent unimmunized lymphocytes within less than 60 min,[21] which is difficult to explain by the inhibition of DNA synthesis.

The fact that the best time to administer a single dose of azathioprine or 6-MP is 24 hours after the antigen has been considered a particularly important argument in favor of an antiproliferative effect of these drugs.[36] In fact, this argument is not absolute, and it is also possible that azathioprine acts on the first phases of the immune response. This possibility is corroborated by the fact that thiopurine action is rapidly reversible in vivo, first because it is rapidly metabolized and second because its cellular activity is not long-lasting, as has been shown for the MLR and rosette formation.[21, 26] The immunosuppressive effect of antibodies administered passively until day 30 after antigen administration suggests that antigen recognition continues during the first 2 to 3 days after antigen administration. Thus, it is possible that thiopurines are not active if given before the antigen because their activity has disappeared while the antigen is still recognized and can still induce an immune response which is nearly normal. The fact that azathioprine inhibits the MLR only when added to the culture during the first 24 hours, while no DNA synthesis is yet detectable, supports such an interpretation.[26]

Thus, the effect of azathioprine on the proliferation of immunocompetent cells through the inhibition of DNA synthesis does not seem to be the exclusive mode of action. Other biochemical effects and cellular activity, such as suppression of antigen recognition, as suggested by inhibition of rosette formation, can also be considered.

The question of the target cell of thiopurines has been extensively investigated. Macrophages are probably not the preferential target for azathioprine since thiopurines do not alter labeled antigen clearance and phagocytosis in vitro. The only evidence of a thiopurine effect on macrophage function is the monocytopenia noted in the rat after treatment with low doses of azathioprine.[274] This observation remains to be confirmed in other species. The anti-inflammatory effect of azathioprine does not seem essential for its immunosuppressive action. Among lymphocytes, T lymphocytes appear to be the preferential target cells.[14] This is suggested by the action of azathioprine on cell-mediated immune responses depending on T cells, such as the MLR, cell-mediated lympholysis, rejection of organ and skin grafts and delayed hypersensitivity, an action much more clear-cut than that on antibody production, both in rodents and in man. (Azathioprine does not readily suppress antibody production in man, as tested for influenza antibodies, for example.) In the rodent, at certain doses 6-MP suppresses delayed hypersensitivity but is inactive on antibody production. Moreover, in in vitro experiments, it has been shown that 6-MP does not suppress in vitro response to flagellin, which is a thymus-independent antigen, at concentrations active on the primary in vitro response toward sheep red blood cells or allogeneic cells, two thymus-dependent responses.[14]

Azathioprine selectively inhibits T rosette forming cells which are long-lived T cells in the mouse.[19] It should also be noted that thymectomy is associated with the loss of rosette forming cell sensitivity to inhibition by azathioprine and that treatment of the spleen cells of such mice with purified thymic hormone reconstitutes the sensitivity of the cells to azathioprine.

This selective effect of azathioprine on T cells explains the efficacy of this drug in renal transplantation, where, at the relatively low doses used, the anti-T cell activity probably predominently accounts for the suppression of cell-mediated rejection without alteration of antibody production. This effect may be useful in the defense against bacteria and viruses, as well as for the production of blocking factors.

Metabolism of Azathioprine

The metabolism of azathioprine has been elucidated in three ways: 1) by *isotope* techniques, using azathioprine labeled by ^{35}S or ^{14}C (in the imidazole moiety); 2) by *chemical* methods, analyzing the various metabolites in blood and urine; 3) by *biologic* methods such as the rosette inhibition test,[21] which is sufficiently sensitive to detect azathioprine in the blood of animals or man. This test can in fact be used to evaluate the serum concentration of the metabolites that are responsible for preventing graft rejection, as there is close correlation between rosette inhibition activity and the degree of inhibition of graft rejection.[21] A similar correlation is found with the inhibition of cell transformation in mixed lymphocyte culture (MLC).[162]

In comparing the results of various tests, the basic fact has emerged that some of the products of azathioprine metabolism, and not azathioprine itself, are responsible for the depression of graft immunity.

Absorption of Azathioprine. Azathioprine is absorbed very rapidly and completely (more than 80%). Significant amounts appear in the blood within 15 min after oral administration.

Transformation of Azathioprine Into 6-MP. Azathioprine is partially transformed into 6-MP. Some workers consider that this 6-MP is responsible for in vivo activity so that it makes no difference which is given, 6-MP or azathioprine. However, it has been shown that azathioprine is a more effective immunosuppressor than is 6-MP in kidney grafts in dogs[57] and in skin grafts in mice.[94] Furthermore, azathioprine is effective in lower concentrations than 6-MP in the various in vitro tests in which it has been tried (rosette inhibition,[21] inhibition of hemolytic plaque formation[6, 231] and inhibition of protein synthesis.[105]) In practice, azathioprine is only marginally better than 6-MP, and even this is doubted by some workers. If azathioprine is more effective, it may be due to better cell penetration by azathioprine than by 6-MP or to the fact that the metabolism of azathioprine may produce other active immunosuppressors in addition to 6-MP.

In Vivo Production of Active Derivatives. Azathioprine and even 6-MP have little or no intrinsic activity. Their activity depends on their metabolites. When azathioprine is given intravenously, no rosette inhibiting activity is seen for 15 min and, here again, it takes an hour to reach maximum. It follows that there must be an activation process.

There is still a great deal to be learned about the metabolic changes which make the drug active in the body, but the following information gives some idea of the processes involved. Chemical studies suggest that the active metabolite may be thioinosinic acid.[93] The production of active metabolites is greatly diminished in liver failure.[18] There are no active metabolites in patients with gout who are deficient in hypoxanthineguanine phosphoribosyltransferase. In cultures of lymphocytes from these patients, azathioprine no longer inhibits cell transformation in the presence of phytohemagglutinin;[53] there is no rosette inhibiting activity in the serum of such patients after administration of azathioprine.[16]

We have also shown that it is possible to create an in vitro model of this metabolic activation of azathioprine by incubating the drug with sheep red cells. The optimum incubation is 20 min at 37°C with 5 ml of sheep red cells for 1 mg of azathioprine.[14, 16]

An attempt has been made in Figure 5.2 to indicate the various possible

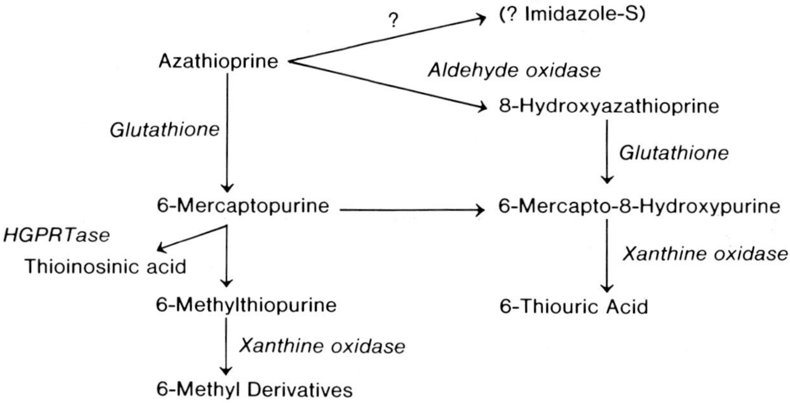

Fig. 5.2. Diagram of azathioprine metabolism. *HGPRTase,* hypoxanthine-guanine phosphoribosyltransferase.

pathways of metabolic activation of azathioprine. Although this scheme may be helpful, it is certainly not exhaustive and by no means represents all the metabolic pathways.

Degradation of Azathioprine and Its Active Metabolites. Aza-

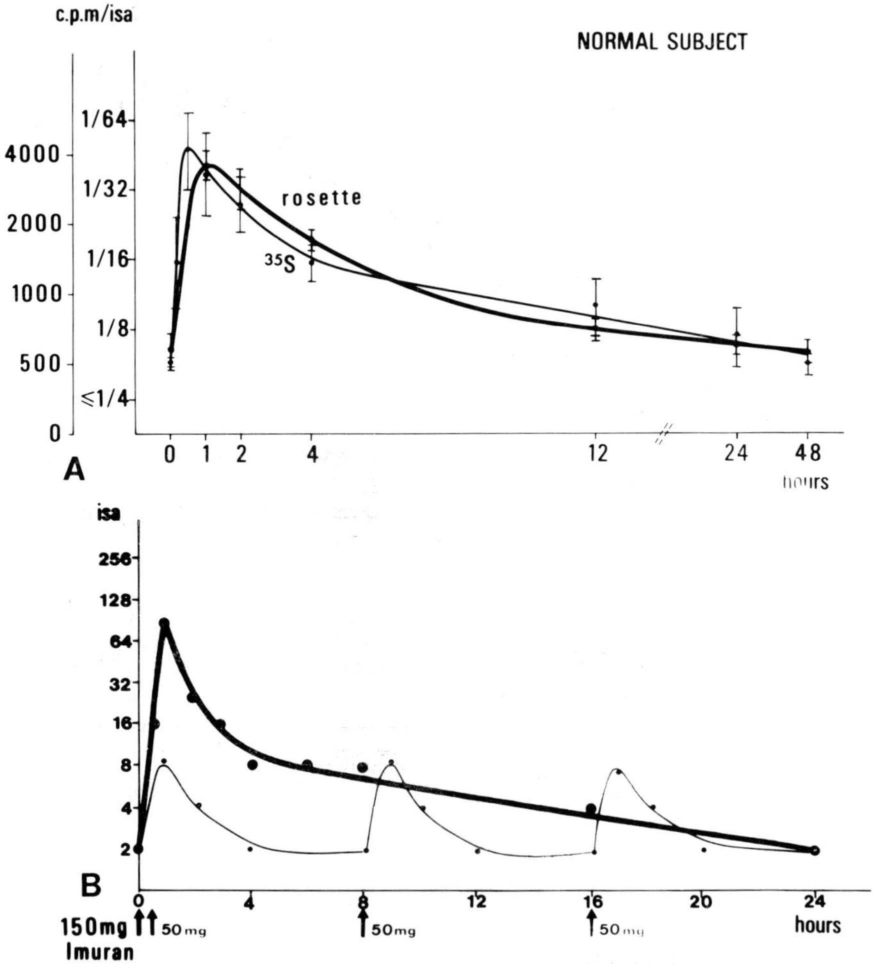

Fig. 5.3. Plasma immunosuppressive activity (isa) measured by the rosette inhibition test after administration of ^{35}S labeled azathioprine. *A*, metabolism of azathioprine in a normal subject. ^{35}S activity (*solid line*) and rosette-inhibiting activity (*dotted line*) in the serum of a normal subject after taking 3 mg/kg of ^{35}S labeled azathioprine by mouth. *B*, rosette-inhibiting activity in the plasma of a normal subject after taking 3 mg/kg of azathioprine by mouth in a single dose (*solid line*) or in three divided doses (*dotted line*) per 24 hours. *C*, azathioprine metabolism in renal failure. ^{35}S activity and rosette-inhibiting activity in a patient with renal failure after taking 3 mg/kg of ^{35}S labeled azathioprine by mouth. *D*, azathioprine metabolism in liver failure. ^{35}S activity and rosette-inhibiting activity in a patient with acute viral hepatitis after administration of 3 mg/kg of ^{35}S labeled azathioprine.

thioprine and its active metabolites are degraded very rapidly, in less than 4 hours. This rapid degradation explains why there is no summation of activity in renal failure, because the drug, although not excreted, is promptly transformed into inactive products.[17]

Xanthine oxidase is involved in the degradation of azathioprine after this has been transformed into 6-MP. If allopurinol, an inhibitor of xanthine oxidase, is given with azathioprine, both the immunosuppressive activity and the toxicity of azathioprine are increased.[97]

Excretion of Azathioprine. Azathioprine and its metabolites are

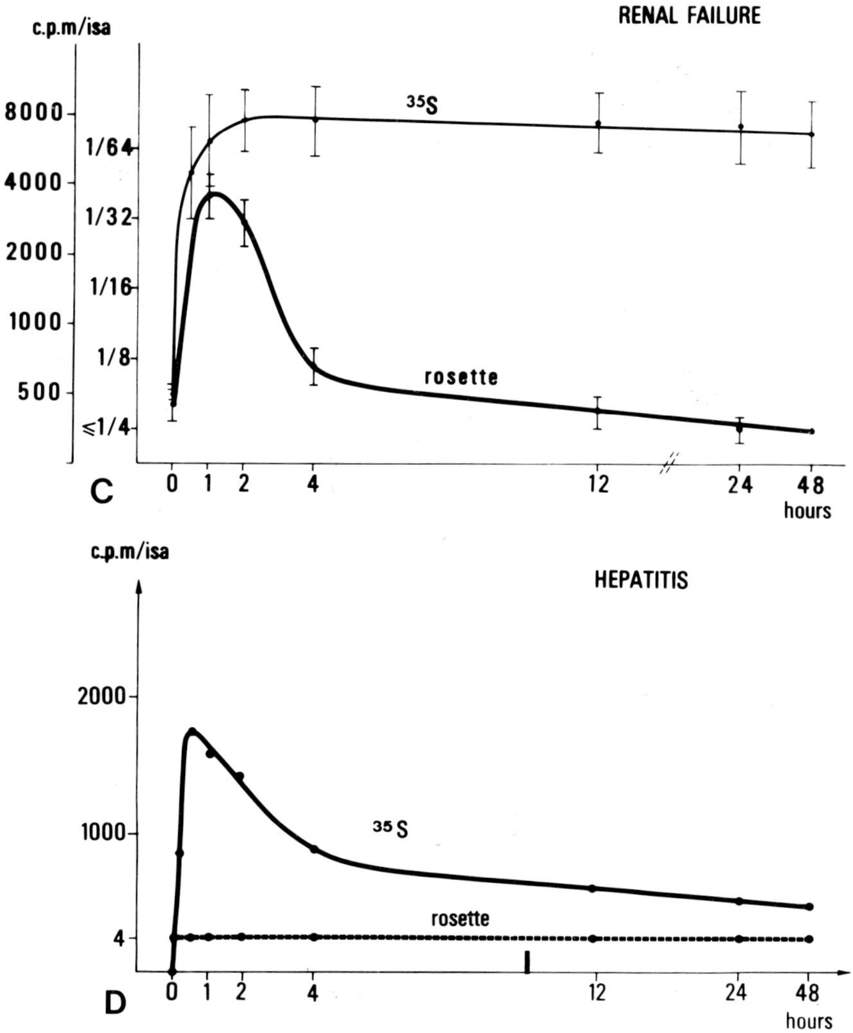

Fig. 5.3

essentially excreted by the kidney. However, very little azathioprine or 6-MP is excreted intact in the urine, where only the metabolites are found.[93] These metabolites are biologically inactive and renal failure does not modify the biologic activity of azathioprine (Fig. 5.3*C*).[17]

Dosage of Azathioprine

Dosage of Azathioprine in Normal Subjects. *Basic Data.* The therapeutic dose generally advised in man is 3 mg/kg/day. This is significantly lower than the dose tolerated by rodents. But in man, doses greater than 3 mg/kg/day often produce a troublesome bone marrow depression: first leukopenia, then thrombocytopenia and anemia. In fact, hematologic tolerance varies in an apparently unpredictable way from one patient to another. Severe bone marrow hypoplasia may be due in some cases to abnormal azathioprine metabolism. Using the rosette inhibition test, it was found in two patients that there was considerable delay in the disappearance of this activity (Fig. 5.4).[13a]

Practical Application. Except where a major abnormality of drug metabolism indicates otherwise, the drug is sometimes given in high dosage (5 mg/kg) for the first 3 days following transplantation and thereafter in normal dosage (3 mg/kg); this maintenance dose is not reduced for at least 2 years. (Details are in Ch. Six, "Indications for Kidney Transplantation.")

Azathioprine is presented in 50-mg or 100-mg tablets. It is generally given in one daily dose, before the noon meal. This method of administration has the advantage of simplicity for the patient, but it is open to

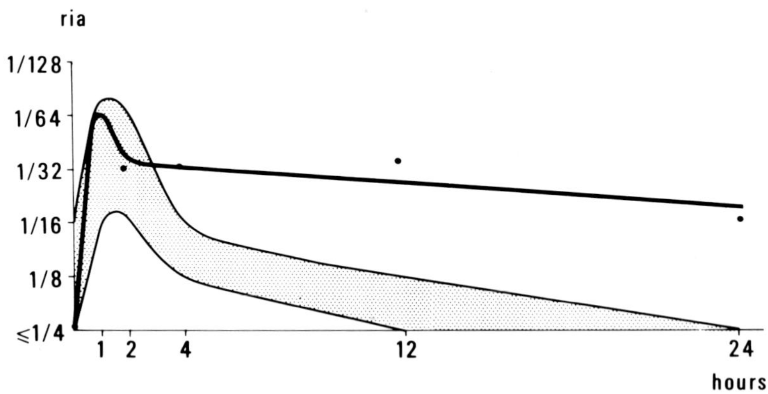

Fig. 5.4. Azathioprine metabolism in a case of early bone marrow aplasia. The rosette-inhibiting activity (*solid line*) is compared with the maximum values found in patients with no hematologic hypersensitivity to azathioprine (*dotted area*). Although the peak of rosette-inhibiting activity (*ria*) is normal at 1 hour, the activity disappears very slowly in comparison with the normal.

the objection that, as described above, more than three-quarters of its activity has disappeared from the blood at the end of 4 hours (Fig. 5.3*B*). However, to date no serious comparative study has been made to determine whether the same quantity given in divided doses would be more effective. Such a study is certainly needed because the mode of administration might affect either the immunosuppressive efficiency or the toxicity, i.e., the therapeutic index.

When oral administration is impossible, for example, in cases of stomach upset, the drug may be given intravenously. A commercial preparation presented in ampoules of 50 mg is available for intravenous injection. Studies using the rosette inhibition test show that the intravenous dose should be the same as that given orally.

Dosage of Azathioprine in Patients with Renal Insufficiency. *Basic Data.* Renal failure does not alter the incidence of leukopenia. We have shown that the hematologic tolerance of azathioprine in patients treated with the drug for more than 1 year after kidney transplantation is the same whatever the level of renal function. This correlates with our observation that the pattern of rosette inhibiting activity in the serum after administration of azathioprine is the same in patients with renal failure and in normal subjects (Fig. 5.3).[17]

Practical Application. From the above data it is apparent that azathioprine dosage should not be altered during renal failure, whether it is acute, as during rejection crises or acute tubular necrosis following prolonged ischemia of the donor kidney, or chronic, due to chronic rejection or recurrent glomerulonephritis.

It is important to emphasize this point. Lowering the drug dosage during renal failure after transplantation is in fact reducing the intensity of immunosuppression at a time when rejection is likely and when good immunosuppression is indispensable. In our experience, leukopenia is no more severe during episodes of renal failure than in patients with good kidney function, and it is rapidly reversible. However, leukocyte counts should be very carefully monitored in patients with renal failure since they may present with overall bone marrow fragility, as compared to other patients exposed to identical azathioprine doses.

Dosage of Azathioprine in Patients with Liver Insufficiency. *Basic Data.* Azathioprine metabolism has been studied by the rosette inhibition test in patients with liver disorders.[18] After administration of azathioprine, complete absence of rosette inhibiting activity was found in all cases with major liver disorder, whether there was significant necrosis (acute or chronic hepatitis) or not (cirrhosis) (Fig. 5.3*D*). Bile duct obstructions do not affect the activity of Imuran.

It is not known why azathioprine metabolism is abnormal in patients with liver disease. The most likely explanation is an absence of activation or an excess of degradation. Intestinal absorption is unchanged and the conversion of azathioprine into 6-MP is not at issue in view of the fact that 6-MP is affected in the same way as azathioprine.

These results, which have been confirmed by Mitchell and associates[195] in liver transplant patients, are in line with the mediocre results of liver transplantation when azathioprine is used alone.

Practical Application. The above data indicate that azathioprine may lose part of its activity when the transplant recipient has hepatitis.

Complications of Azathioprine Therapy

Compared with other immunosuppressive agents, azathioprine is relatively well tolerated. Nonetheless, it can cause complications of varying degrees. It may predispose to infection and especially to viral diseases, hepatitis, bone marrow aplasia and certain malignant diseases.

Infectious and Viral Complications. It is remarkable that the immunosuppressive activity of azathioprine has little effect on the development of bacterial diseases, at least those due to extracellular bacteria (essentially gram-positive). This is probably due to the fact that azathioprine has relatively little effect against humoral activity. We have found, for example, that this drug does not affect the levels of pre-existing circulating antibodies such as antityphoid antibody. In our own series, there have been only a few isolated cases of septicemia, typhoid fever or tuberculosis in patients receiving azathioprine without steroids. The same cannot be said for viral diseases, whose incidence is clearly increased during azathioprine therapy. Herpes simplex, herpes zoster and viral hepatitis are common.

Hepatitis. At some stage after transplantation, 18% of our patients have had hepatitis. Epidemiologic studies and the detection of Australia antigen suggest that a large number of these hepatites are of viral origin. Cholestatic jaundice may also be induced directly by azathioprine.

Bone Marrow Aplasia. Bone marrow aplasia is rare because it is usually possible to stop treatment in time when a significant drop in white cell count occurs. Aplasia is usually seen between the 4th and 9th weeks of treatment. These early aplasias are rapidly reversible, whereas those developing later are much more severe and persistent.

Malignant Diseases. Azathioprine, like other immunosuppressive agents, may favor the appearance of malignant tumors. The incidence of tumors varies very significantly from one group to another (2 to 24%). According to Penn,[220] who has established the International Transplant Tumor Registry, the incidence of tumors is approximately 100 times greater than in the general population in the same age range. It is remarkable that the types of tumors observed in transplant patients are different from those observed in the general population: essentially lymphomas (particularly reticulum cell sarcoma) and skin and lip cancer. However, the high incidence of carcinomas of the cervix of the uterus should be noted. The direct responsibility of azathioprine-induced immunosuppression is highly probable, although all patients also received steroids and some of them antilymphocyte serum. Conversely, the role of alloantigen stimulation seems minimal since similar tumor incidence is observed in autoimmune patients treated with chemical immunosuppressors and in children with congenital immunodeficiency. All these data support the highly debated concept of immunosurveillance,[198] which does not necessarily involve only T cells as initially thought; NK cells, macrophages and K cells, the other candidates for immunosurveillance, are also chronically altered by the immunosuppressive treatment.

Corticosteroids

Action of Corticosteroids on Delayed Hypersensitivity and Grafts

Cortisone was first shown to have immunosuppressive activity in 1950 by Germuth and Ottinger,[114] who found that the Arthus reaction, following injection of albumin, could be prevented by treatment with cortisone beginning at the time of albumin injection. The immunosuppressive effect of corticosteroids in preventing antibody production was confirmed for other antigens and other species, but in some species, especially in man, the effect was often much less marked than in the rabbit.[194a]

In 1951, Billingham et al[43] showed that high doses of cortisone would prolong skin allograft survival, but they and subsequent workers found that the prolongation was slight. Similar results were obtained with organ allografts.[299] Corticosteroids are most effective in association with other immunosuppressive agents, whose activity they potentiate. This has been demonstrated for thiopurines,[188] nitrogen mustards[27] and antilymphocyte sera (ALS).[138a] As noted at the beginning of this chapter, in considering the action of substances such as corticosteroids in allograft rejection, it is difficult to separate the respective roles played by true immunosuppressive activity and by the powerful anti-inflammatory action.

Mode of Action of Steroids

Corticosteroids produce various biochemical lesions in lymphocytes. It is likely, although not definitely established, that these effects are secondary to the binding of the steroids to highly specific cytoplasmic receptors.[14, 98, 193] The steroid receptor complexes interact with DNA and lead to modifications of protein synthesis. This link between the interaction of DNA and ulterior biochemical events is, however, still poorly understood. It is therefore difficult to explain the mechanism of lymphocyte lysis observed in corticosensitive species. It is also difficult to say whether the decrease in glucose uptake observed after steroid treatment is primary or, more likely, secondary to a change in protein synthesis. Cellular lysis is not the only effect of steroids on lymphocytes, since they also induce inhibition of cellular metabolism and seem to alter lymphocyte circulation.

The steroid target cell has not been precisely defined. The action on macrophages and polymorphs plays a major role in the suppression of immune responses, perhaps through lysosome stabilization.[14]

A preferential action of corticosteroids on B and T cells has not been clearly established.[14] Hydrocortisone suppresses the graft-versus-host reaction when administered before the induction of the reaction but has no clear-cut effect on precursor cells. Interestingly, hydrocortisone depresses lymphoid cytotoxicity[254] but does not, here either, destroy the precursors of lymphocytotoxic cells. The effect of steroids on T cells is, in fact, extremely complex. Among quiescent T lymphocytes (not engaged in a specific immune response) only the lymphocytes of the thymic cortex are sensitive to the action of steroids as well as perhaps, a subpopulation of spleen cells sensitive to phytohemagglutinin (PHA). Among lymphocytes engaged in an immune response, cytotoxic lymphocytes seem to be a relatively selective target, which might explain some actions of steroids in organ transplantation.[254] With regard to B cells, it seems that precursor cells are not altered by corticosteroids but rather that steroids act on precursor differentiation into antibody forming cells.

Lastly, it should be noted that steroids have major effects on the traffic of polymorphs (granulocytosis), monocytes (monocytopenia) and lymphocytes (lymphocytopenia)[98] and they interfere with a number of metabolic pathways, some of which might contribute to the immunosuppressive effect (e.g., prostaglandins).

Special Indications for Steroid Therapy in Kidney Transplantation

The action of steroids in rejection crises was demonstrated in 1960.[117, 130] Since then, the main indications for steroid therapy are in rejection crises, for the prevention of chronic rejection and in treating the complications of ALS therapy. Spectacular results are achieved in rejection crises, provided the dose is adequate. Where the crisis produces anuria, diuresis returns in a few hours after beginning treatment; we have seen early crises respond in less than 2 hours after instituting high dose steroid therapy.[127] The results of long-term treatment are much less clear-cut, and we do not give steroids routinely unless there is a rejection crisis.

However, we very often continue long-term steroid therapy at low dosage after a crisis to prevent relapse. We have found that rejection crises recur in 30% of cases after stopping steroid therapy, and almost one-third of all crises are initiated by lowering steroid dosage.[25]

Steroid Metabolism

Corticosteroids are not in a free state in the blood but are 90% bound to plasma proteins, chiefly to glycoprotein, transcortin and albumin. In low concentrations the main linkage is with transcortin, for which steroids have a very great affinity.[10, 193]

Corticosteroids undergo considerable metabolic transformation in the body. The liver is the key factor in these transformations. The metabolites are excreted mainly through the kidney, but the metabolites found in urine are, to a large extent, biologically inactive. In consequence, renal failure produces no summation of the biologic effects of steroid therapy.[271a]

Choice of Steroid and Dosage

Prednisone was the first and is still the most commonly used corticosteroid in transplantation. Other steroids are also used, particularly the fluoride derivatives which diminish the risk of certain side effects, especially sodium retention and diminished carbohydrate tolerance. Prednisone, prednisolone and β-methasone are given orally, and there is no evidence to indicate which of these products is best. Methylprednisolone (Medrol) is generally used for intravenous therapy.

The *optimum dose* is often difficult to assess. For certain biologic actions there seems to be a threshold dose and also a ceiling above which no greater effect is obtained. In addition, it has been shown that for certain effects the dose is less important than the chemical structure. For example, Fauve and Pierce-Chase[99] have shown that even at high doses products with a succinate group produce no diminution of resistance to infection in mice. In practice, it is difficult to find the optimum dose sufficient to obtain the desired therapeutic effect without undesirable side effects. In general, prednisone is used at a dose of 3 to 4 mg/kg/day for short periods in the treatment of rejection crises and at a dose of 0.25 to 0.5 mg/kg/day for long-term treatment. The choice of dosage is largely arbitrary and more precise pharmacologic studies on this point are needed.[10, 193] Many groups use high doses of steroids in the treatment of rejection crises, for example, in the form of intravenous injection of 1 g methylprednisolone (Solumedrol). The rationale is to increase dramatically the serum concentration of free steroids. Although this procedure has seemingly proven useful in some clinical situations, its superiority over less high oral doses is not established. It may be hypothesized that when concentrations are above a certain threshold the steroid receptors are saturated, whatever the concentration.[193]

Another important problem is *dose distribution*. Many authors have suggested that steroids should be given in a single dose every other day.[2] This has the advantage of less interference with the daily rhythm of endogenous physiologic adrenocorticotropic hormone (ACTH) secretion and a lower incidence of adrenal functional insufficiency[189] without lessening the anti-inflammatory action of the steroids. Administration of the drug every other day is less likely to produce Cushing syndrome. However, the action of corticosteroids on delayed hypersensitivity tuberculin skin reactions is less marked with administration every other day than with daily dosage.[186] Interrupted steroid administration should preferably be reserved to long-term therapy, where it has been proved effective and well tolerated in transplant recipients.[226]

For the *practical application* in human kidney transplantation, the reader is referred to Chapter Six, where the indications and dosage of steroid therapy are discussed in detail.

Side Effects of Steroid Therapy

The complications of steroid therapy are the same in kidney transplantation as in other circumstances where this family of drugs is used. It is not necessary to describe these complications in detail but merely to underline the fact that they are often serious. Steroids encourage microbial and viral infections. They may cause gastrointestinal hemorrhage and perforation of gastric ulcers, severe diabetes and bone disorders, especially bilateral aseptic necrosis of the femoral head, which may be crippling. They may also cause serious psychologic disorders which may persist after therapy is stopped. This list of complications suffices to show that, although essential in a large number of cases, steroid therapy represents one of the most serious hazards of kidney transplantation.

Withdrawal of steroids, or lowering the dose, may also present difficulties by provoking a rejection crisis or persistent fever.

Other Drugs

Cyclophosphamide

Cyclophosphamide (Endoxan, Cytoxan) is an alkylating agent. It is one of the most powerful immunosuppressive agents in mice. Its ability to prolong skin allograft survival varies from one species to another. Cyclophosphamide has been used alone in kidney transplantation in man[106] with a certain measure of success, but the number of cases treated is too small to provide the basis for definite conclusions. Overall results appear poorer than with azathioprine (especially because of greater toxicity), although some very long survivals have been reported. When azathioprine is poorly tolerated, especially because of bone marrow depression, cyclophosphamide may certainly be advantageously substituted.

Cyclophosphamide acts on lymphoid cells by fixing alkyle groups on their DNA.[14] This alkylation does not necessarily lead to cell death or inactivation when it occurs before the cell enters DNA synthesis, hence the particular sensitivity of rapidly proliferating cells: B lymphocytes, suppressor T lymphocytes[46, 230] and lymphocytes (B or T) engaged in an immune response during the first 2 days following antigen stimulation. The effect on suppressor T cells may be at the origin of unexpected effects such as enhancement of antibody formation or of T cell-mediated cytotoxicity[46, 230] when given at low doses that do not alter effector cells.

Methylhydrazine

Methylhydrazine (Natulan) and its derivatives have a very spectacular immunosuppressive activity in mice. Methylhydrazine has been used to obtain, in this animal, specific tolerance across the major barrier of the H-2 locus.[102] Unfortunately, the results in dogs are very disappointing; the few studies in man are also discouraging.

Cyclosporin A

Cyclosporin A is a cyclic peptide (11 amino acids) which was initially used as an antifungal agent. By routine screening, Borel et al at Sandoz[49] discovered that cyclosporin A exerts a variety of immunosuppressive activities in rodents and guinea pigs. It inhibits antibody formation against thymus-dependent (not against thymus-independent) antigens, and it depresses mitogen- and alloantigen-induced lymphocyte proliferation. Above all, it is a potent suppressor of allograft rejection, as shown for skin, heart and kidney grafts in various species.[58, 91, 123, 140, 158] In the rabbit it has even been shown that some tolerance was induced since a second graft from the same donor was selectively retained long after cessation of the treatment.[91, 123] It should be noted, however, that the specificity of this latter observation has been questioned.[75, 91, 140]

The mode of action of cyclosporin A has not been determined. It is known, however, that the drug shows strong selectivity of action for proliferating T cells. In particular, it inhibits T cell proliferation induced by T cell mitogens but not that induced by B cell mitogens.[58, 59]

Cyclosporin A has already been used in a limited series of patients undergoing renal transplantation (without azathioprine)[58, 59] or bone marrow transplantation.[224] The immunosuppressive effect was at least as good as that obtained with conventional treatment and permitted decrease of the steroid dosage. At variance with other chemical immunosuppressors, cyclosporin A is not toxic for the bone marrow, but it has other drawbacks that have made the extension of its clinical use difficult. It is highly nephrotoxic at the highest doses used (24 mg/kg/day), and lower doses (10 mg/kg/day), while not nephrotoxic, are much less efficient. There is also some liver toxicity and especially risk of induction of lymphoma (3 cases out of 29 patients).[59] Thus, fuller experimental and clinical investigation must be made before it can be determined whether the very promising results given by cyclosporin A will lead to a clinically useful drug.

Additional Drugs

There are other chemical immunosuppressive agents which will prolong allograft survival in animals but little is known of their action in man: amethopterin[36, 132] especially associated with folinic acid;[37] salicylates,[239] indomethacin,[71] ϵ-aminocaproic acid[115] and adamantoyl cytarabine.[120]

There is a continual search for new products because of the imperfections of current immunosuppressive therapy, and hence the interest in products such as α-globulins,[153] polyribonuclease[50] and asparaginase.[237] However, these are biologic products and synthetic chemicals would certainly be preferable, chiefly because they are easier to standardize.

ANTILYMPHOCYTE SERA

It was at the end of the last century that the idea was first conceived of making therapeutic use of heterologous antibodies to attack human cells. After his discovery of the phenomenon of phagocytosis at the Pasteur Institute, Metchnikoff[194] made the first antileukocyte serum by injecting extracts of rat and rabbit lymph nodes and spleen into guinea pigs. But the immunodepressive effect of ALS was not discovered until 1955, after it had been shown that lymphocytes were involved in immune reactions. Earlier, in 1951, Woodruff and associates[294] had suggested that antilymphocyte sera might be helpful in transplantation. In 1961, Waksman et al[278] obtained a slight but significant increase in the survival of skin grafts in guinea pigs. The first really long survival of a skin allograft was achieved in 1963 by Woodruff and Anderson.[292]

The volume of subsequent work on ALS is far too great to recount here. We shall confine ourselves to the facts relevant to the transplantation of organs, especially the kidney, and the reader who desires further information is referred to the many general surveys of the field.[12, 14, 33, 148, 192]

Preparation of Antilymphocyte Sera

Antilymphocyte sera are heterologous sera prepared by immunizing an animal against the lymphoid cells of an animal from another species. We shall consider the choice of animal, the antigen, the method of immunization, absorption techniques and the fractionation of the serum.

Choice of Animal to Produce Serum

To be effective, serum must be given in relatively large amounts. The bigger the animal treated, the greater the quantity of serum that will be required. For treating dogs or man, serum is usually produced from large animals, generally horses, but also cows, sheep and goats and especially rabbits, where promising results have been achieved.[30, 179, 225] However, a problem in using rabbits is that the ratio of the dose of antigen required to the amount of antibody harvested is much higher than in the horse.

The Antigen

A great variety of antigens has been used: lymphocytes from normal blood, leukemic lymphocytes, lymphocytes from the thoracic duct, lymph node cells, spleen cells and cells from the thymus. Both living and dead cells have been used. It is very difficult to compare the results of various workers because of the variety of antigen and of immunization protocols. It is possible, however, to draw several general conclusions.[14]

The most active sera of low toxicity are obtained with *lymphocytes from the thoracic duct* and the *thymus*. It is not yet known whether the high activity of these cells as immunizing agents is due to the fact that they carry specific antigens (possibly thymus-dependent) or simply to the greater purity of the cell preparations.

Lymph nodes and blood lymphocytes can give effective sera, but sera from the latter are often destructive to platelets. This is no doubt because of the difficulty in avoiding contamination of the lymphocytes by platelets.

Most authors regard the *spleen* as unsuitable, as it gives rise to antibodies which have little activity or are toxic.[30, 85]

Many authors have used as antigen lymphoblasts obtained by *continuous culture of normal human lymphocytes*.[213, 222] This source of antigen is attractive because it can be standardized and adapted to mass production. However, many cell lines are of B origin (and probably unsatisfactory for this reason), and, in fact, the overall activity of ALS produced against cell lines is still dubious.

Lyophilized or frozen or even heated cells can produce immunization of a quality comparable with that obtained with living cells.[22, 150]

What makes it difficult to compare the various suggested methods is the large number of details that differ from series to series: the particular reactivity of the animals, the total mass of antigen injected in a given period, the timing of the injections, the route of administration (subcutaneous, intravenous, intradermal or mixed), the duration of immunization and the use of adjuvants. Details on all these parameters will be found in several general reviews.[12, 83, 140, 179, 204, 246, 267]

In addition to antilymphocyte antibodies, ALS usually contain antibodies against red cells, against platelets, or even against organs such as the kidney. It is customary to remove by absorption at least the anti-erythrocyte antibodies. The sera may have antitissue and particularly antikidney[8] activity, and it would seem desirable to absorb these antibodies also. But this technique, which is rarely used, may lead to a loss of antilymphocyte activity.

In many animal experiments, ALS is used in the crude state or absorbed only by red cells. For clinical use, the sera are fractionated with the aim of reducing the amount of inactive protein. In earlier work, the fractionation was achieved by one or more precipitations with ammonium sulfate. Later, batch chromatography on DEAE-cellulose or DEAE-Sephadex was used, sometimes combined with the absorption of hemagglutinins by columns of erythrocyte stroma.

To diminish the toxicity of ALS preparations, it has been suggested that the globulins should be digested by pepsin. The $F(ab')_2$ fragments resulting from this digestion contain the two sites of antibody combination but are free of the Fc fragment which is liable to fix complement. By reduction, the univalent Fab′ fragment can be obtained, and this has only one antibody fixing site. It has been shown that the $F(ab')_2$ fragments can agglutinate and transform lymphocytes and that Fab′ fragments can transform lymphocytes without agglutinating them, but neither of these fragments has the immunosuppressive effect of undigested globulin.[148, 295] The inefficacy of digested globulin is a weighty argument in favor of the role of complement in the action of ALS.

Influence of Antilymphocyte Sera on Grafts

General Characteristics of the Effect on Grafts

The first results showing the action of ALS in transplantation were those of Woodruff and Anderson in 1963 and 1964 in skin allografts in rats.[292, 293] Following their work, many other authors reported significant prolongation of skin graft survival in many different animal species. We should mention in particular the work of Levey and Medawar,[180] Lance[163] and Monaco et al[202] in mice, of Balner et al in monkeys[28, 29, 31] and of Lucke and associates[185] in pigs. Most of the work in analyzing the immunosuppressive activity of ALS has been done with skin grafting in mice. The following points, which seem particularly important, are worth underlining.

The Effect of the Dosage of ALS. The efficacy of ALS is closely linked to the dose injected, to its distribution in time and to the duration of treatment.[181] For a given serum, the greater the dose the longer the survival of skin grafts. For optimal immunosuppressive activity, it is preferable to give small and repeated doses rather than larger doses at longer intervals.[164]

Potency. ALS is more active against transplantation immunity than all other known immunosuppressive agents (possibly except cyclosporin A). In fact, ALS not only gives a spectacular prolongation of primary allografts, but in mice it may even erase the immunologic memory, with the result that mice sensitized by a first skin graft react in first set fashion to a second graft.[163] The more powerful ALS can prolong the survival of xenografts, as shown by Lance and Medawar[167] in grafting skin from guinea pigs, rabbits and even man to mice, and by Monaco et al[68, 202] in skin grafts from rats to mice.

Association of Other Immunodepressive Agents. The action of ALS is generally augmented when associated with other immunodepressive methods. This is particularly true of the steroids[171] and other chemotherapeutic agents such as 6-MP and methotrexate. Sera which are virtually ineffective when given alone may become active if used with another immunodepressive agent.

Antilymphocyte sera may also be potentiated by other methods of immunodepression such as total body irradiation,[181] drainage of the thoracic duct[293] and thymectomy in adults.[149, 205] True immunological tolerance may be obtained when the treatment with ALS is followed by the intravenous injection of lymphoid cells or cell extracts, as shown by Lance and Medawar,[168–170] and Monaco.[199]

Selective Activity on Graft Immunity. ALS produces preferential inhibition of graft immunity. It has a much less spectacular effect on all other types of immune reactions. It cannot, for example, abolish a preestablished immunity against heterologous erythrocytes or protein, and it must be injected *before* the immunizing antigens to produce an immunosuppressive effect on primary immunization.[7, 39]

Results in Animals

The immunosuppressive effect of ALS alone has been shown in the transplantation of many different organs. Particular attention has been devoted to *renal allografts in dogs.*[1, 9, 70, 84, 135, 196, 200] Some series have shown prolonged mean survival, and in some, animals have survived more than 1 year. In most cases the sera have been given by subcutaneous injection but sometimes intravenously. It is established that the sera must be given *before* transplantation,[216, 238] although the optimal period of preparation has not been defined. In some cases[238] the graft survived for a long time after treatment was stopped, as may happen with animals treated with azathioprine. Chemical immunosuppressors potentiate the action of ALS, but the results are not improved by thymectomy.[252]

The effect of antithymus globulins has also been studied in *renal allografts in the rat.*[126] As in the dog, graft survival is definitely improved by ALS. With a single dose of 10 mg of IgG given intravenously 3 or 4 days before transplantation, the majority of animals have normal renal function on the 7th day and a certain number survive as long as 8 months.

Results in Man

It is in kidney grafting that the greatest amount of experience has been gained with ALS in man. Many patients have been treated with ALS in many centers, and in some there has been long follow-up.

Starzl et al[251, 253] have used antilymphocyte globulins (ALG) since June 1966. Their first patients were treated with relatively small doses and for less than 4 months. The results were better than their previous series, the number of rejection crises was less and the dosage of azathioprine and corticosteroids required was less in patients treated with ALG.

Traeger and his colleagues[270, 271] used ALG obtained by immunizing horses with thoracic duct lymphocytes. Within a few days the globulins suppressed delayed hypersensitivity reactions to tuberculin or other antigens. In 71 cases with long follow-up,[110] there were 37 transplants from living related donors and 34 from cadavers or unrelated living donors; 80% of the first group and 35% of the second group survived at 1 year. The number of rejection crises diminished (only 19% of patients had crises in the first 3 months), as did the requirement for steroids (24 mg/day prednisone, on the average, in the first 3 months). On the other hand, the late pathologic lesions were similar to those found in patients who were not treated with ALG, with the exception that vascular changes were less common.

Antilymphocyte serum has now been used clinically for more than 15 years, and yet its clinical effect is still debated. Many reports[33, 55, 60, 78, 159, 173, 178, 190, 203, 240, 268, 279, 280] have shown favorable effects, as assessed by kidney survival, number of rejection crises, decrease in steroid dosage and even regression of established rejection.[131] Some of these clinical trials have been randomized, well conducted and are a priori quite convincing, even though the improvement brought by ALS is partial and is particularly clear-cut and significant in transplantation groups showing poor results in the control series. It should be noted, however, that negative results have also been reported.[272, 273] These differences are probably related to variations in the source of antigen used for ALS preparation and the immunosuppressive potency of the batch utilized. It is also apparent that centers differ in their clinical protocols and mode of evaluation of results. Progress may be expected in the use of ALS in renal transplantation. Better sera may be selected and produced by using pure T cell antigen sources (thymus, T lymphoblastoid cell lines), perhaps by fractionating the antigen preparation (based on recent knowledge of the chemistry of the various antigens responsible for the induction of ALS antibodies) and especially the production of homogeneous "monoclonal" antibodies by hybridomas. More precisely, one could imagine the use of monoclonal antibodies selectively directed at the T cell subset which is potentially the most harmful to the graft.

Toxicity and Side Effects

Local and General Signs

Most ALS produce pain at the site of injection and an inflammatory reaction.[154, 270] These generally occur 2 to 6 hours after injection and fade within a few hours. Fever is common, especially in the early stages of treatment. Pain and fever often, but not always, tend to diminish as treatment progresses. The severity of these local and general effects varies considerably from one serum to another and even with different batches of the same serum.

The mechanism of these side effects is unknown. Directly or indirectly, the injected antibodies are responsible for the local signs because these signs are found equally with pure IgG and with cruder preparations, and they do not occur with an identical heterologous nonimmune serum. There are several possible explanations for these local reactions: fixation of complement on the aggregates of γ-globulin, the presence of antibodies against muscle and connective tissue and so forth. In patients who become immunized to horse globulin, as described below, the local reactions may become serious and are then similar to the Arthus phenomenon.

The main reason for giving globulins intravenously is to diminish pain and local reactions so that a higher dosage is possible.

Action on Platelets

In man, some sera provoke thrombocytopenia,[151, 154] others produce thrombocytosis[151] and yet others have no appreciable effect on the number or function of the platelets. The findings depend not only on the nature of the ALS, but also on the dosage. A serum which is thrombocytopenic in high dosage loses this effect when the dose is lowered, and there is often a phase of thrombocytosis when treatment is stopped.

Many in vitro tests[151] have been used to investigate the antiplatelet activity of ALS: immunologic tests (thromboagglutination, fixation of complement); coagulation tests (the recalcification time of plasma in the presence of intact platelets, lysed platelets or some other source of phospholipids; thromboelastography; tests of thrombin formation; photometric recording of platelet aggregation; estimation of antiheparin activity); and the inhibition of the incorporation by platelets of serotonin labeled with ^{14}C.

The coagulation tests are the least sensitive. The immunologic tests (thromboagglutination, complement fixation) are the most generally used. These tests correlate well with the onset of thrombocytopenia in man.[23] Both agglutination and complement fixation should be used for in vitro evaluation of the antiplatelet activity of ALS, and if these tests are positive with an ALS diluted more than 1:8 or 1:6, this ALS is likely to be thrombocytopenic in vivo. On the other hand, too much importance should not be attached to a high titer of complement fixation if there is no comparable titer of thromboagglutination, particularly in sera with a high titer of antilymphocyte antibodies.

Antiplatelet antibodies present in ALS are due mainly to platelet contamination of the cell suspensions used to immunize the animals producing the serum, hence the high incidence in ALS produced from spleen and blood lymphocytes. It can also be explained in part, as noted above, by cross-antigenicity between lymphocytes and platelets. The evidence for this is the observation of antiplatelet activity even in ALS prepared from pure lymphocytes in continuous culture.[246]

Sensitization to Horse Proteins

Experimentally, the administration of antilymphocyte sera always sensitizes animals to heterologous proteins, and particularly to the γ-globulins of the animal producing the serum. This has been demonstrated in mice,[166] in rats,[69] in dogs[86, 172] and in monkeys.[170] Howard et al[141] have shown that this immunization is particularly easy to produce by giving, instead of the globulin itself, lymphocytes coated by the antibodies. These lymphocytes then behave as adjuvants to immunization.

It has been shown in mice that the induction of tolerance to normal rabbit IgG, by the injection of unaggregated IgG, increases the efficacy of subsequent treatment by ALS and, conversely, preliminary sensitization to rabbit IgG diminishes the effectiveness of ALS.[142, 286] It has also proved possible in monkeys[170] and dogs[172] to prevent immunization against horse ALS by the preliminary administration of normal horse IgG free of aggregates.

In man, sensitization to horse protein is common. It may lead to complications such as urticaria, malaise with hypotension, sometimes major anaphylactic shock with collapse and respiratory embarrassment and, exceptionally, serum sickness.[250, 270] These complications respond rapidly to the intravenous administration of corticosteroids.

With in vitro tests it is possible to detect the antibodies against horse globulin before clinical complications appear. Hence, these tests should be performed at regular intervals. The simplest test is hemagglutination by the patient's serum of group O human red cells coated with horse immunoglobulin. At a late stage, patients may develop precipitins as well as various heterologous hemagglutinins, especially against sheep and horse immunoglobulin-coated red cells.

The proportion of patients who become immunized against horse immunoglobulin is variously reported, and it is difficult to compare the published statistics because of the great differences in technique. We have seen this phenomenon in at least 50% of patients in the 1st month. Other authors find it in practically every case.[54, 63]

Not only may this sensitization cause complications, but it probably renders ineffective any further treatment with ALS. For this reason, attempts have been made in man to induce prior tolerance to normal horse IgG,[54, 213, 266] and a certain amount of success has been claimed. But if tolerance or nonresponse to horse IgG is not obtained, the patient tends, on the contrary, to become immunized against horse globulin; hence, some authors[212] feel that this technique should be abandoned.

It has been suggested that rather than discontinue treatment in patients who have become sensitized to horse globulin, it may be preferable to change to an ALS prepared in a different animal species such as sheep, rabbit or goat. Rabbit ALS is said to be preferable as the risk of crossreaction with horse serum is less than with larger species.[5]

Kidney Toxicity

Antilymphocyte sera may be toxic for the kidney in two ways: a direct action on the kidney of nephrotoxic antibodies producing a Masugi nephritis, or the intrarenal deposition of antigen-antibody complexes when the patient becomes immunized against heterologous protein. Renal lesions of one or another type have been seen occasionally in mice[22, 150] and rats.[124]

Starzl and his colleagues[147, 253] have found deposits of horse globulin, complement and host γ-globulin in some kidney grafts in dogs. Orr et al[215] found in vitro, in a horse antidog lymphocyte serum, antibodies giving a crossreaction with dog glomeruli; these antibodies also fixed on the glomeruli in vivo, provided the injection was given intravenously or directly into the renal artery. Nonetheless, none of these animals developed a nephritis of the Masugi type. This is explained by the authors as being due to the small amount of antibody giving a crossreaction with the renal glomeruli and to the ability of such antibodies to disappear from the kidney rapidly after they become fixed.

In man, there is so far little evidence that ALS is nephrotoxic. Starzl et al[253] and Traeger et al[270] have failed to find horse globulin in renal biopsies studied by immunofluorescence. Carpenter et al[63] found linear deposits of horse globulin in the glomeruli of two patients with normal renal function. Unfortunately, no absolute conclusion is possible because nephrotoxicity may vary greatly from one batch of serum to another, and this variation is difficult to evaluate in vitro. Moreover, nephrotoxicity may become more common in the future because of the ever increasing use of high doses given intravenously.

Development of Malignant Tumors

It has been shown in mice that ALS may increase the incidence and reduce the time of induction of tumors by oncogenic viruses[4, 174] or by methylcholanthrene.[64] Furthermore, ALS encourages the take and the growth of transplantable tumors.[64]

In man, ALS, like azathioprine,[220] may encourage the development of malignant tumors, whether pre-existing or grafted with a transplant.[82] Everyone agrees on this point. The only question is whether ALS increases the incidence of new tumors, especially of the lymphoid system. This problem is obscured by the fact that all patients showing tumors had also received azathioprine and steroids, which, given alone, may also promote tumorogenesis.[220]

Tests of Activity

Tests in Vivo

Because of the difficulties of direct study in man, a good deal of work has been done with a model that, although not human, is thought to be comparable to man. This is the study of prolongation of skin allograft survival in the macaque or the chimpanzee treated with antihuman ALS. This test was developed by Balner et al,[28-32] who have tested more than 50 sera of worldwide origin.

The assay is not very sensitive and may fail to recognize sera of average quality but will not miss very good sera. In the author's view, it is now possible to use only macaques for the test because the results in these animals tally well with those in chimpanzees. This will make it much easier to test each ALS on many animals because the macaque is much less costly and much easier to obtain than is the chimpanzee. Thus, errors due to chance compatibility and the individual reaction of the recipient will be minimized.

Tests in Vitro

In several animal species and in man, a poor correlation has been found between leukoagglutination or lymphocytotoxicity tests and the immunosuppressive effects of ALS.[12, 83, 149] A large number of other in vitro properties of ALS have been studied in mice and compared with the immunodepressive effect.[11, 83] It is not possible to analyze these studies in detail, but suffice it to say that so far there are two tests which seem capable of predicting in vitro the immunosuppressive activity of an antimouse ALS: the opsonization of lymphocytes[122] and the inhibition of spontaneous rosette formation in the presence of complement.[15, 20]

For the study of antihuman ALS, four main tests have been subjected to detailed analysis and attempted correlation with immunodepressive ability: opsonization in vitro,[92, 229] inhibition of spontaneous rosette formation,[11, 20] inhibition of lymphocyte stimulation in culture[227] and a passive hemagglutination assay.[119] It should be emphasized that in all cases the immunodepressive capacity has been defined by the ability of the ALS to prolong skin allograft survival in monkeys, the only practical criterion currently available.

The spontaneous rosette inhibition test had a particularly good correlation with the immunosuppressive effect evaluated by skin allografting in monkeys.[13, 24, 30] It is interesting to note retrospectively that the rosette inhibition test was described before it was known that E rosettes represent a selective marker of T cells, the selective target of ALS. A satisfactory, although less striking, correlation has also been found with inhibition of antigen-induced lymphocyte proliferation[92] and with the passive hemagglutination assay.[28]

In conclusion, many tests in vitro correlate with the immunosuppressive activity of ALS, but with most methods the correlation is imperfect because a small number of sera react in an unexpected manner. The correlation with the rosette inhibition test is the most satisfactory, with only few individual exceptions, and this test thus gives an accurate prediction of the effectiveness of any given serum.

Mode of Action

The mode of action of ALS is not yet fully understood, but certain important points have been established. The reader is referred to a number of other publications for more details.[14, 165, 182, 197a, 221, 291]

Most of the known facts are derived from experiments on mice treated with rabbit ALS. The same mechanisms are postulated in man but are not proved.

Target Cell of Antilymphocyte Sera

Although it has been suggested that ALS could act by coating the allograft antigenic sites,[125] most authors agree that its main target is the immunocompetent cell. It is possible that ALS acts on the macrophages,[291] which are known to play a part in certain immune reactions. But most of the evidence points to the lymphocytes, and selectively, to the thymus-dependent lymphocytes, as the essential point of impact.[177] Following are some of the arguments for this statement. The histology of lymph nodes from animals receiving ALS is similar to that of neonatally thymectomized animals (depletion of the paracortical zones); in transfer experiments, the thymus is capable of restoring immunocompetence to animals receiving ALS; the inhibiting effect of ALS is much greater on cellular immunity than on humoral immunity; the θ antigen, specific for the thymus, disappears from the spleen of mice treated with ALS. More precisely, ALS depletes the subpopulation of mature, long-lived and recirculating T cells, leaving intact, at least at small doses, the subset of adult thymectomy-sensitive immature T cells.[61]

Site of Action of Antilymphocyte Sera on Lymphocytes

It has been shown that there is poor penetration of ALS into the central lymphoid organs, spleen and lymph nodes, even when there is a high level of antibody in the circulating blood. It has thus been assumed that the ALS reached the thymus-dependent cells in the circulating blood and that the elective depletion of this group of cells could be explained simply by their very rapid recirculation. This explanation may not be, in fact, the only one, or even the best. ALS might also act on thymus-dependent lymphocytes because of the particular sensitivity of these cells to attack by antilymphocyte antibodies.

Mechanism of Immunosuppression of Cellular Processes

Some cells may be destroyed, either by direct cytotoxicity (if the concentration of ALS is very high) or, more often, by opsonization followed by phagocytosis by the reticuloendothelial cells. Cytotoxicity requires the presence of all the factors of complement while the first four factors are necessary for opsonization. Other cells are not destroyed but inhibited, probably reversibly. This inhibition could be due to coating of the receptors on the surface of the thymus-dependent cells, receptors which are specialized in the recognition of antigens. This goes back to the blindfolding hypothesis suggested by Levey and Medawar.[182] Coating can be effective even with low concentrations of ALS and requires only the concurrence of the first two factors of complement, C1 and C4. This explains why ALS is active in mice deficient in C5.

In conclusion, ALS acts mainly on the lymphocytes and especially on thymus-dependent lymphocytes. This action can be explained either by the rapid recirculation of these long-surviving cells, which exposes them to ALS in the circulating blood, or by a particular sensitivity of these lymphocytes to ALS and other immunodepressive agents. The lymphocytes are destroyed by the reticuloendothelial system after opsonization by the ALS, or they may be temporarily inactivated, rather than destroyed. This inactivation is due to coating of the receptors of the cell surface by the antibody and the first two components of complement.

OTHER METHODS OF NONSPECIFIC IMMUNOSUPPRESSION

Total Body Irradiation

Total body irradiation in high dosage produces a temporary depression of the immune responses. A dose of 500 rads reduces considerably the ability of the rabbit to form antibodies against sheep red cells.[81]

In 1950 Dempster et al[77] suggested that this technique might be applied to transplantation. To avoid death from bone marrow aplasia, it was suggested that the radiation should be combined with a bone marrow graft, but the immunologically competent cells of the grafted marrow react against the host antigens and this graft-versus-host reaction produces a dangerous "secondary disease," which is very difficult to control. For this reason, lethal doses of x-rays were soon replaced by a more moderate dosage which would permit patient survival without a marrow graft. The method was improved still further by dividing the x-ray dose over several sessions in order to diminish the general toxic effect without too much diminution of the effect on lymphoid tissue.[210]

In man, total body irradiation was the first method of immunosuppression used in kidney transplantation. It was used at Necker Hospital in 32 patients between 1959 and 1963.[262] In 26 patients receiving transplants from living related donors, a total dose of 350 rads was given at a rate of 3 to 5 rads/min in two sessions, respectively, 5 days and 28 hours before grafting. Two patients who received cadaver kidneys were given a single dose of 350 rads immediately before transplantation. Four patients received 75 rads the day before the operation and azathioprine was begun 1 week before grafting.

Unfortunately, there was a significant number of cases of septicemia due to infection by the patient's own bacteria, as shown by comparing the preoperative flora with the organisms grown from the blood. This is why, like in most other groups, total body irradiation was abandoned in favor of chemical immunosuppression. And yet, the long-term results were better in irradiated patients than in those who received azathioprine alone, to judge by the lower incidence of late rejection where immunosuppressive medication was temporarily withdrawn.[129] The first irradiated patient in our series has never had any other immunosuppressive treatment, and his kidney allograft is functioning well 22 years after transplantation.

Total Lymphoid Irradiation

Total irradiation of the lymphoid system has been used for 15 years in the treatment of Hodgkin's disease and nonHodgkin's lymphomas.[257] It had been noted that patients receiving this treatment showed profound immunosuppression that was selective for T cells (assessed by various markers and functions).[257] The Stanford group which made these important observations decided to investigate in a more systematic fashion the immunosuppressive effects of total lymphoid irradiation (TLI) in mice. The results obtained so far indicate that TLI is one of the most potent methods of preventing allograft rejection and inducing tolerance to alloantigens in adult animals.[244, 245, 257, 296]

The radiotherapy regimen consisted of 17 fractions of 200 rads administered to two large fields (supra and subdiaphragmic, involving the whole abdomen). The skull, lungs, tail, hindlimbs and forelimbs were shielded with lead. All the major lymph nodes, the spleen and the thymus were in the radiation fields. The procedure was generally well tolerated. TLI induces lymphocytopenia (particularly bearing on T lymphocytes) and depressed response to T cell mitogens [more marked to PHA than to Concanavalin (Con A)].[257] TLI also suppresses MLC and provides a nonspecific depression of allograft immunity (about 50 days in control, in a strain combination crossing the H-2 barrier). Suppression of antibody production is also observed, particularly clear-cut for IgG antibodies. TLI may induce tolerance, in particular to allografts, if donor bone marrow cells are injected.[244] Such tolerance, both to soluble antigen and to allogeneic cells, appears to be due to the appearance of suppressor T cells which apparently regenerate first after irradiation.[257, 296] In the case of bone marrow graft, mutual tolerance is observed, possibly due to the presence of suppressor cells of host and donor origin. Suppressor cells seem to be essentially antigen-specific, but nonspecific suppressor cells also exist. Similar data have been obtained in rats and in dogs.[245] Results of the first clinical trials recently started in man are awaited with high interest.

Irradiation of the Blood

Cronkite and associates,[65] who were the proponents of current techniques of extracorporeal irradiation, first suggested radiating the lymph in a shunt between the thoracic duct and the jugular vein. So far, this technique has been employed only in animal experiments. Prolonged renal allograft survival in goats can be obtained by radiating the blood passing through a jugulocarotid shunt.[66]

Local Irradiation

Irradiation of the kidney allograft has been suggested by many authors, particularly for the treatment of crises.[155] The dose usually recommended is 100 to 600 rads, or even more, in one or more sessions. We are reluctant to use this technique because of the danger of inducing radiation damage in the kidney, although it is true that in the published accounts of radiation nephritis, the dose has been much higher.

Drainage of the Thoracic Duct

In theory, drainage of the thoracic duct removes a large number of lymphocytes from the body, and especially the long-lived lymphocytes which are important in allograft immunity. In rats, thoracic duct drainage prolongs skin allograft survival.[293] In man, the chief proponents of the method have been Tilney and Murray[269] in the United States and Revillard and Traeger[226a] in France. The latter authors, in 85 attempts at drainage in man, had one-third technical failures, and in the remaining two-thirds a mean duration of drainage of 12 days, during which time 17 liters of lymph and 50×10^9 lymphocytes were recovered. It is difficult to judge the effect of this procedure on allograft tolerance. At best, it can only be an auxiliary method.

Thymectomy

Starzl[249] carried out thymectomy at the same time as kidney transplantation in several cases. No favorable effect was demonstrated, as might have been expected from the experimental data described in Chapter One. In 1970, Starzl et al[252] reviewed 24 patients submitted to thymectomy before transplantation in 1965 and 1966. They found no improvement in survival, in dosage of immunosuppressive drugs required or in renal function, compared with a control group. The only difference was that pathologic changes in the grafted kidney were less common and less severe in the thymectomized patients. As far as we know, thymectomy is no longer used.

We submitted 24 of our patients to irradiation of the thymus with 1500 rads divided into three sessions, but we found no evidence that this treatment improved transplant prognosis.

Splenectomy

We performed splenectomy in 19 cases for the following reasons. 1) According to unconfirmed work by Ungar (cited by Krohn,[161]) there was reason to think that splenectomy, by diminishing the mass of lymphoid tissue, might increase graft tolerance and diminish the rejection reaction.[160] In fact, in human kidney transplantation there has been no evidence that immunosuppressive drugs are more effective in splenectomized patients.[116, 144, 275] 2) It was also hoped that the leukocytosis induced by splenectomy would increase tolerance to immunosuppressive drugs,[76] but this has not been confirmed.[275] 3) Progressive splenomegaly (also reported by Hume et al[144]) led us to carry out secondary splenectomy in eight of our patients; we thought that this splenomegaly might be a reaction by immunologically competent tissues called on to coexist with a transplanted organ.[128] However, all our cases of splenomegaly occurred during the period 1959 to 1964, when our patients were prepared by total body irradiation; since then we have not seen enlargement of the spleen in patients treated only with azathioprine.[176] It is possible that the radiation may have had something to do with the splenomegaly, although enlargement of the spleen has not been reported after accidental total body irradiation.[139]

Since there is no real proof that splenectomy is effective, the practice has now been abandoned, especially since its use increases postoperative problems and the risk of thromboembolic complications.[143]

Plasmapheresis

The use of plasmapheresis in the treatment of acute rejection has recently been suggested by several groups.[228] It is too early to evaluate the possible benefit of this therapy. Its main mechanism of action is related to removal of circulating antibodies and potentially harmful immune complexes. The effect on macrophages (which lose their immune complex load) and especially the action of the active principles brought by the fresh plasma should also be taken into consideration.

INDUCTION OF SPECIFIC UNRESPONSIVENESS

Unlike the preceding pages, which were concerned with immediately practical applications, this section remains purely theoretical. There is still no practical method available for inducing specific tolerance to an allografted organ. There may possibly be "adaptation" of the transplant in certain cases, to quote the term suggested by Pierce et al.[223] Murray and associates[208] found that some dogs did not reject a kidney after immunosuppression was stopped. This result can be achieved regularly in dogs after 1 year of immunosuppression, provided that the donor animal has been chosen carefully for histocompatibility by MLC.[157] Our first patient, who received no immunosuppression after initial total body irradiation, has tolerated his kidney for 22 years without the slightest sign of rejection (except for one reversible crisis in the early months). But results of this sort are rare and impossible to predict.

Nevertheless, there is so much likelihood that the final solution to the problem of organ transplantation will lie in the creation of a state of specific tolerance, that we must give an account of the current state of our knowledge of this subject. This raises some of the most interesting and most hotly debated fundamental questions in the whole of graft immunology.

The lasting and specific absence of immune response to an antigen can be seen in many situations. Three of these will be considered below: 1) immunologic tolerance, properly so-called; 2) enhancement; and 3) "adaptation."

Immunologic Tolerance

Mitchison,[197] who is one of the leading experts in this field, thinks that we should now regard as synonymous the terms immunologic tolerance and immunologic paralysis, and he defines this situation as "a deletion, to a variable extent, of a specific range of immunological responses brought about by treatment with antigen."

Perinatal Immunologic Tolerance

We owe the concept of immunologic tolerance to the famous experiments of Medawar, which showed that administration of an antigen immediately before or immediately after birth renders the animal incapable of subsequent response to that antigen.[192a] If the antigen is administered in the form of allogeneic cells, a skin graft taken from the animal donating these cells will not be rejected. An example of this phenomenon is found in nature. Dizygotic twins in cattle have a communicating circulation in embryo and, as Owen[219] has shown, this often results in hematologic chimerism, a condition in which the animal carries two types of red cells, those of its twin alongside its own. Kidney grafts from the twin were tolerated by 8 out of 12 such animals for more than 10 months.[73]

A similar hematologic chimerism has sometimes been seen in man.[47, 49] Furthermore, Lejeune[175] studied children who had undergone exchange transfusion at birth and found that they tolerated indefinitely a skin graft from the donor of the blood.

A related mechanism is generally invoked to explain why an individual tolerates his own cells, a tolerance that is thereafter maintained indefinitely by the permanent coexistence of the individual's antigens and his lymphoid system. This recognition of "self" is never dimmed except in the case of autoimmune disease (due, for example, to altered tissue antigenicity) and possibly in structural changes associated with cell aging.

The mechanism of the immune tolerance that can be induced at birth is not entirely clear, but there is no reason to think that it differs in any fundamental way from the mechanism of immune tolerance acquired in adult life.

Immune Tolerance Acquired in Adult Life

Contrary to what was once believed, the same phenomenon of immune tolerance may be observed, under certain conditions, throughout life. But it is much more difficult to produce experimentally and so far has been obtained only with pure and well defined antigens.

Role of the Amount of Antigen: Double Zone of Tolerance. In his studies in mice using bovine serum albumin as antigen, Mitchison[197] found that moderate doses of this antigen (about 100 μg) had a strong immunizing effect, whereas very large doses (more than 1000 μg) or minute doses (less than 10 μg) produced immune paralysis. This *double zone* of dosage, one high and one low, capable of inducing tolerance instead of immunity, has been reproduced with many other antigens, notably by Shellam and Nossal[242] using the flagellin of certain spirochetes, which is one of the most violently "immunogenic" antigens in moderate doses, whereas it is remarkably "tolerogenic" in low doses.

Role of the Physical State of the Antigen. Only soluble forms of antigen can generate tolerance. If there are any aggregates of antigenic molecules in the preparation, immunity is induced instead of tolerance. If, for example, as shown by Dresser and Mitchison,[87a] solutions of bovine globulin are ultracentrifuged, the supernatant may induce tolerance in mice, whereas the sediment provokes immunity in all cases.

The tolerogenic and immunogenic forms of a given preparation can also be separated by passage in vivo. Frei et al[107] injected a massive dose of antigen into an animal. Twenty-four hours later they recovered the fraction of this antigen which remained free in the animal's blood and found that this fraction had the ability to induce tolerance. The liver may play an important part in this selection within the body, since an antigen injected into the portal circulation may become tolerogenic when it reaches the systemic circulation, as if some immunogenic fractions had been taken up by the Küpffer cells.[35]

It might also be noted here that if the antigen is mixed with lipids or other macromolecules contained in certain "adjuvants," the tolerance effect is immediately replaced by an immune effect.

Role of Associated Immunosuppressive Therapy. Rabbits given human albumin and treated with 6-MP two weeks after administration of the antigen no longer react by antibody formation to subsequent injection of the same antigen.[236] This effect of inducing tolerance by associating antigen and immunosuppression can also be achieved in rabbits previously sensitized to the same antigen. Other immunosuppressive agents, such as cyclophosphamide, can also induce tolerance. This tolerance is specific for the particular antigen. A similar result can be obtained with more complex antigens such as heterologous red blood cells. Exact dosage of the immunosuppressive agent (which must be high) and of the antigen is essential for success in this type of experiment.

Mechanism of Immune Tolerance. One fact that is certain is that the change provoked by the antigen to induce tolerance involves the lymphocytes. In 1956 Billingham et al[42] demonstrated this point by abolishing tolerance (induced at birth in mice) simply by refurnishing the mice with normal lymphoid tissue derived from isogenic animals. Even more conclusive is the work of Gowans and associates,[118] who showed in 1963 that a pure population of lymphocytes from the thoracic duct of the rat rendered tolerant at birth to another strain of rats loses its ability to produce a graft-versus-host reaction when injected into this second strain of rats. Further, lymphocytes from the tolerant animal, cultured in the presence of the antigen, have lost their normal ability to react in vitro.

This whole behavior suggests that immune tolerance is due to the disabling of the lymphocyte population capable of reacting against the particular antigen or to the mechanical elimination of the small number of lymphocytes capable of recognizing the antigen.

What then is the mechanism whereby these lymphocytes are disabled in vivo under the influence of the antigen? Some immunologists, such as Nossal (cited by Mitchison[197]), hold the view that the lymphocytes are simply killed by a cytotoxic reaction such as that seen when one mixes serum complement, an antigen and an immunologically competent cell carrying the corresponding specific antibody (or, in the present case, carrying specific receptors that, as described in Chapter One, have characteristics related to those of antibodies). It may be, however, that the lymphocyte does not die but is simply inhibited, as suggested by the loss of tolerance that may occur under the influence of radiation,[187] small doses of immunosuppressive agents[236] or administration of another antigen endowed with the property of cross reacting with the tolerogenic antigen.[126a] Suppressor T cells and anti-idiotypic antibodies probably play a major role in this inhibition.

It is far from clear why an antigen exposed to cells will in some circumstances provoke the violent upheaval of an immune reaction and in other circumstances induce tolerance. Why are some dosages, some modes of administration and some physical states of the antigen tolerogenic rather than immunogenic? This is a crucial question but as yet there is no definitive answer. We would merely note in passing that many studies indicate that macrophages are associated with lymphocytes in the production of immunity. It is possible that, when the antigen is taken up by a macrophage before reaching the lymphocyte, factors are produced that increase the immune response of the lymphocyte. The importance of this macrophage-lymphocyte association has been clearly established for antigens such as bacteriophage,[101] *Shigella,*[100] serum albumin[197] and erythrocytes (J.L. Gowans, cited by Mitchison[197]). It may indeed have some part to play in allograft immunity, but so far there is no evidence that this part is essential. It is definitely proven that perfusion of a kidney for a very short time by a pure population of lymphocytes is sufficient to sensitize these lymphocytes.[256]

Tolerance to Allografts

Cells, tissues and organs lend themselves much less readily than soluble antigens to the induction of a state of tolerance. Some degree of tolerance has, however, been achieved in experimental skin and kidney transplantation.[51]

In experiments performed mainly in mice, prolonged survival of skin allografts was obtained after administration of very small numbers of lymphoid cells[197] or after allografting an ovary from an animal isogenic with the donor.[183] The simultaneous use of a powerful nonspecific immunosuppressive agent facilitates the establishment of immune tolerance.[52, 80, 103, 169] By combined administration of ALS and lymphoid cells, it has been shown that the origin, dose, time and site of administration of the cells are essential factors for the induction of tolerance.[287, 289] In mice, bone marrow cells are the most tolerogenic. In this animal, small numbers of cells (10×10^6) are more tolerogenic than amounts 10 times larger. The best time of administration is 4 to 8 days after the graft from a C_3H/He mouse to an A/He mouse; accelerated rejection is produced by administering the cells 1 day after grafting, and there is no effect if the cells are given 16 to 23 days after the graft. Finally, the route of administration is crucial since cells which induce tolerance when given intravenously into the spleen, into the liver or, better still, simultaneously into liver and spleen, have no tolerogenic effect when given intraperitoneally, subcutaneously or into the kidney.[201]

Subcellular fractions of spleen or liver cells have also been used successfully to prolong allograft survival. Here again the effect is easier to demonstrate with associated ALS administration, comparing the results with control animals receiving only ALS. Extracts of cell membranes of spleen and liver administered 16 to 26 days before a skin allograft in mice receiving ALS 2, 4 and 6 days after grafting give significantly better survival than in control animals.[51]

Kidney allografts also have provided evidence of some degree of immunologic tolerance achieved by previous administration of antigen preparations coming from the donor. These experiments have been performed in dogs[297] and in rabbits.[218] The association of a small dose of immunosuppressive drugs is essential to bring out the tolerogenic effect.[285] In some of these experiments, however, it is difficult to distinguish the part played by true immunologic tolerance from that played by enhancement, which is described below. The device for obtaining, by in vivo passage, antigenic fractions that are more specifically tolerogenic has been applied to kidney grafts in rats. One milliliter of serum from a Lewis rat (L), injected 48 hours previously with tissue homogenate from (LxBN)F_1 rats, is given to other Lewis rats 2 hours before, 1 hour after and then every other day for 10 days following a renal allograft from an (LxBN)F_1 rat. Graft survival is prolonged to the point of indefinite tolerance in some cases.[264]

Even kidney xenografts can be prolonged by the intravenous injection of 0.5 μg/kg/day of an extract of liver tissue (obtained by open biopsy of the donor) for 5 weeks before and some days after transplantation of a guinea pig kidney into a rabbit or a pig kidney into a dog.[217]

In man, most authors are still of the opinion that in the present state of our knowledge the risk of inducing preimmunization instead of tolerance is much too high to justify the use of such a technique.

Many immunologists hope that the problem will be solved as soon as histocompatibility antigens are available in a pure and soluble state. Prolonged skin allograft survival can be obtained in mice with very high (many milligrams) or very low (micrograms) doses of more or less purified H-2 antigens.[104] "In my view," writes Mitchison,[197] "the immunologic facts are sufficiently clear to pass the ball into the court of the chemists." But when we recall the complexity of graft antigens and that it is enough for the body to be immunized against a single antigenic determinant (or even against a contaminant substance) to prevent tolerance to all the other determinants, we may well hesitate to predict when and how the dream of producing specific immunologic tolerance to an organ allograft will be translated into practical reality.

Mechanisms of Unresponsiveness to Alloantigens

There are many methods for inducing unresponsiveness to alloantigens and accordingly several postulated mechanisms. We shall now review the three main aspects of allograft tolerance: enhancement, suppression by T cells and anti-idiotypic immunization.[255]

Enhancement

The growth of some tumor grafts is enhanced by previous intraperitoneal or intravenous injection of a lyophilized extract of the tumor (active enhancement).[152, 243, 276, 284] The same phenomenon can be produced by injecting either the serum of an animal that has been given this tumor extract or even a graft of the tumor (passive enhancement). It is now known that the agent in either active or passive enhancement is an antibody (or several antibodies) differing to a certain extent from cytotoxic antibodies,[265, 277] probably because the class of immunoglobulin to which they belong does not fix complement. A further distinction between enhancing antibodies and immune antibodies is that, chronologically, the former appear after the latter.[243, 283]

There have been many reports of considerable prolongation of kidney allograft survival in experimental animals by passive or active enhancement. The vast majority of these experiments was carried out in rats.[108, 214, 233, 260, 264] Thus, kidneys from (BN $\times$ L)F_1 rats grafted to L rats (differing at the principal histocompatibility locus Rt-1 or AgB) survive indefinitely if the recipients are treated by an ALS from the donor (anti-BN rat serum from the Lewis rat).[202] It can be shown that this is, in fact, a peripheral action on the graft and not a central deletion or inactivation of the host lymphocytes, because the latter can still be stimulated normally in mixed culture by the donor cells. In similar passive enhancement experiments between Le and Buffalo (Buf) rats (differing at the principal H-1 histocompatibility locus), it can be shown that only the IgG of the anti-Buf serum of the Le rat is enhancing, whereas the IgM is ineffective or may even accelerate rejection.[207] Active enhancement has also been studied experimentally. It may be induced by the injection of ultrasonicated allogeneic spleen cells. Ideally, the best protocol associates simultaneous injection of cells and enhancing serum 7 to 10 days before grafting (perhaps the time necessary for the appearance of anti-idiotypic antibodies; see below).

The rat is particularly suitable for successful enhancement of kidney grafts. In fact, preimmunization of a rat practically never leads to hyperacute rejection of a kidney allograft, unlike the results in other species.[68] Thus, it is particular to kidney allografts in rats that they are more easily enhanced than rejected under the influence of passive or active preimmunization; only xenografts (rabbit kidney transplanted into a rat) are rejected in a hyperacute fashion, within 10 to 20 min, after specific active or passive immunization. Furthermore, it should be noted that, in certain combinations incompatible at the Rt-1 locus, for example, kidney grafts from AS2 rats to AS rats, the graft may survive spontaneously for as long as 200 days without any preparation, doubtless due to specific tolerance because a skin graft from the donor is tolerated by the rats carrying one surviving kidney graft, at least until the kidney is rejected; in addition, the recipient lymphocytes become less easily stimulated in vitro by donor cells in mixed lymphocyte culture.[235]

Thus, the special features of the rat kidney allograft model are such that it is unwise to extrapolate too hastily to other species the results of enhancement experiments. In dogs, prolonged survival is obtained only with the addition of small doses of azathioprine or methylprednisolone.[284]

The mechanisms of enhancement have been thoroughly studied. The specificity of enhancing antibodies is a matter of controversy: some authors claim that they are essentially directed at Ia antigens,[247, 248] others that antibodies specific of "sero-defined" (SD) antigens (H-2D and H-2K in the mouse) are at least as good as enhancers.[74, 88, 113] Complement fixation is not required since IgGl and possibly IgA antibodies are very active,[276] but the presence of the Fc fragment is necessary. Fab and $F(ab')_2$ fragments seem essentially inactive.[34, 109] The recent use of anti-MHC (major histocompatibility complex)[259] monoclonal antibodies[113, 259] has confirmed that anti-SD antibodies can enhance; in the near future it should provide more definitive information on the fine characteristics of enhancing antibodies.

The site of action of enhancing antibodies is not clear.[34, 62, 109, 206, 259] A peripheral action on the target must be taken into consideration; it could intervene by preventing recipient sensitization or by opposing the action of cytotoxic T cells. It has been shown that enhanced animals possess vigorous cytotoxic cells[41, 282] and that such cells are functionally blocked by the animal's serum, at least in the microcytotoxicity assay[133, 258] (but not in the chromium release assay). A central inactivation, possibly through the formation of immune complexes, could also play a role. The cytotoxic cells of enhanced allograft recipients do not show exaggerated activity after multiple immunization and do not express T cell memory.[281, 282] Such action could involve the opsonization by macrophages of antigen-reactive cells that have bound the complex of the antigen and of the enhancing antibody.[146]

Lastly, enhancing antibodies might interfere with other regulatory mechanisms. They might stimulate suppressor cells (as suggested by the decrease of their activity observed in adult thymectomized mice known to have lost part of their suppressor T cells).[276] They might also induce anti-idiotypic antibody.[44, 45, 191]

Suppressor T Cells

An alternative way to enhance antibodies, explaining the active inhibition of antigraft response observed in various experimental settings, involves the suppressor T cells that are generated in most allograft recipients. The first hint of the existence of suppressor T cells derived from the experiments of Kilshaw and Brent,[156] showing that one may transfer tolerance to normal mice with lymphoid cells. This finding fits with the other observation that tolerance could not be abolished by a mere transfer to tolerant animals of normal or immune syngeneic spleen cells.[137] Recently, suppressor cells have been found in various types of tolerance states, in particular those induced by ALS, hydrocortisone[134, 137, 288] and total lymphoid irradiation.[257] Their presence has also been demonstrated in tolerance induced by neonatal injection of allogeneic cells.[87, 232] This latter finding is interesting because it provides a new interpretation of neonatal tolerance: the newborn are probably exquisitely sensitive to tolerance induction because of their particular capacity to produce suppressor T cells and not because of their relative immunoincompetence. Lastly, it should be noted that suppressor T cells have also been observed in specific and nonspecific suppression of the in vitro generation of cytotoxic T cells.[138] All these data argue in favor of the involvement of suppressor T cells in allograft tolerance, even if some results have not always been reproducible.[109, 259]

Anti-Idiotypic Immunization

The antigen binding sites of antibodies express antigens, the idiotypes, that are characteristic of the antibody specificity. The injection into an animal of anti-idiotypic antibodies will suppress, if adequate protocols are used, the production of antibodies showing the corresponding idiotypes.[72] It was first thought that anti-idiotypic antibodies acted by binding to the receptors of the B cell type precursor of antibody forming cells.[72] The demonstration of the presence of common idiotypes on B and T cell receptors[44, 45] (see p. 5) suggests that anti-idiotypic antibodies could also act at the T cell level and inhibit cell-mediated immunity. Indeed, passive injection of anti-idiotypic antibodies or, better, autoimmunization of a mouse or a rat against its own idiotypes corresponding to a precise donor-recipient combination, specifically prevents skin allograft rejection or inhibits in vitro manifestation of cell-mediated immunity (such as MLC or CML).[44, 45] Similar data have been reported in monkeys, at least for in vitro tests.[211] However, negative results have also been published.[259] Lastly, it should be noted that anti-idiotypic antibodies are observed in the serum of animals repeatedly immunized with alloantigens,[191, 261] and prolongation of renal allograft survival may be obtained by injecting Lewis rats with l × l (L × BN)F_1 spleen cells plus Lewis anti-BN antibody, the degree of enhancement of graft survival being correlated to the level of serum anti-idiotypic antibodies.[261]

Adaptation

An allograft which has been tolerated incompletely for a long time may survive longer than a second graft from the same donor. Renal allografts, tolerated by virtue of immunodepressive chemotherapy, may continue to be tolerated by the recipient after all medication has been stopped.[208, 223] Nevertheless, the recipient does not lose his immune activity, as shown by his capacity for rapid rejection of another kidney. Neither has there been any fundamental change in the antigenic structure of the grafted kidney, since if it is reimplanted into the donor from which it was taken, it is tolerated perfectly.[208] This behavior suggests that, in the long term, the kidney may acquire a specific defense against the immunologic attacks by the host. A similar phenomenon can be seen in man, but it can be neither foreseen nor controlled.

We can find no evidence to contradict the view that this phenomenon of adaptation, to recall the term used by Woodruff,[290] is very closely related to the phenomenon of active enhancement. There is an ingenious hypothesis that adaptation may equally result from repopulation of the vascular endothelium of the graft by host endothelial cells, but no such phenomenon has been demonstrated so far except in experimental grafts of aorta segments.[259, 283]

Summary and Clinical Perspectives

Unresponsiveness to alloantigens may be induced by a number of methods, and several mechanisms have been proposed to explain the prolonged survival of allografts with which it is associated. It should be recognized, however, that it is still difficult to reconcile all the data reported so far. It is generally agreed that unresponsiveness represents a balance between aggressor mechanisms which tend to destroy the graft and regulatory mechanisms which oppose the attacker cells. Three main regulatory mechanisms have been proposed: blocking antibodies, anti-idiotypic antibodies and suppressor cells. It is still impossible to choose any of these mechanisms in a given case. It is in fact possible that the intervention of each mechanism varies with clinical conditions, although they are derived from similar therapeutic protocols.

None of the methods that has been described has reached clinical use. Some of them have been tried in pilot studies but so far have not been successful (enhancing antibodies, and ALS); others have not yet been tested (total lymphoid irradiation, cyclosporin A and anti-idiotypic immunization in conjunction with donor cells). It may be hoped that these latter techniques will be applicable to human renal transplantation in the near future and will fulfill the promise they have raised in animal experimentation.

CONCLUSIONS

Numerous methods are available for suppressing the immune response of the recipient to the renal allograft. Although it remains true that not much practical progress has been made since the discovery of azathioprine and steroids, it is fair to say that such progress may reasonably be predicted for the near future. The time has come when one may hope for more selective immunosuppression altering the lymphocyte subsets involved in rejection and/or induction of specific unresponsiveness. It will then be possible to obtain indefinite organ graft survival without such side effects as infections and neoplasias which are still observed today.

REFERENCES

1. Abaza, H. M., Nolan, B., Watt, J. G., and Woodruff, M. F. A. Effect of antilymphocytic serum on the survival of homotransplants in dogs. Transplantation, *4:*618, 1966.
2. Ackerman, G. L., and Nolan, C. M. Adrenocortical responsiveness after alternate day corticosteroid therapy. N. Engl. J. Med., *278:*405, 1968.
3. Alexandre, G. P., Murray, J. E., Dammin, G. J., and Nolan, B. Immunosuppressive drug therapy in canine renal and skin homografts. Transplantation, *1:*432, 1963.
4. Allison, A. C. Effect of antilymphocytic serum on bacterial and viral infections and virus oncogenesis. Fed. Proc., *29:*167, 1970.
5. Amemiya, M., Kashiwagi, N., Putnam, C. W., and Starzl, T. E. Cross-reactivity studies of horse, goat and rabbit antilymphocyte globulin. Clin. Exp. Immunol., *6:*279, 1970.
6. Amiel, J. L., and Doré, J. F. Etude expérimentale des immunodépresseurs chimiques. In *Advance in Transplantation*, edited by J. Dausset, J. Hamburger and G. Mathé, p. 163. Munksgaard, Copenhagen, 1968.
7. Anderson, N. F., Clark, J. G., James, K., Reid, B. L., and Woodruff, M. F. A. Biological properties of antilymphocytic antibody and antibody fragments. In *Advance in Transplantation*, edited by J. Dausset, J. Hamburger and G. Mathé, p. 103. Munksgaard, Copenhagen, 1968.
8. Antoine, B., Neveu, T., Bach, J. F., and Dardenne, M. Activité immunoprécipitante de sérums antilymphocytes. Corrélations avec d'autres effets. In *Advance in Transplantation*, edited by J. Dausset, J. Hamburger and G. Mathé, p. 123. Munksgaard, Copenhagen, 1968.

9. Attai, M., and Kelly, W. Preparation of an effective heterologous antilymphocyte serum for use in the dog. Surg. Forum, *17:*249, 1966.
10. Axerold, L. Glucocorticoid therapy. Medicine, *55:*39, 1976.
11. Bach, J. F. In vitro assay for antilymphocyte serum. Fed. Proc., *29:*120, 1970.
12. Bach, J. F. Les sérums antilymphocytes. Eur. J. Clin. Biol. Res., *15:*28, 1970.
13. Bach, J. F. Mechanism and significance of rosette inhibition by antilymphocyte serum. In *International Symposium on Antilymphocyte Serum, Versailles, 1970,* edited by J. F. Bach, J. Dormont, A. Eyquem and M. Raynaud, p. 189. Karger, Basel, 1970.
13a. Bach, J. F. Immunosuppression by chemical agents. Transplant. Proc., *3:*27, 1971.
14. Bach, J. F. *The Mode of Action of Immunosuppressive Agents,* 379 p. American Elsevier, New York, 1975.
15. Bach, J. F., and Antoine, B. In vitro detection of immunosuppressive activity of antilymphocyte sera. Nature, *217:*658, 1968.
16. Bach, J. F., and Dardenne, M. Etudes sur le métabolisme de l'azathioprine. C.R. Acad. Sci., *271:*453, 1970.
17. Bach, J. F., and Dardenne, M. The metabolism of azathioprine in renal failure. Transplantation, *12:*253, 1971.
18. Bach, J. F., and Dardenne, M. Serum immunosuppressive activity of azathioprine in normal subjects and patients with liver disease. Proc. R. Soc. Med., *65:*260, 1972.
19. Bach, J. F., and Dardenne, M. Antigen recognition by T-lymphocytes. II. Similar effects of azathioprine, antilymphocyte serum and antitheta serum on rosette-forming lymphocyte in normal and neonatally thymectomized mice. Cell Immunol., *3:*11, 1972.
20. Bach, J. F., Dardenne, M., Dormont, J., and Antoine, B. A new in vitro test evaluating ALS potency. Transplant. Proc., *1:*403, 1969.
21. Bach, J. F., Dardenne, M., and Fournier, C. In vitro evaluation of immunosuppressive drugs. Nature, *222:*998, 1969.
22. Bach, J. F., Dardenne, M., Galanaud, P., Watchi, J. M., and Antoine, B. Etude analytique de 69 sérums de lapin antilymphocytes de souris. I. Activités in vivo. Pathol. Biol. (Paris), *18:*471, 1970.
23. Bach, J. F., and Dormont, J. Evaluation of immunosuppressive activity and toxicity of antihuman ALS. In *Propriétés Immunodépressives et Mécanisme d'Action du Sérum Antilymphocytaire,* edited by B. Halpern, p. 157. C.N.R.S., Paris, 1971.
24. Bach, J. F., Dormont, J., Dardenne, M., and Balner, H. In vitro rosette inhibition by antihuman ALS. Correlation with skin graft prolongation in primates. Transplantation, *8:*265, 1969.
25. Bach, J. F., and Leski, M. The rejection crisis in human renal transplantation. Eur. J. Clin. Biol. Res., *15:*1048, 1970.
26. Bach, M. A., and Bach, J. F. Activities of immunosuppressive agents in vitro. II. Different timing of azathioprine and methotrexate in inhibition and stimulation of mixed lymphocyte reaction. Clin. Exp. Immunol., *11:*89, 1972.
27. Baker, R., Gordon, R., Huffer, J., and Miller, G. H. Experimental renal transplantation. I. Effect of nitrogen, cortisone and splenectomy. Arch. Surg., *65:*702, 1952.
28. Balner, H. In vivo evaluation of antihuman lymphocyte sera. Fed. Proc., *29:*117, 1970.
29. Balner, H., and Dersjant, H. Effect of antilymphocyte serum in primates. In *Antilymphocytic Serum, a Ciba Foundation Study Group,* edited by G. E. W. Wolstenholme and M. O'Connor, p. 85. Churchill, London, 1967.
30. Balner, H., Dersjant, H., Betel, I., and Van Bekkum, D. W. Current state of evaluating antihuman lymphocyte sera by in vivo testing. In *International Symposium on Antilymphocyte Serum, Versailles, 1970,* edited by J. F. Bach, J. Dormont, A. Eyquem and M. Raynaud, p. 179. Karger, Basel, 1970.
31. Balner, H., Dersjant, H., and Van Bekkum, D. W. Testing of antihuman lymphocyte sera in chimpanzees and lower primates. Transplantation, *8:*281, 1969.

32. Balner, H., Eijsvoogel, V. P., and Cleton, F. J. Testing of antihuman lymphocyte sera in champanzees and lower primates. Lancet, *i:*19, 1968.
33. Barna, A. D. The clinical use of antilymphocyte globulins. In *Recent Advances in Clinical Immunology*, edited by R. A. Thompson, p. 203. Churchill Livingstone, Edinburgh, 1977.
34. Batchelor, J. R., and Welsh, K. I. Mechanisms of enhancement of kidney allograft survival. A form of operational tolerance. Br. Med. Bull., *32:*113, 1976.
35. Battisto, J. R., and Miller, J. Immunological unresponsiveness produced in adult guinea pigs by parenteral introduction of minute quantities of hapten or protein antigen. Proc. Soc. Exp. Biol. Med., *111:*111, 1962.
36. Berenbaum, M. C. Prolongation of homograft survival in guinea pigs with amethopterin. Nature, *198:*606, 1963.
37. Berenbaum, M. C. Prolongation of homograft survival by methotrexate with protection against toxicity by folinic acid. Lancet, *ii:*1363, 1964.
38. Berenbaum, M. C. Immunosuppressive agents and the cellular kinetics of the immune response. In *Immunity, Cancer and Chemotherapy*, edited by E. Mihic, p. 217. Academic Press, New York, 1967.
39. Berenbaum, M. C. Time-dependent immunosuppressive effects of antilymphocyte serum. Nature, *215:*1481, 1967.
40. Berenbaum, M. C. Immunosuppressive agents: the design of selective therapeutic schedules. *The Immune Response and Its Suppression, International Symposium, Davos, 1968*, p. 155. Karger, Basel, 1969.
41. Biesecker, J. L., Fitch, F. W., Rowley, D. A., and Stuart, F. P. Cellular and humoral immunity after allogeneic transplantation in the rat. The effect of passive antibody on cellular and humoral immunity after allogeneic rat transplantation. Transplantation, *16:*432, 1973.
42. Billingham, R. E., Brent, L., and Medawar, P. B. Quantitative studies in tissue transplantation immunity. III. Actively acquired tolerance. Philos. Trans. R. Soc. Lond., *239:*357, 1956.
43. Billingham, R. E., Krohn, P. L., and Medawar, P. B. Effects of cortisone on survival of skin homografts in rabbits. Br. Med. J., *i:*1157, 1951.
44. Binz, H., and Wigzell, H. Antigen-binding, idiotypic T lymphocyte receptors. Contemp. Top. Immunobiol., *7:*113, 1977.
45. Binz, H., and Wigzell, H. Induction of specific transplantation tolerance in adult animals. Transplant. Proc., *11:*914, 1979.
46. Bonavida, B., Hutchinson, I. V., and Thomas, A. Cyclophosphamide-sensitive and cyclophosphamide-resistant suppressor cells in the immune response to alloantigens. Transplant. Proc., *11:*874, 1979.
47. Booth, P. B., Plaut, G., James, J. D., Ikin, E. W., Moores, P., Sanger, R., and Race, R. R. Blood chimerism in a pair of twins. *Br. Med. J. 1:*1456, 1957.
48. Borel, J. F., Feurer, C., Magnee, C., and Staheln, H. Effects of the new antilymphocyte peptide cyclosporin A in animals. Immunology, *32:*1017, 1977.
49. Borel, Y., and Schwartz, R. S. Inhibition of immediate and delayed hypersensitivity in the rabbit by 6-MP. J. Immunol., *92:*754, 1964.
50. Boylston, A. W., Mowbray, J. F., and Ackermann, J. R. W. Immunosuppression by ribonucleases. In *Advance in Transplantation*, edited by J. Dausset, J. Hamburger and G. Mathé, p. 189. Munksgaard, Copenhagen, 1968.
51. Brent, L., Hansen, J. A., and Kilshaw, P. J. Unresponsiveness to skin allografts induced by tissue extracts and antilymphocytic serum. Transplant. Proc., *3:*684, 1971.
52. Brooke, M. Immunological paralysis in mice exposed to sublethal irradiation or treated with 6-mercaptopurine. Transplantation, *4:*1, 1966.
53. Brown, R., Kelley, W. N., Seegmiller, J. E., and Carbone, P. P. The action of

thiopurines in lymphocytes lacking hypoxanthine-guanine phosphoribosyltransferase. J. Clin. Invest., *47:*12a, 1968.

54. Butler, W. T., Rossen, R. D., Hersh, E. M., et al. Prevention of rapid immune elimination of antilymphocytic globulin in transplant patients. Nature, *224:*856, 1969.
55. Butt, K. M. H., Zielinski, C. M., Parsa, I., Elberg, A. J., Wechter, W., and Kountz, S. L. Trends in immunosuppression for kidney transplantation. Kidney Int., *13:*S-95, 1978.
56. Calne, R. Y. The rejection of renal homografts. Inhibition in dogs by 6-MP. Lancet, *i:* 417, 1960.
57. Calne, R. Y. Inhibition of the rejection of renal homografts in dogs by purine analogues. Transplant. Bull., *28:*65, 1961.
58. Calne, R. Y. Immunosuppression for organ grafting. Observations on cyclosporin A. Immunol. Rev., *46:*113, 1979.
59. Calne, R. Y. Cyclosporin A in renal transplantation. In *Advances in Nephrology*, edited by J. Hamburger, J. Crosnier, J. P. Grünfeld and M. H. Maxwell, vol. 10. Year Book Medical Publishers, Chicago, 1980.
60. Calne, R. Y., Williams, R., Dawson, J. L., Ansell, I. D., Evans, D. B., Flute, P. T., Herbertson, P. M., Joysey, V., Keates, G. H. W., Knill-Jones, R. P., Mason, S. A., Millard, P. R., Pena, J. R., Pentlow, B. D., Salaman, J. R., Sells, R. A., and Cullum, P. A. Liver transplantation in man. II. A report of two orthotopic liver transplants in adult recipients. Br. Med. J., *1:*541, 1968.
61. Cantor, H., and Weissman, I. Development and function of subpopulations of lymphocytes and T lymphocytes. Prog. Allergy, *20:*1, 1976.
62. Carpenter, C. B., d'Apice, A. J. F., and Abbas, A. K. The role of antibodies in the rejection and enhancement of organ allografts. In *Advances in Immunology*, edited by F. J. Dixon and H. G. Kunkel, vol. 22, p. 1. Academic Press, New York, 1976.
63. Carpenter, C. B., Rashid, A., Busch, G. J., Katz, A. I., Sheffer, A. L., Valentine, M. D., Birtch, A. G., Kay, R. G., Levine, L., Murray, J. E., Austen, K. F., and Merrill, J. P. A clinical trial of horse antihuman lymphocyte globulin in renal and hepatic transplantation. In *International Symposium on Antilymphocyte Serum,* edited by J. F. Bach, J. Dormont, A. Eyquem, M. Raynaud and R. H. Regamey, p. 641. Karger, Basel, 1971.
64. Cerilli, G. J., and Treat, R. C. The effect of antilymphocyte serum on the induction and growth of tumor in the adult mouse. Transplantation, *8:*774, 1969.
65. Chanana, A. D., Cronkite, E. P., Joel, D. D., Schiffer, L. M., and Schnappauf, H. Studies on lymphocytes. XII. The role of immunologically committed lymphocytes in rejecting skin allografts. Transplantation, *7:*459, 1969.
66. Chanana, A. D., Cronkite, E. P., Joel, D. D., and Stevens, J. B. Prolonged renal allograft survival: Extracorporeal irradiation of blood. Transplant. Proc., *3:*838, 1971.
67. Chanmougan, D., and Schwartz, R. S. Enhancement of antibody synthesis by 6-mercaptopurine. J. Exp. Med., *124:*363, 1966.
68. Chavez-Peon, F., Monchik, G., Winn, H. J., and Russell, P. S. Humoral factors in experimental renal allograft and xenograft rejection. Transplant. Proc., *3:*573, 1971.
69. Clark, J. G., James, K., and Woodruff, M. F. A. Elimination of normal horse IgG labelled with iodine-131 in rats receiving horse antirat lymphocytic IgG. Nature, *215:* 869, 1967.
70. Clunie, G. J. A., Nolan, B., James, K., Watt, J. G., and Woodruff, M. F. A. Prolongation of canine renal allograft survival with antilymphocytic serum. Transplantation, *6:*459, 1968.
71. Coppola, E. D., Hemstreet, G. P., and Villegas, G. R. Suppression of allogenic skin graft rejection by indomethacin. In *Pharmacological Treatment in Organ and Tissue Transplantation,* edited by A. Bertelli and A. P. Monaco, p. 79. Excerpta Medica, Amsterdam, 1970.

72. Cosenza, H., and Kohler, H. Specific suppression of the antibody response by antibodies to receptors. Proc. Natl. Acad. Sci. USA, *69:*2701, 1972.
73. Cragle, R. G., Stone, W. H., Short, C. E., Mewborn, W. B., Wykoff, M. H., and Hall, R. F. Prolonged function of reciprocally transplanted kidneys in chimeric cattle twin. In *Advance in Transplantation,* edited by J. Dausset, J. Hamburger and G. Mathé, p. 379. Munksgaard, Copenhagen, 1968.
74. Davis, W. C. Enhancement of heart allograft survival across H-2 complex. Transplant. Proc., *9:*937, 1977.
75. Deeg, H. J., Storb, R., Gerhard-Miller, L., Sluelman, H. M., Weiden, P. L., and Thomas, E. D. Cyclosporin A, a powerful immunosuppressant in vivo and in vitro in the dog, fails to induce tolerance. Transplantation, *29:*230, 1980.
76. Demetz, A., Herter, F. P., and Evans, S. The role of the spleen in prevention of nitrogen mustard toxicity. Surg. Forum, *11:*45, 1960.
77. Dempster, W. J., Lennox, B., and Boag, J. W. Prolongation of survival of skin homotransplants in rabbit by irradiation of host. Br. J. Exp. Pathol., *31:*670, 1950.
78. Diethelm, A. G., Blackstone, E., Whelchel, J. D., Pass, R. F., Chambers, L., Phillips, S. J., and Thiry, C. The adjunctive value of equine antithymocyte membrane globulin in a randomized study of patients undergoing cadaver renal transplantation. Transplant. Proc., *11:*27, 1979.
79. Dimitriu, A., and Fauci, A. S. Differential sensitivity of human lymphocyte subpopulations to azathioprine. Transplant. Proc., *11:*878, 1979.
80. Dixon, F., and Maurer, P. Immunologic unresponsiveness induced by protein antigens. J. Exp. Med., *245:*101, 1955.
81. Dixon, F. J., Talmage, D. W., and Maurer, P. H. Radiosensitive and radioresistant phases in antibody response. J. Immunol., *68:*693, 1952.
82. Doak, P. B., Montgomerie, J. Z., North, J. D. K., and Smith, F. Reticulum cell sarcoma after renal homotransplantation and azathioprine and prednisone therapy. Br. Med. J., *1:*719, 1968.
83. Dormont, J., Debray-Sachs, M., and Bach, J. F. Sérums antilymphocytes et transplantation d'organes. In *Actualités Néphrologiques de l'Hôpital Necker,* p. 23. Med. Flammarion, Paris, 1969.
84. Dormont, J., Eyquem, A., Lavergne, M., Bach, J. F., Dimitriu, D., Watchi, J. M., Lamy, R., and Raynaud, M. Etude de sérums de chevaux antilymphocytes de chien. Prog. Immunobiol. Stand., *4:*230, 1970.
85. Dormont, J., Eyquem, A., Lavergne, M., Lamy, R., Bach, J. F., de Montera, H., Wallon, C., and Raynaud, M. Allogreffes rénales chez les chiens traités par des sérums antilymphocytes. Comparaison entre les tests in vitro et l'effet immunodépresseur des sérums. Pathol. Biol. (Paris), *17:*807, 1969.
86. Dormont, J., Josso, F., Hors, J. Jungers, P., and Bach, J. F. Toxicité et effets secondaires des sérums antilymphocytes. J. Urol. Néphrol. (Paris), *75:*589, 1969.
87. Dorsch, S., and Roser, B. Recirculating suppressor T cells in transplantation tolerance. J. Exp. Med., *145:*1144, 1977.
87a. Dresser, D. W., and Mitchison, N. A. The mechanism of immunological paralysis. In *Advances in Immunology,* edited by F. J. Dixon and H. G. Kunkel, vol. 8, p. 129. Academic Press, New York, 1968.
88. Duc, H. T., Kinsky, R. G., and Voisin, G. A. Ia versus K and D antigens in immunological enhancement of tumor allograft. Transplantation, *25:*182, 1978.
89. Duclos, H., Maillot, M. C., Kreis, H., and Galanaud, P. T-suppressor cell function impairment in peripheral blood lymphocytes from transplant recipients under azathioprine and corticosteroid. Transplantation, *28:*437, 1979.
90. Dumonde, D. C. The role of the macrophage in transplantation immunity. Symposium on Tissue Organ Transplantation. J. Clin. Pathol. (Suppl.) *20:*430, 1967.

91. Dunn, D. C., White, D. J. G., Herbertson, B. M., and Wade, J. Prolongation of kidney survival during and after cyclosporin A therapy. Transplantation, *27:*359, 1979.
92. Eijsvoogel, V. P., Van Der Hart, M., Du Bois, M. J. G. J., and Van Loghem, J. J. The specificity of antilymphocyte serum in vitro and its possible implications in vivo. In *International Symposium on Antilymphocyte Serum, Versailles, 1970*, edited by J. F. Bach, J. Dormont, E. Eyquem and M. Raynaud, p. 291. Karger, Basel, 1970.
93. Elion, G. B. Biochemistry and pharmacology of purine analogues. Fed. Proc., *26:*898, 1967.
94. Elion, G. B. Personal communication, 1970.
95. Elion, G. B., Bingi, E., and Hitchings, G. H. Study on condensed pyrimidine systems. IX. The synthesis of some 6-substituted purine. J. Am. Chem. Soc., *74:*411, 1952.
96. Elion, G. B., Callahan, S., Bieber, S., Hitchings, G. H., and Rundles, R. W. A summary of investigations with 2-amino-6-[methyl-4-nitro-5-imidazolythio]purine (B. Z. 57-322). Cancer Chemother. Pharmacol. *14:*93, 1961.
97. Elion, G. B., Callahan, S., Rundles, R. W., and Hitchings, G. H. Potentiation by inhibition of drug degradation: 6-substituted purines and xanthine-oxidase. Biochem. Pharmacol., *12:*85, 1963.
98. Fauci, A. S. Mechanisms of the immunosuppressive and anti-inflammatory effects of gluco-corticosteroids. J. Immunopharmacol., *1:*1, 1979.
99. Fauve, R. M., and Pierce-Chase, C. H. Comparative effects of corticosteroids on host resistance to infection in relation to chemical structure. J. Exp. Med., *125:*807, 1967.
100. Feldman, M., and Gallily, R. Cell interactions in the induction of antibody formation. Symp. Quant. Biol., *32:*415, 1967.
101. Fishman, M., and Adler, F. L. The role of macrophage-RNA in the immune response. Symp. Quant. Biol., *32:*343, 1967.
102. Floersheim, G. L. Drug-induced tolerance for skin allografts across the H2 barrier in adult mice. Science, *156:*951, 1967.
103. Floersheim, G. L., and Brune, K. Tolerance to skin allografts by immunosuppressive "pulse of methylhydrazine derivatives and antilymphocyte serum." Transplant. Proc., *3:*688, 1971.
104. Florentin, I. Effet, selon la dose, du prétraitement chez la souris receveur d'homogreffes de peau par des préparations lipoprotéiques, hydrosolubles et purifiées d'antigènes H-2. Rev. Fr. Etud. Clin. Biol., *14:*690, 1969.
105. Forbes, I. J., and Smith, J. L. Effects of anti-inflammatory drugs on lymphocytes. Lancet, *ii:*334, 1967.
106. Fox, M. Suppression of tissue immunity by cyclophosphamide. Transplantation, *2:*475, 1964.
107. Frei, P. C., Benacerraf, B., and Thorbecke, G. J. Phagocytosis of the antigen, a crucial step in the induction of the primary response. Proc. Nat. Acad. Sci. USA, *53:*20, 1965.
108. French, M. E., and Batchelor, J. R. Immunological enhancement of rat kidney grafts. Lancet, *ii:*1103, 1969.
109. French, M. E., and Batchelor, J. R. Enhancement of renal allografts in rat and man. Transplant. Rev., *13:*115, 1972.
110. Fries, D., Traeger, J., Bansillon, V., Dubernard, J. M., Touraine, J. L., Betuel, H., and Mamelle, C. Critères cliniques biologiques et histologiques de l'activité des globulines antilymphocytaires en transplantation rénale. In *International Symposium of Antilymphocyte Serum, Versailles, 1970*, p. 363. Karger, Basel, 1970.
111. Gabrielsen, A. E., and Good, R. A. Chemical suppression of adaptive immunity. In *Advances in Immunology*, edited by F. J. Dixon and H. G. Kunkel, vol. 6, p. 91. Academic Press, New York, 1967.
112. Galanaud, P., Crevon, M. C., Duclos, H., and Dormont, J. New data on the effect of

azathioprine at the cellular level. In *Advances in Nephrology*, edited by J. Hamburger, J. Crosnier, and M. H. Maxwell, vol. 6. Year Book Medical Publishers, Chicago, 1976.

113. Gallico, G. G., Butcher, G. W. and Howard, J. C. The role of subregions of the rat major histocompatibility complex in the rejection and passive enhancement of renal allografts. J. Exp. Med., *149:*244, 1979.
114. Germuth, F. G., and Ottinger, B. Effects of 17-hydroxy-11-dehydrocorticosterone (compound E) and of ACTH on Arthus reaction and antibody formation in the rabbit. Proc. Soc. Exp. Biol. Med., *74:*815, 1950.
115. Gillette, R. W., Findley, A., and Conway, H. Prolonged survival of homografts in mice treated with EACA. Transplantation, *1:*116, 1963.
116. Gleason, R. E., and Murray, J. E. Report from the Kidney Transplant Registry: Analysis of variables in the function of human kidney transplants. I. Blood group compatibility and splenectomy. Transplantation, *5:*343, 1967.
117. Goodwin, W. E., Kaufman, J. J., Mims, M. M., Turner, R. D., Glassock, R., Goldman, R., and Maxwell, M. H. Human renal transplantation. I. Clinical experiences with 6 cases of renal homotransplantation. J. Urol., *89:*13, 1963.
118. Gowans, J. L., McGregor, D. D., and Cowen, D. M. The role of small lymphocytes in the rejection of homografts of skin. In *The Immunologically Competent Cell. Ciba Foundation Study Group*, edited by G. E. W. Wolstenholme and J. Knight, p. 20. Churchill, London, 1963.
119. Gozzo, J. J., Wood, M. L., and Monaco, A. P. Studies on heterologous antilymphocyte serum in mice. IX. In vitro assay by indirect leukoagglutination. Transplantation, *14:* 358, 1972.
120. Gray, G. D., and Mickelson, M. M. The immunosuppressive effects of adamantoyl cytarabine. II. Effects of skin allograft rejection by rats and mice. Transplantation, *9:* 176, 1970.
121. Gray, G. D., Perper, R. J., Mickelson, M. M., Crim, J. A., and Zukoski, C. F. The immunosuppressive activity of aracytidine (cytarabine). Transplantation, *7:*183, 1969.
122. Greaves, M. F., Tursi, A., Playfair, J. H. R., Torrigiani, G., Zamir, R., and Roitt, I. M. Immunosuppressive potency and in vitro activity of antilymphocyte globulin. Lancet, *i:*68, 1969.
123. Green, L. J., and Allison, A. C. Extensive prolongation of rabbit kidney allograft survival after short-term cyclosporin A treatment. Lancet, *i:*1182, 1978.
124. Guttmann, R. D., Carpenter, C. B., Lindquist, R. R., and Merrill, J. P. Treatment with heterologous antithymus sera: Nephritis associated with modification of renal allograft rejection and the immune status of the host to the foreign protein. Transplantation, *5:* 1115, 1967.
125. Guttman, R. D., Carpenter, C. B., Lindquist, R. R., and Merrill, J. P. An immunosuppressive site of action of heterologous antilymphocyte serum. Lancet, *i:*248, 1967.
126. Guttman, R. D., Lindquist, R. R., and Ockner, S. A. Renal transplantation in the inbred rat. XII. A mechanism of long term survival of allografts after antithymocyte immunoglobulin treatment. Transplantation, *8:*837, 1969.

126a. Halpern, B. Facteurs biologiques modifiant la synthèse des anticorps. Presse Méd., *77:* 539, 1969.

127. Hamburger, J. Renal transplantation. In *Organ Transplantation Today*, p. 276. Excerpta Medica, Amsterdam, 1969.
128. Hamburger, J., Crosnier, J., and Dormont, J. Observations in patients with a well tolerated homotransplanted kidney: possibility of a new secondary disease. Ann. NY Acad. Sci., *120:*558, 1964.
129. Hamburger, J., Crosnier, J., and Dormont, J. Experience with 45 renal homotransplantations in man. Lancet *i:*985, 1965.
130. Hamburger, J., Vaysse, J., Crosnier, J., Auvert, J., Lalanne, C. M., and Hopper, J., Jr.

Renal homotransplantation in man after radiation of the recipient. Am. J. Med., *32:* 854, 1962.

131. Hardy, M. A., Nowygrod, R., Elberg, A., and Appel, G. Use of ATG in treatment of steroid-resistant rejection. Transplantation, *29:*162, 1979.
132. Hechtman, M. B., Blumenstock, D. A., Thomas, E. D., and Ferrebee, J. W. Prolongation of canine skin homografts by antimetabolites. Surg. Forum, *13:*55, 1962.
133. Hellstrom, K. E., and Hellstrom, I. Lymphocyte-mediated cytotoxicity and blocking serum to tumor antigens. In *Advances in Immunology*, edited by F. J. Dixon and H. G. Kunkel, vol. 18, p. 209. Academic Press, New York, 1974.
134. Hendry, W. S., Tilney, N. L., Baldwin, W. M., Graves, M. J., Milford, E., Strom, T. B., and Carpenter, C. B. Transfer of specific unresponsiveness to organ allografts by thymocytes. Specific unresponsiveness by thymocyte transfer. J. Exp. Med., *149:*1042, 1979.
135. Herman, A. H., and Schloer, P. R. The effect of thoracic duct lymphocyte antiserum on canine renal allografts. Transplantation, *5:*732, 1967.
136. Hersh, E. M., Carbone, P. P., and Freireich, E. J. Recovery of immune responsiveness after drug suppression in man. J. Lab. Clin. Med., *67:*566, 1966.
137. Hilgert, I. The involvement of activated specific suppressor T cells in maintenance of transplantation tolerance. Immunol. Rev., *46:*27, 1979.
138. Hodes, R. J., and Hathcock, K. S. In vitro generation of suppressor cell activity: Suppression of in vitro induction of cell-mediated cytotoxicity. J. Immunol., *116:*167, 1976.

138a.Hoelm, R. J., and Simmons, R. L. Immunosuppressive drugs combined with heterologous antilymphocyte serum for allograft prolongation. Transplantation, *5:*1409, 1967.

139. Hollingsworth, J. W. Delayed radiation effects in survivors of the atomic bombings. N. Engl. J. Med., *263:*481, 1960.
140. Homan, W. P., Falne, J. W., and Morris, P. J. Nature of the unresponsiveness induced by cyclosporin A in rats bearing renal allografts. Transplantation, *28:*439, 1979.
141. Howard, R. R. S., Asfis, N., and Woodruff, M. F. A. Comparative immunogeneicity of antilymphocytic globulin in solution and absorbed on lymphocytes. Nature, *220:*816, 1968.
142. Howard, R. J., Dougherty, S. F., and Mergenhagen, S. E. Prolongation of skin homografts by rabbit antimouse lymphocyte serum in mice rendered tolerant to rabbit gammaglobulin. J. Immunol., *101:*301, 1968.
143. Hume, D. M. Kidney transplantation. In *Human Transplantation*, edited by F. T. Rapaport and J. Dausset, p. 110. Grune and Stratton, New York, 1968.
144. Hume, D. M., Magee, J. H., Prout, G. R., Jr., Kauffman, H. M., Jr., Cleveland, R. H., Bower, J. D., and Lee, H. M. Studies of renal homotransplantation in man. Ann. NY Acad. Sci., *120:*578, 1964.
145. Hurd, E. R., and Ziff, M. Studies on the anti-inflammatory action of 6-MP. J. Exp. Med., *128:*785, 1968.
146. Hutchinson, I. V., Antigen-reactive cell opsonization (ARCO) and its role in antibody-mediated immune suppression. Immunol. Rev., *49:*167, 1980.
147. Iwasaki, Y., Porter, K. A., Amend, J. R., Marchioro, T. L., Zuhlke, V., and Starzl, T. E. The preparation and testing of horse antidog and antihuman antilymphoid plasma or serum and its protein fractions. Surgery, *124:*1, 1967.
148. James, K. Antilymphocytic antibody: A review. Clin. Exp. Immunol., *2:*615, 1967.
149. Jeejeebhoy, H. F. The relationship of lymphopenia production and lymphocyte agglutinating and cytotoxic antibody titers to the immunosuppressive potency of heterologous antilymphocyte plasma. Transplantation, *5:*1121, 1967.
150. Jooste, S. V., Lance, E. M., Levey, R. H., Medawar, P. B., Ruszkiewicz, M., Sharman,

R., and Taub, R. N. Notes on the preparation and assay of antilymphocyte serum for use in mice. Immunology, *15:*697, 1968.

151. Josso, F., Hors, J., Bach, J. F., Kamoun, P., and Dormont, J. Activité antiplaquettaire des sérums antilymphocytes. In *International Symposium on Antilymphocyte Serum, Versailles, 1970,* edited by J. F. Bach, J. Dormont, A. Eyquem, and M. Raynaud, p. 333. Karger, Basel, 1970.
152. Kaliss, N. Immunological enhancement of tumor homografts in vivo. A review. Cancer Res., *18:*992, 1958.
153. Kamrin, B. B. Successful skin homografts in mature nonlittermate rats treated with fractions containing α-globulins. Proc. Soc. Exp. Biol. Med., *100:*58, 1959.
154. Kashiwagi, N., Brantignan, C. O., Brettschneider, L., Groth, C. G., and Starzl, T. E. Clinical reactions and serologic changes after the administration of heterologous antilymphocyte globulin to human recipients of renal homografts. Ann. Intern. Med., *68:*275, 1968.
155. Kauffman, H. M., Jr., Cleveland, R. J., Dwyer, J. J., Lee, H. M., and Hume, D. M. Prolongation of renal homograft function by local graft radiation. Surg. Gynecol. Obstet., *120:*49, 1965.
156. Kilshaw, P. J., Brent, L., and Pinto, M. Suppressor T cells in mice made unresponsive to skin allografts. Nature, *255:*489, 1976.
157. Kisken, W. A., and Daouk, A. A. Host acceptance of well-matched kidney allograft. Transplant. Proc., *3:*693, 1971.
158. Kostakis, A. J., White, D. J. G., and Calne, R. Y. Prolongation of the rat heart allograft survival by cyclosporin A. IRCS Med. Sci. Surg. Transplant., *5:*280, 1977.
159. Kountz, S. L., Butt, K. H. M., Rao, T. K. S., Zielinski, C. M., Rafi, M., Schultz, J. R. Antithymocyte globulin (ATG) dosage and graft survivial in renal transplantation. Transplant. Proc., *9:*1023, 1979.
160. Kountz, S. L., and Cohn, R. Prolonged survival of a renal homograft by simultaneous splenectomy and homotransplantation. Surg. Forum., *13:*59, 1962.
161. Krohn, P. The influence of the spleen on the homograft reaction. Transplant. Bull., *1:* 21, 1953.
162. Laborde, M. A., and Bach, J. F. Inhibition et stimulation par l'azathioprine de l'incorporation de thymidine par les lymphocytes en culture mixte. C.R. Acad. Sci. *272:*509, 1971.
163. Lance, E. M. Erasure of immunological memory with antilymphocyte serum. Nature, *217:*557, 1968.
164. Lance, E. M. The effects of chronic ALS administration in mice. In *Advance in Transplantation,* edited by J. Dausset, J. Hamburger and G. Mathé, p. 107. Munksgaard, Copenhagen, 1968.
165. Lance, E. M. The selective action of antilymphocyte serum on recirculating lymphocytes. Clin. Exp. Immunol., *6:*789, 1970.
166. Lance, E. M., and Dresser, D. W. Antigenicity in mice of antilymphocyte gammaglobulin. Nature, *215:*488, 1967.
167. Lance, E. M., and Medawar, P. B. Survival of skin heterografts under treatment with antilymphocytic serum. Lancet, *i:*1174, 1968.
168. Lance, E. M., and Medawar, P. B. Induction of tolerance with antilymphocyte serum. Transplant. Proc., *1:*429, 1969.
169. Lance, E. M., and Medawar, P. B. Immunosuppressive effects of heterologous antilymphocyte serum in monkeys. Lancet, *i:*167, 1970.
170. Lance, E. M., and Medawar, P. B. Antilymphocyte serum and the induction of tolerance to transplantation antigens. Fed. Proc., *29:*151, 1970.
171. Lance, E. M., Medawar, P. B., Nehlsen, S. L., Cooper, S., and Gunn, A. Synergistic effects of antilymphocyte serum and hydrocortisone on lymphoid populations. In

International Symposium on Antilymphocyte Serum, Versailles, 1970, edited by J. F. Bach, J. Dormont, A. Eyquem and M. Raynaud, p. 231. Karger, Basel, 1970.

172. Land, W., Brendel, W., Seifert, J., Fateh-Moghadam, A., and Pichlmayr, R. Induction of immunological tolerance to xenogenic IgG in adult dogs. In *Pharmacological Treatment in Organ and Tissue Transplantation*, edited by A. Bertelli and A. P. Monaco, p. 215. Excerpta Medica, Amsterdam, 1970.
173. Launois, B., Campion, J. P., Fauchet, R., Kerbaol, M., and Cartier, F. Prospective randomized clinical trial in patients with cadaver-kidney transplants. Transplant. Proc., *9:*1027, 1977.
174. Law, L. W. Effect of antilymphocyte serum on the induction of neoplasms of lymphoreticular tissues. Fed. Proc., *29:*171, 1970.
175. Lejeune, G. *Homogreffes Cutanées, Étude Expérimentale,* p. 165. Maloine, Paris, 1962.
176. Leski, M., Kreis, H., Descamps, B., and Crosnier, J. Les complications extra-rénales des transplantations de rein. In *Actualités Néphrologiques de l'Hôpital Necker*, p. 229. Med Flammarion, Paris, 1969.
177. Leuchars, E., Wallis, V. J., and Davies, A. J. S. Mode of action for antilymphocyte serum. Nature, *219:*1325, 1968.
178. Levey, R. H. Workshop on immunosuppression by biologic methods. Transplant. Proc., *11:*1179, 1979.
179. Levey, R. H., Burleson, R., Lucas, D., and Parke, P. Notes on the preparation and assay on antilymphocytic serum for use in man. In *International Symposium on Antilymphocyte Serum, Versailles, 1970*, edited by J. F. Bach, J. Dormont, A. Eyquem and M. Raynaud, p. 9. Karger, Basel, 1970.
180. Levey, R. H., and Medawar, P. B. Some experiments on the action of antilymphoid antisera. Ann. NY Acad. Sci., *129:*164, 1966.
181. Levey, R. H., and Medawar, P. B. Nature and mode of action of antilymphocyte antiserum. Proc. Natl. Acad. Sci. USA, *56:*1130, 1966.
182. Levey, R. H., and Medawar, P. B. The mode of action of antilymphocytic serum. In *Antilymphocytic Serum, a Ciba Foundation Study Group*, edited by G. E. W. Wolstenholme and M. O'Connor, p. 72. Churchill, London, 1967.
183. Linder, O. E. A. Comparisons between the survival of grafted skin, ovaries and tumors in mice across histocompatibility barriers of different strength. J. Natl. Cancer Inst., *27:*351, 1961.
184. Lipinski, M., Tursz, T., Kreis, H., Finale, Y., Amiel, J. L. Dissociation of natural killer cell activity and antibody-dependent cell-mediated cytotoxicity in kidney allograft recipients receiving high-dose immunosuppressive therapy. Transplantation, *29:*214, 1980.
185. Lucke, J. N., Immelman, E. J., Symes, M. O., and Hunt, A. C. Use of horse antipig leucocyte serum to suppress the homograft reaction in pigs. Nature, *217:*560, 1968.
186. MacGregor, R. R., Sheagren, J. N., Lipsett, M. B., and Wolff, S. M. Alternate day prednisone therapy. Evaluation of delayed hypersensitivity responses, control of disease and steroid side effects. N. Engl. J. Med., *280:*1427, 1969.
187. Makela, O., and Nossal, G. J. V. Accelerated breakdown of immunological tolerance following whole body irradiation. J. Immunol., *88:*613, 1962.
188. Marchioro, T. L., Extell, H. K., La Via, M. F., Waddell, W. R., and Starzl, T. E. The role of adrenocortical steroids in reversing established homograft rejection. Surgery, *55:*412, 1964.
189. Martin, M. M., Gaboardi, F., Podolsky, S., Raiti, S., and Calcagno, P. L. Intermittent steroid therapy. Its effect on hypothalamic-pituitary-adrenal function and the response of plasma growth hormone and insulino-stimulation. N. Engl. J. Med., *279:*279, 1968.
190. Mathé, G., Amiel, J. L., Schwarzenberg, L., Schneider, M., Cattan, A., Schlumberger, J. R., Hayat, M., Vassal, F. de, Jasmin, C., Rosenfeld, C., Choay, J., and Trolard, P.

Greffe de moelle osseuse allogénique chez l'homme prouvée par six marqueurs antigéniques après conditionnement du receveur et du donneur par le sérum antilymphocytaire. Rev. Fr. Etud. Clin. Biol., *13:*1025, 1968.

191. McKearn, T. J., Stuart, F. P., Fitch, F. W. Anti-idiotypic antibody and rat transplantation immunity. I. Production of anti-idiotypic antibody in animals repeatedly immunized with alloantigens. J. Immunol., *113:*1876, 1974.

192. Medawar, P. B. Biological effects of heterologous antilymphocyte serum. In *Human Transplantation*, edited by F. T. Rapaport and J. Dausset, p. 501. Grune and Stratton, New York, 1968.

192a. Billingham, R. E., Brent, L., and Medawar, P. B. Quantitative studies on tissue transplantation immunity. Philos. Trans. R. Soc. Lond., *239:*357, 1956.

193. Melby, J. C. Systemic corticosteroid therapy: Pharmacology and endocrinologic considerations. Ann. Int. Med., *84:*304, 1974.

194. Metchnikoff, E. Etudes sur la résorption des cellules. Ann. Inst. Pasteur, *13:*737, 760, 1899.

194a. Mirick, G. S. The effects of ACTH and cortisone on antibodies in human beings. Bull. Johns Hopkins Hosp., *88:*332, 1951.

195. Mitchell, C. G., Eddleston, A. C. W., Smith, M. G. M., and Williams, R. Serum immunosuppressive activity due to azathioprine and its relation to hepatic function after liver transplantation. Lancet, *i:*1196, 1970.

196. Mitchell, R. M., Sheil, A. G. R., Slafsky, S. F., and Murray, J. E. The effects of heterologous immune serum on canine renal homografts. Transplantation, *4:*323, 1966.

197. Mitchison, N. A. Immunological tolerance. Symposium on Tissue and Organ Transplantation, J. Clin. Pathol. (Suppl.), *20:*451, 1967.

197a. Mitchison, N. A. Mechanism of action of antilymphocyte serum. Fed. Proc., *29:*222, 1970.

198. Moller, G., and Moller, E. Immunologic surveillance revisited. Transplant. Proc., *11:* 1041, 1979.

199. Monaco, A. P. Use of antilymphocyte serum in the induction of immunological tolerance to tissue allografts. Fed. Proc., *29:*153, 1970.

200. Monaco, A. P., Abbott, W. M., Othersen, H. B., Simmons, R. L., Wood, M. L., Flax, M. H., and Russell, P. S. Antiserum to lymphocytes: Prolonged survivals of canine renal allografts. Science, *153:*1264, 1966.

201. Monaco, A. P., Gozzo, J. J., Wood, M. L., and Liegeois, A. Use of low doses of homozygous allogeneic bone marrow cells to induce tolerance with antilymphocyte serum (ALS): Tolerance by intraorgan injection. Transplant. Proc., *3:*680, 1971.

202. Monaco, A. P., Wood, M. L., Gray, J. G., and Russell, P. S. Studies on heterologous antilymphocyte serum in mice. II. Effect on the immune response. J. Immunol., *96:* 229, 1966.

203. Monaco, A. P., Wood, M. L., and Russell, P. S. Some effects of purified heterologous antihuman lymphocyte serum in man. Transplantation, *5:*1106, 1967.

204. Monaco, A. P., Wood, M. L., Van Der Werf, B. A., and Russell, P. S. Effects of antilymphocyte serum in mice, dogs and man. In *Antilymphocyte Serum, a Ciba Foundation Study Group*, edited by G. E. W. Wolstenholme and M. O'Connor, p. 111. Churchill, London, 1967.

205. Morris, R., and Lucas, Z. J. Immunologic enhancement of rat kidney grafts: Evidence for peripheral action of homologous antiserum. Transplant. Proc., *3:*697, 1971.

206. Morriss, P. J. Suppression of rejection of organ allografts by alloantibody. Immunol. Rev., *49:*93, 1980.

207. Mullen, Y., and Hildemann, W. H. Kidney transplantation genetics and enhancement in rats. Transplant. Proc., *3:*669, 1970.

208. Murray, J. E., Sheil, A. G. R., Moseley, R., and Knight, G. J. Analysis of mechanism of immunosuppressive drugs in renal homotransplantation. Ann. Surg., *160:*449, 1964.

209. Murray, J. E., Sheil, A. G. R., Moseley, R., Knight, P., McGarie, J. D., and Dammin, G. J. Analysis of the mechanism of immunosuppressive drugs in renal homotransplantation. Ann. Surg., *160:*449, 1964.
210. Murphy, J. B., and Sturm, E. A. A comparison of the effects of X-ray and dry heat on antibody formation. J. Exp. Med., *41:*245, 1925.
211. Myburgh, J. A., and Smit, J. A. Autoantiidiotypic immunization and transplantation tolerance in the primate. Transplant. Proc., *11:*923, 1979.
212. Najarian, J. S., Moberg, A. W., Gewurz, H., Jetzer, T., and Simmons, R. L. Forced flow electrophoretic purification of antihuman antilymphoblast globulin. In *International Symposium on Antilymphocyte Serum, Versailles, 1970*, edited by J. F. Bach, J. Dormont, A. Eyquem and M. Raynaud, p. 49. Karger, Basel, 1970.
213. Najarian, J. S., Simmons, R. L., Gewurz, H., Moberg, A., Merkel, F., and Moore, G. E. Antihuman lymphoblast globulin. Fed. Proc., *29:*197, 1970.
214. Ockner, S. A., Guttmann, R. D., and Lindquist, R. R. Renal transplantation in the inbred rat. XIV. Mechanism of the modified rejection produced by bone marrow cell pretreatment. Transplantation, *9:*39, 1970.
215. Orr, W. M., Diethelm, A. G., Birtch, A. G., Dubernard, J. M., Duquella, J., Busch, G., Murray, J. E., and Moore, F. D. Heterologous antilymphocyte serum in canine hepatic and renal allografts. Abstracts of the First International Congress of the Transplantation Society, p. 154, Paris, 1967.
216. Otte, H., and Grosjean, O. Influence du sérum antilymphocyte sur la survie de la greffe rénale allogénique chez le chien. C.R. Soc. Biol., *161:*738, 1967.
217. Owen, E. R. Xenograft protection by low dose, antigen-induced tolerance. Transplant. Proc., *3:*562, 1971.
218. Owen, E. R., Slome, D., and Waterson, D. Prolongation of rabbit kidney allograft survival by "Desensitization." In *Advance in Transplantation*, edited by J. Dausset, J. Hamburger and G. Mathé, p. 385. Munksgaard, Copenhagen, 1968.
219. Owen, R. D. Immunogenetic consequences of vascular anastomoses between bovine twins. Science, *102:*400, 1945.
220. Penn, I. Tumor incidence in human allograft recipients. Transplant. Proc., *11:*1047, 1979.
221. Perper, R. J., Glenn, E. M., Yu, T. Z., Monovich, R. E., and Brunden, M. N. Analysis of the biological activities in antilymphocyte serum. In *Pharmacological Treatment in Organ and Tissue Transplantation*, edited by A. Bertelli and A. P. Monaco, p. 298. Excerpta Medica, Amsterdam, 1970.
222. Perper, R. J., Yu, T. Z., and Kooistra, J. B. The in vitro specificity of antilymphocyte sera produced by either cultured or noncultured lymphocytes. Int. Arch. Allergy, *37:*418, 1970.
223. Pierce, J. C., Varco, R. L., and Good, R. A. Prolonged survival of renal homograft in a dog treated with 6-mercaptopurine. Surgery, *50:*186, 1961.
224. Powles, R. L., Barrett, A. J., Clark, H., Kay, H. E. M., Sloan, J., and McElwain, T. J. Cyclosporin A for the treatment of graft-versus-host disease in man. Lancet *2:*1327, 1978.
225. Prince, G. H., Rabbit antihuman lymphocyte serum. In *International Symposium on Antilymphocyte Serum, Versailles, 1970*, edited by J. F. Bach, J. Dormont, A. Eyquem and M. Raynaud, p. 93. Karger, Basel, 1970.
226. Reed, W. P., Lucas, Z. J., and Cohn, R. Alternate day prednisone therapy after renal transplantation. Lancet, *i:*747, 1970.
226a. Revillard, J. P. Déplétion lymphocytaire par drainage du canal thoracique chez l'homme. Cah. Méd. Lyon., *46:*703, 1970.
227. Revillard, J. P., Brochier, J., Traeger, J., and Balner, H. In vitro assay of suppressive properties of antilymphocyte sera on lymphocyte stimulation. Transplantation, *9:*592, 1970.

228. Rifle, G., Chalopin, J. M., Turc, J. M., Guigner, F., Vialtel, P., Dechelette, E., Chenais, F., and Cordonnier, D. Plasmapheresis in the treatment of renal allograft rejections. Transplant. Proc., *11:*20, 1979.
229. Roitt, I. M., Greaves, M. F., Tursi, A., Torrigiani, G., Playfair, J. H. L., and Verbi, W. Correlation between immunosuppressive potency of antilymphocyte globulin and its activity in an opsonic adherence test in vitro. In *Pharmacological Treatment in Organ and Tissue Transplantation,* edited by A. Bertelli and A. P. Monaco, p. 284. Excerpta Medica, Amsterdam, 1970.
230. Röllinghof, M., Starzinski-Powitz, A., Pfizenmaier, K., and Wagner, H. Cyclophosphamide-sensitive T lymphocytes suppress the in vivo generation of antigen-sensitive T lymphocytes. J. Exp. Med., *145:*455, 1977.
231. Rose, N. R., Haber, J. A., and Calabresi, P. Immunosuppressive effects of selected metabolic inhibitors in vivo and in vitro. Proc. Soc. Exp. Biol. Med., *128:*1121, 1968.
232. Roser, B., and Dorsch, S. The cellular basis of transplantation tolerance in the rat. Immunol. Rev., *46:*55, 1979.
233. Rowely, D. A., Fitch, F. W., Saitoh, T., and Stuart, F. P. Specific suppression of cell-mediated immune responses. Transplant. Proc., *1:*580, 1969.
234. Rowley, M. J., Mackay, I. R., and McKenzie, I. F. C. Antibody production in immunosuppressed recipients of renal allografts. Lancet, *ii:*708, 1969.
235. Salaman, J. R., Elves, M. W., and Festensteil, H. Factors contributing to survival of rats transplanted with kidneys mismatched at major locus. Transplant. Proc., *3:*577, 1971.
236. Schwartz, R. S. Immunosuppressive drug therapy. In *Human Transplantation,* edited by F. T. Rapaport and J. Dausset, p. 440. Grune and Stratton, New York, 1968.
237. Schwartz, R. S. Immunosuppression by L-asparaginase. Nature, *224:*275, 1969.
237a. Schwartz, R. S., Eisner, A., and Dameshek, W. The effect of 6-mercaptopurine on primary and secondary immune responses. J. Clin. Invest. *38:*1394, 1959.
238. Shanfield, I., Ladaga, L. G., Wren, S. F. G., Blennerhassett, J. B., and McLean, L. D. Prolongation of canine renal allograft survival with antilymphoid antisera. Surg. Gynecol. Obstet., *127:*29, 1968.
239. Shehadeh, I. H., Guttmann, R. D., Lindquist, R. R., and Rodriguez-Erdmann, F. Renal transplantation in the inbred rat. XVI. Effects of salicylates and anticoagulant drugs on rejection. Transplantation, *10:*75, 1970.
240. Sheil, A. G. R., Mears, D., Johnson, J. R., Kelly, G. E., May, J., Ibels, L. S., and Stewart, J. H. Antilymphocyte globulin in patients with renal allografts from cadaveric donors. Late results of a controlled trial. Lancet, *2:*227, 1973.
241. Sheil, A. G. R., Mitchell, R. M., Dammin, G. J., and Murray, J. E. Analysis of the mechanism of drug-induced tolerance to renal allografts in dogs. In *Advance in Transplantation,* edited by J. Dausset, J. Hamburger and G. Mathé, p. 599. Munksgaard, Copenhagen, 1968.
242. Shellam, G. R., and Nossal, G. J. V. Mechanism of induction of immunological tolerance. IV. The effects of ultralow doses of flagellin. Immunology, *14:*273, 1968.
243. Sinclair, N. R. StC. Immunoregulation by antibody and antigen-antibody complexes. Transplant. Proc., *10:*349, 1978.
244. Slavin, S., Kaplan, H. S., and Strober, S. Transplantation of allogeneic bone marrow without graft vs. host disease using total lymphoid irradiation (TLI). J. Exp. Med., *147:*963, 1978.
245. Slavin, S., Kaplan, H. S., and Strober, S. Transplantation of bone marrow in outbred dogs without graft vs. host disease using total lymphoid irradiation (TLI). Transplantation, *27:*139, 1979.
246. Sokal, G., Bruyère, M. De, Alexandre, G. P. J., and Zenebergh, A. Preparation and

testing of horse antihuman lymphocyte globulins. In *International Symposium on Antilymphocyte Serum, Versailles, 1970,* edited by J. F. Bach, J. Dormont, A. Eyquem and M. Raynaud, p. 133. Karger, Basel, 1970.

247. Soulillou, J. P., Carpenter, C. B., d'Apice, A. J., and Strom, T. B. The role of nonclassical, Fc receptor-associated Ag-B antigens (k) in rat allograft enhancement. J. Exp. Med., *143:*405, 1976.
248. Staines, W. A., Guy, K., and Davies, D. A. L. The dominant role of Ia antibodies in the passive enhancement of H-2 incompatible skin grafts. Eur. J. Immunol., *5:*782, 1975.
249. Starzl, T. E. *Experience in Renal Transplantation.* Saunders, Philadelphia, 1964.
250. Starzl, T. E., Brettschneider, L., Penn, I., Schmidt, R. W., Bell, P., Kashiwagi, N., Townsend, C. M., and Putman, C. W. A trial with heterologous antilymphocyte globulin in man. Transplant. Proc., *1:*448, 1969.
251. Starzl, T. E., Marchioro, T. L., Porter, K. A., Iwasaki, Y., and Cerilli, G. J. The use of heterologous antilymphoid agents in canine renal and liver homotransplantation and in human renal homotransplantation. Surg. Gynecol. Obstet., *124:*301, 1967.
252. Starzl, T. E., Porter, K. A., Andres, G., Groth, C. G., Putnam, C. W., Penn, I., Halgrimson, C. G., Starkie, S. J., and Brettschneider, L. Thymectomy and renal homotransplantation. Clin. Exp. Immunol., *6:*803, 1970.
253. Starzl, T. E., Porter, K. A., Iwasaki, Y., Marchioro, T. L., and Kashiwagi N. The use of heterologous antilymphocyte globulin in human renal homotransplantation. In *Antilymphocyte Serum, a Ciba Foundation Study Group,* edited by G. E. W. Wolstenholme and M. O'Connor, p. 4. Churchill, London, 1967.
254. Stavy, L., Cohen, I. R., and Feldman, M. The effect of hydrocortisone on lymphocyte-mediated cytolysis. Cell. Immunol., *7:*302, 1973.
255. Steinmuller, D. Methods for induction of permanent graft survival. Transplant. Proc., *11:*1198, 1979.
256. Strober, S., and Gowans, J. L. The role of lymphocytes in the sensitization of rats to renal homografts. J. Exp. Med., *122:*347, 1965.
257. Strober, S., Slavin, S., Gottlieb, M., Zan-Bar, I., King, O. P., Hoppe, R. T., Fuks, Z., Grumet, F. C., and Kaplan, H. S. Allograft tolerance after total lymphoid irradiation (TLI) Immunol. Rev., *46:*87, 1979.
258. Stuart, F. P., Fitch, F. W., Rowley, D. A., Biesecker, J. L., Hellstrom, K. E., and Hellstrom, I. Presence of cell-mediated immunity and serum blocking factors in rat renal allografts enhanced by passive immunization. Transplantation, *12:*331, 1971.
259. Stuart, F. P., McKearn, T. J., Weiss, A., and Fitch, F. W. Suppression of rat renal allograft rejection by antigen and antibody. Immunol. Rev., *49:*127, 1980.
260. Stuart, F. P., Saitoh, T., and Fitch, F. W. Rejection of renal allografts: Specific immunologic suppression. Science, *160:*1463, 1968.
261. Stuart, F. P., Scollard, D. M., McKearn, T. J., and Fitch, F. W. Cellular and humoral immunity after allogeneic transplantation in the rat. V. Appearance of anti-idiotypic antibody and its relationship to cellular immunity after treatment with donor spleen cells and allo antibody. Transplantation, *22:*455, 1976.
262. Surmont, J., Dutreix, A., and Lalanne, C. M. Les irradiations in toto pour greffe de tissu ou transplantation d'organe chez l'homme. J. Radiol. Electrol., *41:*679, 1960.
263. Swanson, M. A., and Schwartz, R. S. Immunosuppressive therapy. The relation between clinical response and immunologic competence. N. Engl. J. Med., *277:*163, 1967.
264. Taguchi, Y., Siddiquie, N., Shepherd, R. R., and MacKinnon, K. J. Inhibition of allograft reaction by biologically filtered antigens. Transplant. Proc., *3:*908, 1971.
265. Takasugi, M., and Hildemann, W. H. Lymphocyte-antibody interactions in immunological enhancement. Transplant. Proc., *1:*530, 1969.

266. Taub, R. N., Kochwa, S., Brown, S. M., Rubin, A., and Dameshek, W. Antigen-induced immunological tolerance in man to equine antihuman thymocyte gammaglobulin. Lancet, *ii:*521, 1969.
267. Taylor, H. E. Clinical trial of antilymphocyte serum. In *International Symposium on Antilymphocyte Serum, Versailles, 1970*, edited by J. F. Bach, J. Dormont, A. Eyquem and M. Raynaud, p. 343. Karger, Basel, 1970.
268. Thomas, F., Thomas, J., Flora, R., Mendez-Picon, G., Peace, K., and Lee, H. M. Effect of antilymphocyte-globulin potency on survival of cadaver renal transplants. Prospective randomised double-blind trial. Lancet, *2:*671, 1977.
269. Tilney, N. L., and Murray, J. E. The thoracic duct fistula as an adjunct to immunosuppression in human renal transplantation. Transplantation, *5:*1204, 1967.
270. Traeger, J., Carraz, M., Fries, D., Perrin, J., Saubier, E., Bernhardt, J. P., Revillard, J. P., Bonnet, P., Archimbaud, J. P., and Brochier, J. Studies of antilymphocyte globulins made from thoracic duct lymphocytes. Transplant. Proc., *1:*455, 1969.
271. Traeger, J., Fries, D., Revillard, J. P., Durix, A., Carraz, M., and Plan, M. Production of human antilymphocyte serum in horse with thoracic duct lymphocytes and peripheral blood lymphocytes. Fed. Proc., *29:*108, 1970.
271a. Travis, R. H., and Sayers, G. Adrenocorticotropic hormone; adrenocortical steroids and their synthetic analogs. In *The Pharmacological Basis of Therapeutics*, edited by L. S. Goodman and A. Gilman, ed. 3, p. 1608. Macmillan, New York, 1967.
272. Turcotte, J. G., Feduska, N. H., Haines, R. F., et al. Antithymocyte globulin in renal transplant recipients. A clinical trial. Arch. Surg., *106:*484, 1973.
273. Uittenbogaart, C. H., Robinson, B. J., Malekzadeh, M. H., Pennisi, A. J., Ettenger, R. B., and Fine, R. N. Use of antithymocyte globulin (dose by rosette protocol) in pediatric renal allograft recipients. Transplantation, *28:*291, 1979.
274. Van Furth, R., Thompson, I., and Gassman, A. E. The kinetics of mononuclear phagocytes during normal steady-state condition, acute inflammation, and the effect of glucocorticosteroid and azathioprine (Imuran). In *Non-specific Factors Influencing Host Resistance*, edited by W. Braun and J. Ungar, p. 79. Karger, Basel, 1973.
275. Veith, F. J., Luck, R. J., and Murray, J. E. The effects of splenectomy on immunosuppressive regimens in dog and man. Surg. Gynecol. Obstet., *212:*229, 1965.
276. Voisin, G. A. Role of antibody classes in the regulatory facilitation reaction. Immunol. Rev., *49:3*, 1980.
277. Voisin, G. A., Kinsky, R., Jansen, F., and Bernard, C. Biological properties of antibody classes in transplantation immune sera. Transplantation, *8:*618, 1969.
278. Waksman, B. H., Arbouys, S., and Arnason, B. G. The use of specific "lymphocytes" antisera to inhibit hypersensitive reactions of the "delayed" type. J. Exp. Med., *114:* 997, 1961.
279. Wechter, W. J., Morrell, R. M., Bergan, J., Rosenberg, X., Turcotte, J., and Schueltz, J. R. Extended treatment with antithymocyte globulin (ATGAM) in renal allograft recipients. Transplantation, *28:*365, 1979.
280. Weiden, P. L., Doney, K., Storb, R., and Thomas, E. D. Antihuman thymocyte globulin for prophylaxis of graft versus host disease. A randomized trial in patients with leukemia treated with HLA-identical sibling marrow grafts. Transplantation, *27:*227, 1979.
281. Weiss, A., Fitch, F. N., McKearn, T. J., and Stuart, F. P. Immunologic memory is regulated in the enhanced rat renal allograft recipient. Nature, *273:*662, 1978.
282. Weiss, A., Stuart, F. P., and Fitch, F. W. Immune reactivity of cells from long term rat renal allograft survivors. Transplantation, *26:*346, 1978.
283. Williams, G. M., Krajewski, C. A., Dagher, F. J., Haar, A. M. ter, Roth, J. A., and Santos, G. W. Host repopulation of endothelium. Transplant. Proc., *3:*869, 1971.
284. Wilson, R. E., Maggs, P. R., Vanwijck, R., Shaipanich, T., Holl-Allen, R. T. J., Lukl,

P., and Simonian, S. J. Active enhancement of renal allografts in dog and rat by subcellular antigen. Transplant. Proc., *3:*705, 1971.

285. Wilson, R. E., Rippen, A., Hayes, C. R., Dagher, R. K., and Busch, G. J. Prolonged renal allograft survival associated with antigen pretreatment. Transplant. Proc., *1:*290, 1969.
286. Wood, M. L. Effect of rabbit antilymphocyte gammaglobulin. Transplantation, *9:*122, 1970.
287. Wood, M. L., and Monaco, A. P. The effect of timing of skin grafts on subsequent survival of ALS-treated, marrow-infused mice. Transplantation, *23:*78, 1977.
288. Wood, M. L., and Monaco, A. P. Suppressor cells in specific unresponsiveness to skin allografts in ALS-treated, marrow-injected mice. Transplantation, *29:*196, 1980.
289. Wood, M. L., Monaco, A. P., Gozzo, J. J., and Liegeois, A. Use of homozygous allogenic bone marrow for induction of tolerance with antilymphocyte serum: dose and timing. Transplant. Proc., *3:*676, 1971.
290. Woodruff, M. F. A. *The Transplantation of Tissue and Organs*, p. 96. Charles C. Thomas Publishers, Springfield, Illinois, 1961.
291. Woodruff, M. F. A. The mode of action of antilymphocyte antibody. In *International Symposium on Antilymphocyte Serum, Versailles, 1970,* edited by J. F. Bach, J. Dormont, A. Eyquem and M. Raynaud, p. 379. Karger, Basel, 1970.
292. Woodruff, M. F. A., and Anderson, N. F. Effect of lymphocyte depletion by thoracic duct fistula and administration of antilymphocytic serum on the survival of skin homograft in rats. Nature, *200:*702, 1963.
293. Woodruff, M. F. A., and Anderson, N. F. The effect of lymphocyte depletion by thoracic duct fistula and administration of antilymphocytic serum on the survival of skin homografts in rats. Ann. NY Acad. Sci., *120:*119, 1964.
294. Woodruff, M. F. A., Forman, B., and Fraser, K. B. The effects of antilymphocyte serum on circulating antibody levels. J. Immunol., *67:*57, 1951.
295. Woodruff, M. F. A., Reid, B., and James, K. Effect of antilymphocytic antibody and antibody fragments on human lymphocytes in vitro. Nature, *215:*591, 1967.
296. Zan-Bar, I., Slavin, S., and Strober, S. Induction and mechanism of tolerance to bovine serum albumin in mice given total lymphoid mediation (TLI). J. Immunol. *121:*1400, 1978.
297. Zimmerman, C. E., Busch, G. J., Stuart, F. P., and Wilson, R. E. Canine renal homografts after pretreatment with subcellular splenic antigens. Surgery, *63:*437, 1968.
298. Zukoski, C. F., Callaway, J. M., and Rhea, W. G. Prolongation of canine renal homograft survival by antimetabolites. Transplantation, *1:*293, 1963.
299. Zukoski, C. F., Callaway, J. M., and Rhea, W. G. Tolerance to a canine renal homograft induced by prednisolone. Surg. Forum, *14:*208, 1963.

CHAPTER SIX

Indications for Kidney Transplantation Preparation, Treatment and Supervision of the Patient

Jean Crosnier

Indications and contraindications for kidney transplantation—Preparation of the hemodialysis patient for transplantation—Immunosuppressive therapy—Supervision of the patient after transplantation.

INDICATIONS AND CONTRAINDICATIONS FOR KIDNEY TRANSPLANTATION[19, 72]

The majority of patients treated by hemodialysis sincerely desire a kidney transplantation. The physician who has to make the decision between hemodialysis and renal transplantation for each patient must consider both the need to offer this patient the longest and most comfortable survival possible and to treat the largest number of patients in the country despite logistical and economic problems. Thus, transplantation is usually proposed to all patients who desire it, except where there are contraindications.

Choice of the Moment for Transplantation in Chronic Renal Disease

The indication for transplantation, as for treatment by hemodialysis, in a patient with chronic renal disease may be stated in Starzl's[91] words, "the patient should have irreversible renal disease from which life expectancy is limited to a few weeks or months," or as perhaps even better put by Merrill[79], the patient should have "exhausted the conservative measures of treatment available" but he "should not be allowed to become critically ill, malnourished or infected."

In practice, these conditions are met in patients whose creatinine clearance is less than 5 ml/min, but earlier recourse to maintenance dialysis or kidney transplantation may be indicated in various circumstances: malignant hypertension that cannot be controlled by medical treatment, development of progressive polyneuritis, hyperparathyroidism and so forth.

Contraindications to Transplantation

There are very few *permanent and absolute contraindications*:

Patient's Age

Upper Age Limit. Age constitutes an important factor in determining the statistical results obtained in transplantation in terms of patient or graft survival, and transplantation failure increases markedly after 50 years.[20, 45] These data have led most groups to consider 50 years as an upper age limit and to transplant beyond this age only patients who, for various reasons, poorly tolerate chronic hemodialysis.

All our transplant patients were under the age of 50 years except 7, who were between 51 and 61 years of age. With regard to the oldest patient, the circumstances were exceptional since the donor was an identical twin; the recipient died from gastric carcinoma 21 months after transplantation. Table 6.1 shows the age range of transplant recipients by decade.

Lower Age Limit. Theoretically, there is no lower age limit for kidney transplantation since grafts have been attempted in infants who were only a few days old.[45] Although transplantation is technically possible in these very young children, successful transplantation remains extremely rare in those under 1 or 2 years of age.[28]

Renal transplantation is more frequently successful with a related living donor (parents, or siblings having attained their majority), but the use of cadaver kidney transplantation in children is increasing.[20, 39]

Transplantation in children raises some special problems. One concerns the size of the kidney to be transplanted: when the recipient's weight is less than 15 kg it is advisable to use a cadaver kidney from a child. Immunosuppressive treatment includes the usual combination of azathioprine, antithymocyte globulin (ATG) and corticosteroids. The growth of children after renal transplantation is not always satisfactory,[47] depending on the age of the child at the time of transplantation, the function of the allograft and the dosage of steroids. The risk of growth retardation may be diminished by giving a double dosage of steroids on alternate days.

TABLE 6.1
Age of transplant recipients

Years of age at transplantation	10–20	20–30	30–40	40–50	≥50
No. of patients	81	188	136	59	7

The overall results of transplantation in children are satisfactory, and actuarial curves show that graft survival is better in recipients who are less than 15 years old, when compared with the total population of graft recipients.[84]

Visceral Lesions Associated with Renal Failure

It could be unreasonable to perform a transplantation in a patient for whom the short-term prognosis is unfavorable because of an evolutive or incurable disease or visceral lesions. In practice, however, this contraindication is not always easy to categorize.

Liver Disease. Transplantation would not be considered in the case of end-stage cirrhosis. Conversely, certain types of chronic hepatitis do not contraindicate transplantation,[109] but a liver biopsy may be useful in some cases. Of course the sole presence of the HB antigen is not a contraindication and even, for some groups, it significantly improves the survival of the transplanted kidney[67, 76] (cf. p. 250).

Cancer. A patient with a malignant spreading tumor would not be considered for transplantation. However, despite the highly abnormal incidence of cancer in transplanted patients treated by immunosuppressive drugs (cf. p. 256), some investigators[60, 70, 79] have not hesitated to perform transplantation in patients with histories of apparently cured cancers treated many years previously. In our opinion, the unpredictable risks in such patients make it preferable to continue treatment by chronic hemodialysis.

General Diseases and Metabolic Disorders

In the first edition of this book, published in 1971, we wrote: "When the kidney disease is but the local expression of a general disease, transplantation should not be considered because of the risk that the disease will spread to the transplanted kidney" (p. 59). In fact, today oxalosis and probably also amyloidosis seem to be the only absolute contraindications.[1] On the other hand, diabetes, systemic lupus erythematosis, necrotizing angiitis, Goodpasture's syndrome, Fabry's disease, hemolytic uremic syndrome and cystinosis sometimes require particular and appropriate therapy and must be carefully followed after transplantation but are practically never contraindications to transplantation.[72]

Some contraindications are *absolute but can be temporary*:

Infectious diseases, tuberculosis or focal infection, for example, which run the risk of being aggravated or complicated by immunosuppressive treatment, must be treated and totally cured before transplantation can be performed.

Some contraindications are *relative*:

In practice, the physical state of each potential recipient must be considered individually to weigh the risk of complications and advantages of transplantation against those of hemodialysis.

Complications Provoked by Immunosuppressive and Corticosteroid Therapy or by Surgery

1. Risk of gastroduodenal hemorrhage or perforations provoked by prednisone in patients with a history of ulcers.
2. Vascular risks in atheromatous patients.
3. Psychiatric risks in patients with a history of neurosis.
4. Risk of infectious complications or aggravation of the metabolic disorders in diabetics.

Nature of the Primary Kidney Disease

Serious, complex disorders of the lower urinary tract can endanger the graft by eventually inducing pyelonephritis in the recipient. Although a certain number of successful transplantations have been performed after intestinoplasty or cutaneous ureterostomy, such patients seem to be better managed by chronic hemodialysis.

Polycystic disease constitutes a particularly difficult problem since these patients are often near the upper age limit for transplantation. Moreover, before transplantation, polycystic disease requires nephrectomy, which is often very difficult to perform. Finally, these patients generally tolerate dialysis very well, as long as they have their own kidneys because of high hematocrit and abundant diuresis.

Glomerular disease involves the risk of recurrence in the transplant, but with a variable rate and severity according to the type of glomerular lesions (cf. p. 217). Cases of rapidly progressive glomerulonephritis with extracapillary proliferation should be carefully considered: when antibasement membrane antibodies are found, it seems advisable not to perform transplantation until the antikidney antibodies disappear from the circulation.[18, 44]

PREPARATION OF THE HEMODIALYSIS PATIENT FOR TRANSPLANTATION

Progress in the fields of organ preservation (cf. p. 70) and histocompatibility (cf. Ch. Three) has permitted the same results with cadaver kidneys as with kidneys from living not HLA-identical (human leukocyte A) donors. This fact explains the wider use of cadaver kidneys. Most transplantation centers restrict living donor transplantation to cases where the patient has a healthy volunteer HLA-identical sibling, or an HLA half-identical sibling or parent when mixed lymphocyte reaction (MLR) between donor and recipient is negative or very weak. At Necker Hospital the percentage of cadaver kidney transplantations, which was less than 20% before 1965, passed 50% in 1970 and has been between 83 and 100% each year since 1972 (Fig. 6.1).

In this chapter only the problems concerning cadaver kidney recipients will be discussed and any peculiarities involving recipients of living donor kidneys will be simply pointed out.

Care of the Hemodialysis Patient before Transplantation

The great majority of transplant patients have been on maintenance dialysis for many months, or even many years, while waiting for a cadaver kidney. This waiting period, in a series of 307 patients transplanted with a cadaver kidney at Necker Hospital between June 1959 and June 1977, ranged from 0 to 86 months with a mean of 23.23 months.

During this time, all our hemodialysis patients waiting for transplantation are seen regularly once a year on an outpatient basis. Our four principal objectives are to:

1. Check that all the preoperative investigations required for successful transplantation have been correctly performed.

2. Detect the occurrence of complications that are frequent in hemodialysis patients and that may be a contraindication to transplantation,

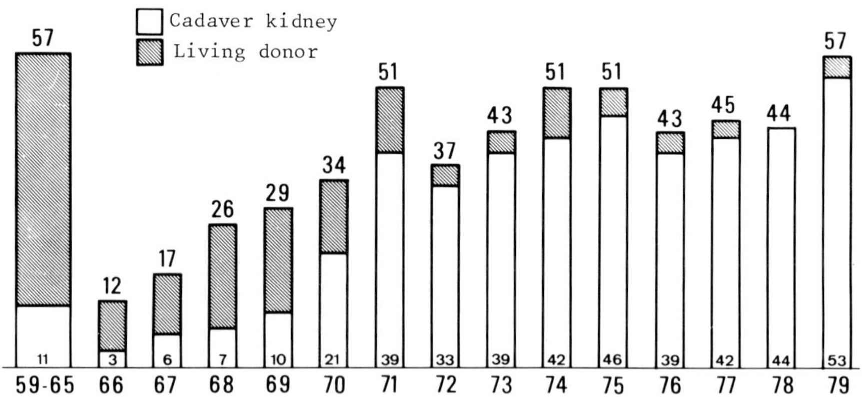

Fig. 6.1. Number of kidney transplantations performed each year at Necker Hospital showing percentage of cadaver donors (open columns) and living related donors (hatched columns).

particularly vascular or heart lesions, infectious diseases or severe chronic hepatitis due to the contamination of hemodialysis centers by the virus of B hepatitis. It may be useful to perform liver biopsy to determine the type of liver lesions. On the contrary, earlier recourse to kidney transplantation may be indicated in various circumstances: accelerated atherosclerosis, uncontrollable hypertension, development of progressive polyneuritis, hyperparathyroidism, etc.

3. Provide psychological support. Frequently discouragement and even anxiety or deep depression occur in patients experiencing a long waiting period for a cadaver kidney. It is necessary to convince them that they are not forgotten and that the long delay is due only to the fact that an appropriate and compatible cadaver kidney has not yet been found and that the successful outcome of their transplantation depends on careful donor-recipient matching.

4. Possibly supervise protocols destined to promote good graft tolerance. These protocols are based on present concepts concerning the effects of preimmunization. The pejorative effect on allograft survival of anti-HLA cytotoxic antibodies is seen only in presensitized HLA incompatible recipients, whereas the best results, on the contrary, are seen in subjects with circulating antibodies but who are HLA compatible.[28, 101] Conversely, the effect of locus A and B antigens of the HLA system is only slight in subjects without circulating antibodies[27, 28, 101] (Fig. 3.2*B*). In past years, in an effort to reduce the risk of preimmunization, blood transfusions were avoided inasmuch as possible in hemodialysis patients awaiting transplantation.[21, 101] Surprisingly enough, and contrary to what had been expected, subjects who had never received blood transfusions before receiving a transplant (nor been pregnant, nor had a previous graft) clearly show a poorer graft tolerance than their counterparts who had received blood transfusions.[23, 101] These data, first described by Dossetor et al,[33] were demonstrated in large series by Terasaki and associates[82] and Van Rood[112] and confirmed by most other workers.[38, 41, 83, 100] Nonetheless, since this phenomenon, established by retrospective studies, was confirmed only by a few randomized prospective protocols,[117] controversy still exists[62, 89] and a fully satisfactory explanation to this better outcome has yet to be found. However, most physicians no longer consider it reasonable to perform renal transplantation in a never transfused patient, and most of the recent data published corroborate Terasaki's[83] view that favorable graft outcome is directly proportional to the number of transfusions received. But a liberal policy of blood transfusions increases the risk of developing polyspecific antibodies against HLA antigens which would make it difficult to find a donor with whom a crossmatch would not be positive. To avoid this possibility, many physicians prefer to prescribe only a few transfusions, particularly because Van

Rood et al[87] have reported that a single transfusion is sufficient to induce these improved post-transplantation results.

At Necker Hospital, each patient awaiting transplantation receives transfusions every 2 weeks, up to a total of 10 units of blood, as long as the previous transfusion has not stimulated the production of antibodies. When antibody production is stimulated, the patient is considered a "responder," the transfusions are interrupted and the transplant is made with the best match possible, particularly for the B locus. If, on the contrary, no anti-HLA antibody is found after 10 units of blood, the patient is considered a "nonresponder" and it is possible to be less strict as to the degree of HLA compatibility required.

Recipient's Own Kidneys

In the early years of transplantation, the principal groups[60, 79, 91] and our own group[54] systematically removed the recipient's own kidneys prior to or during transplantation. Today bilateral nephrectomy is exceptional. Contrary to what has been hypothesized, it has not been confirmed that bilateral nephrectomy would reduce the risk of recurrence of glomerulonephritis in the transplant recipient. Dixon et al[30] have even reported a patient with rapidly progressive glomerulonephritis in whom circulating antibasement membrane antibodies, found after binephrectomy, disappeared from the circulation after transplantation and were found, by immunofluorescence, fixed on the basement membranes of the transplanted kidney.

Our present policy is as follows:

1. Bilateral nephrectomy prior to transplantation is performed: a) In exceptional cases of uncontrolled hypertension in the patient on dialysis; and b) In cases of rapidly progressive glomerulonephritis with circulating antibasement membrane antibodies, but in these cases transplantation is subsequently performed only after several successive investigations indicate the disappearance of these antibodies.

2. Uni- or bilateral nephrectomy prior to transplantation may be performed in cases of untractable kidney infections or large polycystic kidneys (but we have seen, p. 149, that transplantation is rare in the latter case).

3. Unilateral nephrectomy is performed during transplantation, and on the same side, when the ureter of the allograft is directly anastomosed to the recipient's ureter.

4. Uni- or bilateral nephrectomy may, of course, be secondarily performed after transplantation in cases of severe hypertension or of infection of the patient's own kidney.

Prevention of Infection

The necessity of using immunosuppressive drugs, notably high doses of corticosteroids, makes infections an important and frequent cause of failure and of death in transplantation.

To minimize the risk of these complications, it is important: 1) not to transplant any patient who has evidence of local or generalized infection; 2) to carefully seek and to treat vigorously any local infection; and 3) to obtain precise identification and antibiotic sensitivity of oral, cutaneous and fecal bacterial organisms that could potentially cause infection after grafting.

With these precautions, the use of a sterile hospitalization unit prior to and after surgery is no longer required, as it was when total body irradiation was used for immunosuppression. However, during the pre- and postoperative periods each patient is nursed by an individual team.

Immediate Preparation of the Recipient at Time of Transplantation

Recipient treatment in the immediate preoperative period is of the utmost importance in preventing or at least sharply decreasing the number of immediate renal failure episodes and wound infections.

Prevention of Early Anuria

It is now clear that an adequately circulating blood volume and hydration of the recipient play a major role in the post-transplant recovery of renal function. The evaluation of fluid balance in the recipient at the time of surgery is rendered difficult by the fact that the optimum "dry weight" frequently represents a state of hypohydration. The most reliable index of recipient hydration appears to be the pulmonary arterial pressure (PAP). When mean PAP can be maintained at or slightly above 20 mmHg, the incidence of postoperative oliguria is less than 10% when the kidney is in relatively good condition. PAP monitoring is necessary in order to avoid fluid overload and pulmonary edema because a very large amount of fluid is usually required to establish a high blood flow when reopening the kidney.[77] The practice in our group is to insert a polyethylene catheter into the pulmonary artery through a peripheral vein. The course of the catheter is followed on a pressure recorder. ECG and PAP are constantly monitored throughout the surgical procedure. Fluid infusion is stopped whenever PAP rises above 20 mmHg. Saline and macromolecular solution (Plasmion) are both used. In addition, the patient receives an intravenous injection of 500 mg furosemide, 10 to 15 min before the vessels are unclamped.

Prevention of Infection

Wound infection is one of the most frequent risks during the 1st post-transplantation week. It can be the origin of much more severe infection such as septicemia and pulmonary infection, responsible for death of the recipient. Thorough peroperative hemostasis is certainly the most important tool in the prevention of wound infection. It seems, however, that a single high dose of a broad spectrum antibiotic administered at the beginning of anesthesia is effective. In a recent report, the Boston group[107] showed that the incidence of wound infection has been thus reduced from 25 to 2%. The choice of a prophylactic antibiotic must be based on the local past experience of a given center. In our group, *Staphylococcus aureus* and gram-negative enteric bacilli are the most frequent infectious agents encountered during wound infection. Dalacine (20 mg/kg body wt., iv) and Negram (1 g, iv) are given during the first 3 hours following anesthesia. This type of guided prophylactic antibiotic therapy will probably modify the frequency and severity of post-transplantation infectious complications and thus dramatically reduce the mortality rate involved in this method of treating end-stage renal failure.

IMMUNOSUPPRESSIVE THERAPY

Although various protocols have been proposed for experimentally inducing specific unresponsiveness in the host, none is yet usable in clinical practice and it is not yet possible to induce specific tolerance to an allograft in man. The prevention of allograft rejection is thus attempted by immunosuppressive therapy.

Total body irradiation,[24, 98] extracorporeal irradiation of the blood,[116] thoracic duct drainage,[106] splenectomy,[113] thymectomy,[91] etc., have virtually been abandoned, either because they can induce severe complications or because their efficacy is not proven.

A few years ago, Guttmann and Lindquist[49] experimentally showed that it is possible to reduce the immunogenicity of an allograft by killing in the organ what he called "passenger leukocytes." In man, he proposed donor pretreatment by intravenous administration of 5 g of methylprednisolone and 5 g of cyclophosphamide 4 to 12 hours before nephrectomy.[48] Unfortunately, the encouraging results observed by Guttmann have not been confirmed, and the lack in his series of an adequate control group comparable with the treated groups makes it impossible to determine whether the favorable results were unquestionably the consequence of donor pretreatment.

In the past 2 years, great hope was set on a new drug, Cyclosporin A, which was shown to have an immunosuppressive effect.[8]

Animal studies performed in the main laboratory species with a variety of grafts substantiated the powerful and relatively nontoxic immunosuppressive effects of Cyclosporin.[12, 13, 46, 61, 65] These studies showed an extensive prolongation of graft survival in treated animals, the possibility of using Cyclosporin A alone without the association of steroids or any other immunosuppressive drugs and a long allograft survival even after cessation of Cyclosporin treatment.

Calne et al[11] performed a clinical trial of the drug and between June 1978 and October 1979 treated 34 patients, 32 recipients of cadaver kidneys, 1 of them also receiving the pancreas of the kidney donor, and 2 recipients of orthotopically grafted livers (1 of them also given a heterotopic pancreas allograft).

Initially these patients did not receive additional immunosuppressive therapy, but finally most of them also received prednisone and/or cytinium (a cyclophosphamide derivative). The patients must be divided into four groups:

- Group I: 16 patients treated by Cyclosporin alone
- Group II: 8 patients treated by Cyclosporin plus prednisone
- Group III: 3 patients treated by Cyclosporin alone but having received three shots of 1 g Solumedrol,
- Group IV: 7 patients treated by Cyclosporin, prednisone and cytinium.

In *Group I* there are nine recipients with good results (creatinine lower than 200 μmol/liter), but five of these have had their transplant for less than 3 months; there are six cases of renal failure, with creatinine at more than 200 μmol/liter, and one graftectomy, with return to hemodialysis.

In *Group II*, two patients have good function, five have poor function and there has been one death due to septicemia and lung lymphoma.

In *Group III* the three patients have poor graft function.

In *Group IV* two have poor function and there have been five deaths (one septicemia with lymphoma found in the jejunum, three septicemia and one pneumocystis pneumonia).

In conclusion, good results are found in only 32% of recipients, and there was an 18% mortality. In addition, the treatment was totally devoid of steroids in only 47% of patients. The side effects were not negligible, and Calne[11] himself insists on the nephrotoxicity of the drug and on the frequency of infections and abnormalities of liver function when patients receive both Cyclosporin and immunosuppressive drugs and/or prednisone. He also observed three cases of lymphoma. Consequently, it appears that cautious evaluation of the clinical and experimental trials must be made before reaching any definite conclusions on the use of this drug in transplant recipients.

Most groups do not use donor pretreatment or Cyclosporin and treat the recipient essentially with azathioprine, antilymphocyte globulin (and now most particularly antithymocyte globulin) and corticosteroids.

Our lack of knowledge of the mode of action of each drug and of the exact processes involved in graft rejection and the impossibility of determining the immunosuppressive activity of a given dose in man and what dose will provide optimum immunosuppression with least toxicity explain why each group has its own rules for and methods of administration. Variations are legion, and we shall confine ourselves to an account of our own methods at Necker Hospital (Fig. 6.2).

Azathioprine (Imuran)

The patient is given 3 mg/kg a few hours before transplantation, and then, in the absence of complications, 3 mg/kg/day in a single daily dose indefinitely as long as the graft survives.

Any sign of bone marrow toxicity requires a systematic search for infection because bone marrow suppression often occurs in association with infectious episodes,[37] or investigation by the rosette inhibition test to detect any abnormality of azathioprine metabolism producing abnormally high blood levels of active products.[5] When leukopenia occurs, the

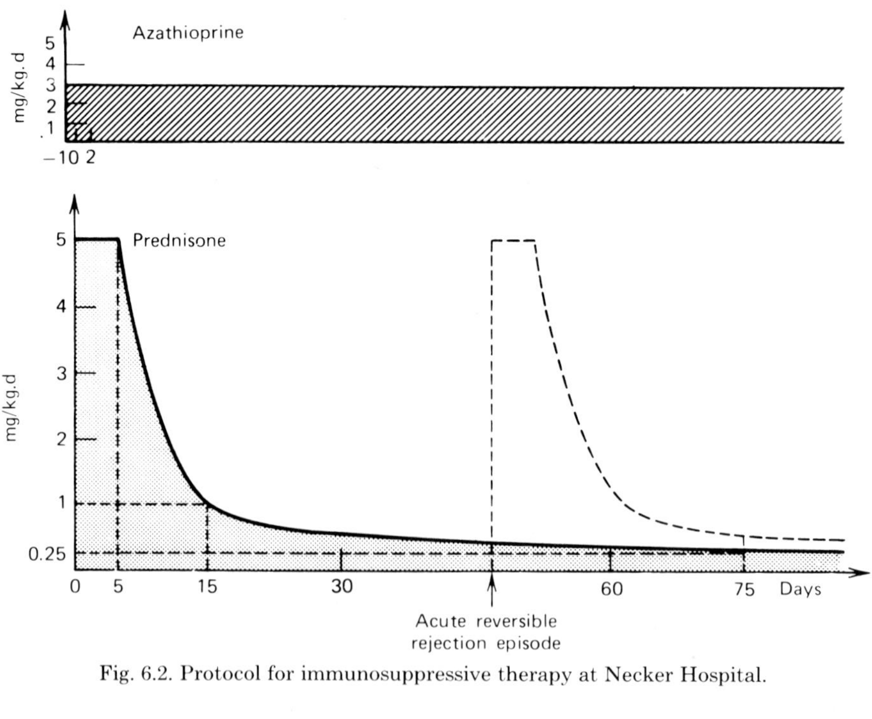

Fig. 6.2. Protocol for immunosuppressive therapy at Necker Hospital.

dose is reduced by 50% at a polynuclear count below 1500 cu mm, and treatment is stopped if the count falls to 1000 cu mm or less.

Since there is no increase in the level of active metabolites or the immunosuppressive activity of serum from patients receiving azathioprine while in renal failure, we have felt that a reduction in the doses of azathioprine is not indicated when the kidney is not functioning totally normally.[3] Actually, the frequency of bone marrow toxicity is considerably higher when renal function is impaired, and in this case the daily dose is markedly reduced in the majority of centers.

The hepatic toxicity of azathioprine, clearly established in experimental animals,[57] is not demonstrated with the doses used in transplant patients (cf. p. 249). Thus, there is no evidence that the use of the drug in transplant recipients who develop hepatitis has any influence on the course of the disease. However, the inhibitory activity of the serum on spontaneous rosette formation is nil in patients having severe hepatitis (Fig. 6.3).[4] The continuation of treatment at the same doses would therefore appear illogical. It would be more consistent either to increase the dose until some immunosuppressive activity is detectable in the serum or discontinue a surely useless and possibly toxic treatment. Increasing the dose would perhaps demonstrate in transplant recipients the favorable action of azathioprine observed in hepatology on chronic hepatitis and subacute necrosis in nontransplanted patients. We have never dared adopt this course and, on the contrary, we discontinue treatment whenever the biologic and histologic course of hepatitis appears severe.[22]

Azathioprine seems to be the principal agent responsible for the high risk of malignancy after transplantation (cf. p. 258). For this reason, the drug should be discontinued if malignancy occurs or in the presence of any disorder associated with a high risk of the development of cancer.

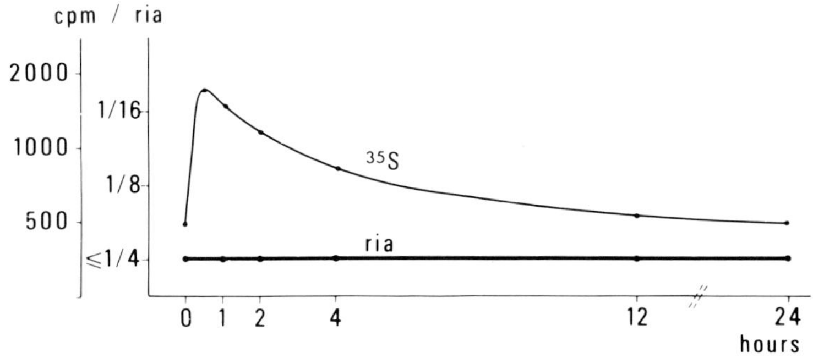

Fig. 6.3. Plasma immunosuppressive activity measured by the rosette inhibition test after administration of 3 mg/kg of ^{35}S labeled azathioprine in a patient with liver disease. ^{35}S activity (*upper line*) and rosette inhibiting activity (*ria*) (*lower line*).

Interruption of azathioprine treatment may be perfectly tolerated during long periods. In our group[22] we have had to discontinue treatment in 21 patients at 1 to 122 months after transplantation. Fourteen of these patients (66.7%) showed no alteration of renal function during an interruption of from 3 months to 3 years (Fig. 6.4). It is tempting to consider discontinuing azathioprine in patients who have perfect renal function several years after transplantation. Studies on tolerance and enhancement have indeed shown that immunosuppression may be interrupted in experimental animals in this manner, but in man it is still impossible to predict the recipient whose graft will tolerate the lack of immunosuppression (cf. p. 169). In the absence of immunologic tests that are able to

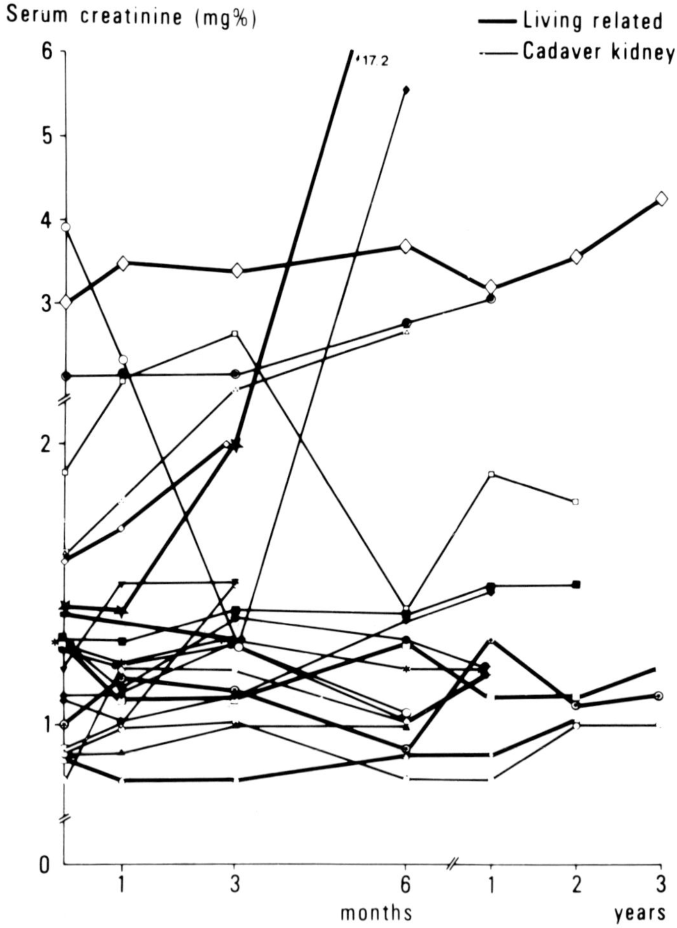

Fig. 6.4. Graft function as related to length of time after azathioprine withdrawal.

identify grafts shielded from rejection, the continuation of the treatment as long as the graft is functioning seems the most reasonable policy.

There is, however, one circumstance in which the continuation of azathioprine is not desirable: when there is evidence of irreversible chronic rejection. In fact, the death of transplanted patients is more often due to severe extrarenal complications provoked by immunosuppressive therapy than to rejection,[80] and these complications are more common and more severe when transplant function is poor.[73] In these circumstances, it is preferable to stop all immunosuppressive therapy in good time with a view to returning the patient to chronic hemodialysis or undertaking a second transplantation.

Corticosteroids

One of the most difficult problems in transplanted patients is the administration of corticosteroids. This is due to several factors:

1. Whereas it has been clearly demonstrated that rejection episodes respond favorably to the acute use of corticosteroids, the benefit of steroid therapy on the long-term survival of the graft, in contrast, is not clearly established. However, as the interruption of steroid treatment may provoke acute rejection,[6, 71] the great majority of transplant recipients is indefinitely treated by steroids.

2. Although most rejection episodes have a spontaneous course toward irreversible lesions of the graft and are reversible only by corticosteroid therapy, it is nevertheless possible that some of these episodes may resolve spontaneously. Unfortunately, as it is generally impossible to distinguish among these various types of rejection, all immunological complications are routinely considered responsive to steroids and are so treated.

3. It is almost impossible to evaluate the optimal dose of corticosteroids because it varies from one individual to another and depends on the type of rejection treated and the interval after transplantation. Moreover, the effective level of immunosuppressive activity is probably not related to the drug level in the blood.[104] For these reasons, usually very large, and surely too large, doses of steroids are administered during the first few months after transplantation, even though it has been clearly demonstrated that corticosteroids are responsible for a considerable number of serious complications during this period (cf. Ch. Eight).

4. Finally, the optimum method of administration has not been determined, and it is unknown whether it is preferable to give a single or a divided daily dose. It is well recognized that the side effects of steroids can be reduced by giving double doses on alternate days, but the use of

this technique is possibly associated with a less satisfactory long-term outcome.[2, 40]

All these uncertainties explain the considerable variations among centers in the dosage of corticosteroids.

Our own administration protocol at Necker Hospital has been modified several times since 1959. Today it is the following (Fig. 6.2):

Corticosteroids are systematically given to *cadaver graft recipients* from the day of the transplantation. During the operation, just before the end of vascular anastomosis, 1 g of methylprednisolone is given intravenously. Then prednisolone is given orally for 5 days at a dose of 5 mg/kg/day; the dose is gradually reduced to reach 1 mg/kg/day at day 15, then 0.25 mg/kg/day at day 75. This dose is continued indefinitely as long as the graft is functional. It is discontinued only in the case of severe infectious complication. Rejection crises are treated in the same way, but if a crisis occurs when the dosage is above the maintenance level of 0.25 mg/kg/day, or if the risk of complication is high (diabetes, visceral complications, Cushing's syndrome, etc.), the daily dose of steroids is continued at the same level but associated with 3 to 5 intravenous boluses methylprednisolone at the dose of 1 g on alternate days.

For *HLA-identical* siblings, because of the lower incidence of rejection episodes, corticosteroids are not systematically administered at the time of transplantation. They are used only in the case of a rejection crisis and then in the same manner as for cadaver kidney recipients.

The maintenance dose of 0.25 mg/kg/day is continued in these patients until the end of the 2nd year. Therapy is then definitively stopped if renal function is normal and if no alterations are seen on renal biopsy.

Thus, 24% of recipients of HLA-identical sibling kidneys have never received corticosteroids, and 36% of those who have received corticosteroids have had their therapy interrupted after the 2nd year without subsequent complications.

Antilymphocyte Globulin

Since the early works of Woodruff et al[118, 119] and Waksman and associates,[114] the effects of antilymphocyte sera in organ grafting and especially in kidney transplantation have been the subject of a large number of works, with various and contradictory results and opinions. There is so far no proof that the use of antilymphocyte globulin (ALG) improves overall survival or the long-term functional or histologic results. The authors who believe that ALG is of value, particularly Starzl et al[92] in the United States and Traeger and associates[110] in France, base their opinion on the improved results, as compared to earlier figures. In the few studies with simultaneous control series[15] there was no significant difference in results between treated and control series. In the first edition of this book (p. 108), we mentioned a study we undertook in 1968 on 31 treated patients and 37 controls; no difference was observed between the two groups.[31]

This diversity in results is certainly due to the fact that many different products are included under the term "antilymphocyte serum" or "antilymphocyte globulin."

More recently, the efficacy of antithymocyte globulin (ATG) has again been suggested, and Cosimi et al[10, 17] have recommended the use of a T cell count to monitor accurately the daily dose of ATG required in a patient in order to maintain an effective therapeutic level. Between March 1977 and August 1978 we participated in an international, multicenter study aimed at determining the actual effectiveness of ATG* in prolonging kidney graft survival.[68]

Fifty consecutive cadaver kidney recipients were randomly assigned to a treatment group or a control group. In both groups, patients received our standard immunosuppressive regimen of prednisolone and azathioprine (cf. above).

In the treated group, ATG was administered intravenously every day for 2 weeks, then every other day for another two weeks; 40 mg of intravenous methylprednisolone sodium succinate (included in the total daily prednisoline dose) was given prior to each ATG infusion. Daily ATG doses were determined by the level of rosette forming cells, with the goal of maintaining this level at 10% of baseline values. Sex, age, total ischemia time of the graft, HLA compatibility, previous preimmunization and blood transfusion status of patients were comparable in the treated and the control groups.

In the treated group we observed a statistically significant decrease in the frequency of rejection episodes (cf. Fig. 7.3, Ch. Seven), a significantly prolonged kidney survival (up to 2 years) (Fig. 6.5), a better level of kidney function during the 1st month post-transplantation and smaller mean daily doses of steroids received by patients during the first 3 months. ATG toxicity was very low, and even the occurrence of fever, often reported in other series, was infrequent. We did not observe an increased incidence of bacterial, viral or fungal infection in the treated group as compared to the control patients. The only severe and life-threatening complication that might be attributed to ATG in our study was an epidermal necrolysis (Lyell's disease) during the first week of treatment and in association with a significant rise in antihorse globulin antibody level in the serum of the patient.

In conclusion, our study demonstrated the effectiveness and the inoc-

* ATG prepared by the Upjohn Company.

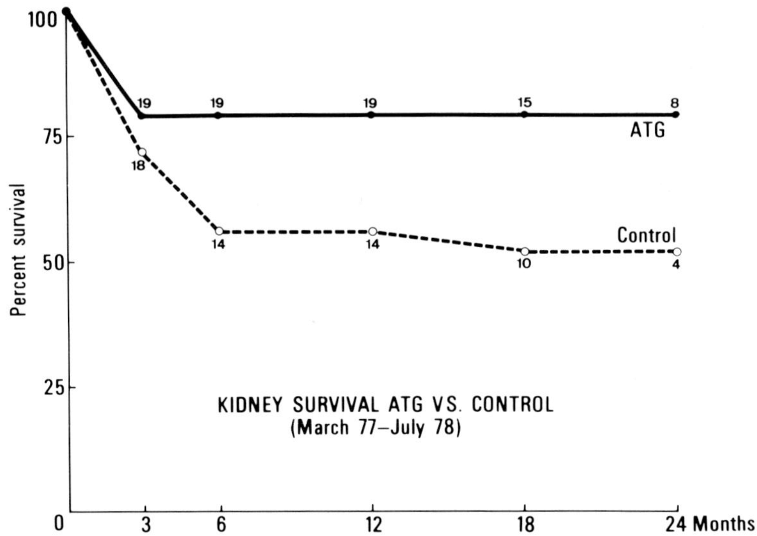

Fig. 6.5. Kidney graft survival in ATG-treated patients compared to a control group of patients receiving conventional immunosuppression.

uousness of the lot of ATG used in a randomized population of transplant patients.

SUPERVISION OF THE PATIENT AFTER TRANSPLANTATION

The objectives of transplant recipient follow-up are to assess the function and anatomical state of the graft, detect as early as possible any iatrogenic complications, which can occur even very late after transplantation and detect early any rejection episodes and to try to better understand their mechanism.

For this purpose we systematically and regularly perform a series of investigations that we will study schematically in two parts, clinical care and immunologic monitoring.

Clinical Care of the Transplant Recipient

In the absence of complications, the patient leaves the hospital during the 3rd postoperative week, when the wound has healed and the daily dose of corticosteroids is below 1 mg/kg/day.

During the period of hospitalization, the condition of the patient and his renal function are monitored by daily clinical assessment and usual blood and urine measurements. Intravenous urography is performed before discharge to establish if the urinary tract is functioning well; the homogeneity of vascularization and volume of the graft may be studied on the early nephrogram phase.

Once discharged, the patient is regularly seen on an outpatient basis by the same team which performed the transplantation. In our group, the patient returns every week for the first 6 months, then every 2 weeks until the end of the 1st year, every month during the 2nd year and every 3 or 6 months after that (Fig. 6.6). Table 6.2 shows the frequency of follow-up biochemical and radiologic examinations. If any problems or complications are observed or even suspected, the patient is immediately hospitalized.

In addition to the initial intravenous pyelogram and regular chest x-ray films, an arteriogram of the graft is performed during the first 2 years to detect arteriolar lesions and any possible renal artery stenosis.

Renal biopsies are systematically made at 6 months, 2 years and 10 years.

In addition to these systematic and regular investigations, a number of others are undertaken in the case of complications. We will study their indications and their results in Chapter Eight, "Extrarenal Complications."

Immunologic Studies

Since the first transplantations in the human, our group at Necker Hospital has been concerned that a range of immunologic tests, inspired by basic research into graft immunity, be introduced into clinical transplantation. Thus, in 1959,[55] we were the first to concentrate our efforts on the immunologic selection of the donor and on discovering the means of assessing the degree of immunologic similarity between donor and recipient (cf. p. 25).

Similarly, in 1969, J. F. Bach et al[5] proposed a rosette inhibition technique for studying the metabolism of azathioprine in the serum of transplant recipients and evaluating the immunosuppressive activity of ALG. During the last 10 years, our group at Necker Hospital has proposed a number of immunologic tests for routine study of the immunologic response of the organ allograft recipient.[50, 52] It was tempting to extrapolate clinical tests from experimental models in order to follow the kinetics of the allograft recipient response. This would supplement clinical follow-up of human allograft recipients by immunologic surveillance of the various factors involved in rejection and would lead to more rational management of these patients. However, it is not yet possible to follow the kinetics of all immunologic events responsible for rejection.[55] In 1975, one of us wrote:

> It is true that in a large number of cases cytotoxic lymphocytes or antibodies appear in the blood at the time of allograft rejection, but this coincidence is not consistent and there are gaps in our knowledge that make it yet impossible to predict impending rejection, to modify our treatment and thereby to assure invariable success in organ transplantation.[51]

TABLE 6.2

Routine follow-up studies at Necker Hospital after kidney transplantation

Examination	Frequency					
	1st Year			2nd Year		3rd Year and After
	Weekly	Monthly	Quarterly	Monthly	Quarterly	Quarterly
Blood						
Plasma urea, creatinine, potassium, blood cell count including platelets, hematocrit	+			+		+
Reticulocytes, hemoglobin, plasma glucose, bilirubin, transaminases, alkaline phosphatases		+		+		+
Plasma iron, plasma calcium, phosphorus, uric acid, complement activity, search for immune complexes by polyethylene glycol, cryoglobulinemia, Australia antigen			+		+	+
Urine						
Tests for protein and glucose, urea, creatinine and sodium concentration	+			+		+
Cytology and bacteriology		+		+		+
Calcium and phosphorus concentration, urinary cell count			+		+	+
Urea and creatinine clearances	+			+		+
Ophthalmoscopy and slit lamp examination of the eyes			+		+	+
Electrocardiogram			+		+	+
X-ray of the thorax and pelvis			+		+	+
Intravenous urography	15 days, 6 months			2 years		
Immunologic studies	+			+		+
Arteriography of the transplant				2 years		
Transplant biopsy	6 months			2 years		4 years 10 years

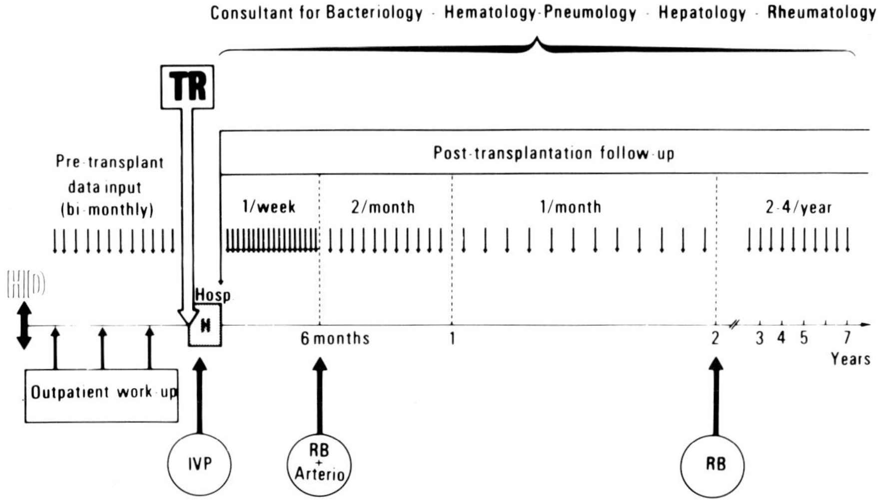

Fig. 6.6. Routine follow-up of transplanted patients at the Necker Hospital. *HD*, hemodialysis; *TR*, transplantation; *H*, hospitalization period; *IVP*, intravenous pyelography and/or ultrasound scan; *RB*, routine renal biopsy.

There are several reasons for the lack of total success in this area, and they are easily understandable:

1. The differing results observed by various groups using the same test are probably due to variations in techniques (differences in incubation time, the culture media, etc.) and to a lack of standardization of in vitro tests, which limits interpretation and comparison.

2. Episodes of renal failure following kidney transplantation are too often assumed to be of immunologic origin when no evident cause of renal failure is detected. Based on the results of renal biopsy, these episodes are considered to be acute rejection. We know, however, that even in uncomplicated cases with normal renal function tests, allograft biopsy reveals latent changes in more than 50% of cases.[52] This means that such alterations, particularly edema and focal cellular infiltration into the interstitial tissue, may be found in patients with renal failure without being the cause of the failure. On the other hand, analyzing retrospectively 91 episodes of renal failure thought to be rejection crises, it was possible to suspect a posteriori a nonimmunologic factor responsible for or contributing to the occurrence of renal failure in 45% of these episodes.[69] Undetected, these factors would strongly bias attempts to use immunologic monitoring to forecast and even recognize rejection episodes.

3. Even when renal failure is actually the result of immunologic rejection, the highly complex and numerous events playing a role in the recipient response are intricately and, above all, variously interlocked.

This explains why in each individual case of clinical rejection the role of cellular and humoral mechanisms, and thus the succession of events, may vary. Consequently, the results of immunologic tests in vitro are not consistent in an overall patient population, whereas their interpretation would perhaps be feasible in well selected patients.[95]

4. While rejection processes occur within the graft itself, by far the great majority of immunologic tests proposed are performed on blood samples. It is possible that the blood imperfectly reflects what actually occurs within the renal parenchyma.

5. Finally, the results of immunologic tests may be modified because they are performed on blood samples taken from patients treated by immunosuppressive drugs.

Despite these difficulties, every transplant team is concerned by the necessity of the "Immunologic follow-up of the renal allograft recipient,"[50] in order to permit:

1. Early detection and even prediction of rejection processes, thus avoiding irreversible alterations of the graft by rapid institution of treatment;[14]

2. Constant adjustment of immunosuppressive therapy to the immunologic response of the recipient, allowing prescription of the optimum dose rather than of the maximum tolerated dose;

3. Detection of patients with a state of tolerance, with specific non-reactivity to graft antigens, in whom immunosuppression could be withdrawn or drastically reduced. We have seen (cf. p. 158) that we have discontinued azathioprine in 14 patients with no deleterious effects but that 7 others in the same conditions experienced a rejection episode.[22] Similarly, we have seen (p. 160) that in most of our HLA-identical recipients, although not in all, we have been able to interrupt corticosteroids after the 2nd post-transplantation year.[26]

This need for immunologic follow-up was reflected by the organization of the First International Symposium on Immunologic Monitoring of the Transplant Patient in London, Ontario[93] and by the large place devoted to this problem during the Seventh International Congress of the Transplantation Society.

Dossetor and Myburgh[34] and Stiller and Sinclair[94] have attempted to summarize data derived from various transplantation groups and their interpretations.

Early Diagnosis of Renal Allograft Rejection

Antibody-Mediated Responses. *Complement-Dependent Cytotoxicity (CDC).* For all authors,[25, 42, 96] CDC in the recipient's serum against donor peripheral blood lymphocytes is associated with rejection. However, there are many false positive and false negative results,[34] and the clinical usefulness of CDC for predicting rejection is lessened by the high variability of its temporal relationship with rejection.[94]

Complement-Dependent Cytotoxicity Against Donor B Cells. Whereas a positive pretransplant B cell cross-match does not appear to indicate poor graft survival,[35, 90] the advent of antidonor B cell antibodies in the post-transplant period is frequently associated with[108] but is not predictive of rejection.

Antibody-Dependent Cell-Mediated Cytotoxicity (ADCC). There is total disagreement on the meaning of the presence of ADCC and its association or not with rejection[103] or tolerance.[25] These discrepancies may be due to technical differences in the assays.[34] The Brigham group pointed out the favorable meaning of the disappearance of ADCC associated with treatment of rejection episodes by high doses of corticosteroids and the unfavorable meaning of its persistence in this case.[42]

Anti-Fc Receptor Antibody. The Brigham group here observed a close correlation between rejection and the occurrence of antidonor Fc receptor antibodies detected by erythrocyte antibody (EA) rosette inhibition,[99] but these results have not been confirmed. The same group has found anti-Ia antibodies by EA rosette inhibition in the eluate of transplanted kidneys nephrectomized after rejection.[43]

Antiendothelial Antibody. In 1977 Cerilli et al[16] reported the association of graft loss with the presence of antiendothelial antibodies against endothelial cells from the donor or another individual. Using immunofluorescence in vascular rejection, the Leyden group showed antibodies bound along the endothelium of the peritubular capillaries of the allograft.[85]

Cell-Mediated Immunity. *Macrophage Inhibition Factor (MIF).* The leukocyte migration inhibition test, proposed by various authors[36] in 1970 as a test of cell-mediated immunity, was extensively used by our group. Using spleen extracts from the cadaver donor (or even less specific antigens), we found that these antigens inhibit the recipient leukocyte migration in practically all rejection episodes when the test is performed before the corticosteroid treatment.[32] The test becomes positive before any detectable clinical manifestations and is predictive of rejection.[32] Unfortunately, there are many false negative results,[34] perhaps due to a lack of standardization of the technique.

Detection of Transformed Lymphocytes in vivo. Response to Mitogens. Pedersen and Morris,[86] in sheep, and one of us,[53] in man, showed that transformed lymphocytes, similar to those observed in vitro in mixed lymphocyte cultures, may be seen in lymph collected from the renal graft when manifestations of rejection are observed (cf. Fig. 6.3, Ch. One). It has been suggested[59] that transformed lymphocytes can be detected in the circulating blood by measuring tritiated thymidine incorporation into mononuclear blood cells. Unfortunately, elevated levels of incorporation are inconsistently associated with rejection.[58, 59] In addition, Dimitriu et al,[29] using autoradiography, found that incorporating cells were not transformed lymphocytes but immature cells of the myeloid series and that the influx of these cells might result from several factors, e.g., infection, or even the administration of high doses of corticosteroids in treating rejection.

Similarly, highly variable results are observed in the response of recipient peripheral blood lymphocytes to various mitogens.[34]

Rosette Forming Cells. There is considerable disagreement on the correlation between the number of T rosettes observed and the immunologic responses of the recipient. For some authors, changes in T cell number are associated with rejection and may even be predictive,[102] but others have not found this association.[9] Our group[111] has shown that the number of rosette forming cells is generally low in rejection but that in some cases it may rise. This inconsistency may perhaps reflect the reactions of various cell populations.[63]

We will see below that this test is useful in estimating the effectiveness of immunosuppressive therapy (cf. p. 169).

Mixed Lymphocyte Culture (MLC) and Cell-Mediated Lymphocytotoxicity (CML). All studies, in animals and man, conclude that after transplantation an MLC nonreactivity consistently occurs, both during rejection and during quiescence.[7, 56, 117] During rejection, this nonreactivity has been explained by a possible sequestration of responder cells in the graft,[57] and during quiescence it has been considered to reflect immunologic tolerance.[7] However, we have shown that when the MLR is studied after a 48-hour interruption of immunosuppressive treatment, specific depression of recipient cell reactivity is less consistent.

More recently, several groups have observed that the CML production specific to donor cells was depressed except during rejection.[117]

Finally, suppressor cells have been reported in association with good graft function by two groups[74, 105] who observed that suppression by recipient lymphocytes of third-party cell CML production specific to the donor is seen in long-term graft survival.

Lymphocyte-Mediated Cytotoxicity (LMC). For groups that have experience with this test,[34, 42, 66, 78, 96] there is a very good correlation between positive LMC and acute rejection. They report that in 70% of cases LMC is positive prior to rejection and thus has a predictive value.[96] Moreover, the effect of rejection therapy on these test results would have a prognostic value, because in those instances in which the LMC became negative post-treatment, graft survival was better than in those patients who remained LMC positive.

Technical problems (incubation time and types of cells used as targets) can be responsible for false positive results.

The Brigham group considers that the most informative assays for early diagnosis of rejection and the prediction of post-treatment outcome are the association of regular determination of LMC and the search for CDC and ADCC.[42]

Assessment of Immunosuppressive Effectiveness

In order to avoid excessive depression of mechanisms responsible for defense against infection, it is necessary to adjust the immunosuppressive dose to the needs of each individual recipient. To accomplish this, reliable parameters are required.

For most groups,[10, 17, 104] the determination of E rosette numbers, first proposed by J. F. Bach,[5] is the most informative test for adjusting azathioprine and ATG dosage. Stinnet et al[97] proposed a monitoring protocol including T cell number determination, phytohemagglutinin (PHA) responsiveness, a study of bactericidal activity by neutrophils for various germs, serum opsonic activity, etc., to predict and then perhaps to avoid infectious complications in the high risk patients treated by immunosuppressive drugs.

There is no way of measuring the immunosuppressive effect of a specific dose of steroids, and the immunosuppressive activity of corticosteroids is not related to the level of the drug in the blood.[88] The biologic significance of serum levels must be considered in the light of steroid binding to carrier proteins, of in vivo half-life of the steroid used and of modifications in its catabolism. In the future, however, the various aspects of individual variations for a given dosage may be covered by using individual steroid blood level determination with the available radioimmunoassays and the evaluation of the density of lymphocyte receptors for steroids.[75]

Detection of Specific Nonreactivity to Graft Antigens

We have seen above that, in a limited number of patients, we did not observe any alteration of renal function in 66% of patients after prolonged withdrawal of azathioprine but we were not able to predict which patients would tolerate this withdrawal and which would undergo rejection.[22] Several tests have been proposed to detect tolerance—the search for ADCC[25] and for complement-dependent anti-B cell antibodies,[81] inhibition of CML[7, 74, 105] and T rosette number[64]—but none of these assays has yet proved to be sufficiently reliable to allow innocuous withdrawal of all immunosuppressive therapy in patients with good clinical allograft tolerance.

REFERENCES

1. ASC/NIH Renal transplant registry. Renal transplantation in congenital and metabolic diseases (A report). JAMA, *232:*148, 1975.
2. Bach, J. F. Recent advances in steroid therapy. In *Advances in Nephrology*, edited by J. Hamburger, J. Crosnier and M. H. Maxwell, p. 176. Year Book Medical Publishers, Chicago, 1975.
3. Bach, J. F., and Dardenne, M. The metabolism of azathioprine in renal failure. Transplantation, *12:*253, 1971.
4. Bach, J. F., and Dardenne, M. Serum immunosuppressive activity of azathioprine in normal subjects and patients with liver disease. Proc. R. Soc. Med., *65:*260, 1972.
5. Bach, J. F., Dardenne, M., and Fournier, C. In vitro evaluation of immunosuppressive drugs. Nature, *222:* 998, 1969.
6. Bach, J. F., and Leski, M. The rejection crisis in human renal transplantation. Rev. Eur. Etud. Clin. Biol., *15:*1048, 1970.
7. Bach, M. L., Engstrom, M. A., Bach, F. H., Etheredge, E. E., and Najarian, J. S. Specific tolerance in human kidney allograft recipients. Cell. Immunol., *3:*161, 1972.
8. Borel, J. F. Comparative study of in vitro and in vivo drug effects on cell-mediated cytotoxicity. Immunology, *31:*631, 1976.
9. Buckingham, J. M., Ritts, R. E., Woods, J. E., and Ilstrup, D. M. An assessment of cell-mediated immunity in acute allograft rejection in man. A prospective study. Mayo Clin. Proc., *52:*101, 1977.
10. Byfield, P. E., Barth, C. L., Brodie, J. A., Cosimi, A. B., Dienst, S. G., Elberg, A. J., Elfing, G. L., Hardy, M. A., Hayashi, H., Kountz, S. L., Lamborn, K. R., Loughaman, B. E., Sakai, A., Satoh, P. S., Zielinski, C. M., and Wechter, W. J. The use of circulating rosette forming cells as a guide to determination of ATG dose (Dose by rosette). Transplant. Proc., *10:*627, 1978.
11. Calne, R. Y., Rolles, K., Thiru, S., McMaster, P., Craddock, G. N., Aziz, S., White, D. J. G., Evans, D. B., Dunn, D. C., Henderson, R. G., and Lewis, P. Cyclosporin A initially as the only immunosuppressant in 34 recipients of cadaveric organs: 32 kidneys, 2 pancreases, and 2 livers. Lancet, *II:*1033, 1979.
12. Calne, R. Y., and White, D. J. G. Cyclosporin A: A powerful immunosuppressant in dogs with allografts. IRCS Med. Sci. Surg. Transplant., *5:*595, 1977.
13. Calne, R. Y., White, D. J. G., Rolles, K., Smith, D. P., and Hebertson, B. M. Prolonged survival of pig orthopic heart grafts treated with cyclosporin A. Lancet, *I:*1183, 1978.
14. Carpenter, C. B. The early diagnosis of renal allograft rejection in man. In *Advances in Nephrology*, edited by J. Hamburger, J. Crosnier and M. H. Maxwell, vol 5, p. 229. Year Book Medical Publishers, Chicago, 1975.
15. Carpenter, C. B., Rashid, A., Busch, G. J., Katz, A. J., Scheffer, A. L., Valentine, M. D., Birtch, A. G., Kay, R. G., Levine, L., Murray, J. F., Austen, K. F., and Merrill, J. P. A clinical trial of horse antihuman lymphocyte globulin in renal and hepatic transplantation. *International Symposium on Antilymphocyte Serum; Symposium Series in Immunological Standardization*, edited by J. F. Bach, J. Dormont, A. Eyquem, M. Raynaud and R. N. Regamey, p. 641. Karger, Basel, 1971.
16. Cerilli, J., Holliday, J. E., and Fesperman, D. P. Role of antivascular endothelial antibody in predicting renal allograft rejection. Transplant. Proc., *9:*771, 1977.
17. Cosimi, A. B., Delmarico, F. L., Burdick, J. F., and Russell, P. S. Individualized management of immunosuppresion according to serial monitoring of immunocompetence. Transplant. Proc., *10:*647, 1978.

18. Couser, W. G., Wallace, A., Monaco, A. P., and Lewis, E. J. Successful renal transplantation in patients with circulating antibody to glomerular basement membrane. Clin. Nephrol., *1:*381, 1973.
19. Crosnier, J. Treatment of terminal renal failure: general concepts of supportive therapy. In *Nephrology*, edited by J. Hamburger, J. Crosnier and J. P. Grünfeld, p. 1193. John Wiley, New York, 1979.
20. Crosnier, J., and Broyer, M. Treatment of chronic renal failure in children. In *Nephrology*, edited by J. Hamburger, J. Crosnier and J. P. Grünfeld, p. 1361. John Wiley, New York, 1979.
21. Curtoni, E. S., Scudeller, G., Mattiuz, P. L., Savi, M., and Ceppellini, R. Anti-HL-A antibody evolution in recipients of planned transfusions. Tissue Antigens, *2:*415, 1972.
22. Dandavino, R., Trunet, P., Descamps, B., and Kreis, H. Prolonged withdrawal of azathioprine in kidney transplantation. Transplant. Proc., *10:*655, 1978.
23. Degott, C., Rueff, B., Kreis, H., Duboust, A., Potet, F., and Benhamou, J. P. Peliosis hepatitis in renal transplant recipients. Digestion, *14:*467, 1976.
24. Dempster, W. J., Lennox, B., and Boag, J. W. Prolongation of survival of skin homotransplants in rabbit by irradiation of host. Br. J. Exp. Pathol. *31:*670, 1950.
25. Descamps, B., Gagnon, R., Debray-Sachs, M., Barbanel, C., and Crosnier, J. Lymphocyte dependent and complement dependent antibodies in human renal allograft recipients. Transplant. Proc., *7:*635, 1975.
26. Descamps, B., Hinglais, M., and Crosnier, J. Renal transplantation between 33 HL-A identical siblings. Transplant. Proc., *5:*231, 1973.
27. Descamps, B., and Kreis, H. Recipient presensitization: a critical survey. In *Advances in Nephrology*, edited by J. Hamburger, J. Crosnier and M. H. Maxwell, vol. 6, p. 443. Year Book Medical Publishers, Chicago, 1976.
28. De Shazo, C. V., Simmons, R. L., Bernstein, D. N., De Shazo, M. M., Willmert, J., Kjellstrand, C. N., and Najarian, J. S. Results of renal transplantation in 100 children. Surgery, *76:*461, 1974.
29. Dimitriu, A., Debrays-Sachs, M., Descamps, B., Sultan, C., and Hamburger, J. Tritiated thymidine incorporation in blood leukocytes of renal allograft recipients. Transplant. Proc., *3:*1577, 1971.
30. Dixon, F. J., McPhaul, J. J., and Lerner, R. A. The contribution of kidney transplantation to the study of glomerulonephritis. The recurrence of glomerulonephritis in renal transplants. Transplant. Proc., *1:*194, 1969.
31. Dormont, J., Kreis, H., Leski, M., and Crosnier, J. A clinical trial of antilymphocyte globulin in renal transplantation. Failure to observe a significant improvement. Eur. J. Clin. Biol. Res., *17:*382, 1972.
32. Dormont, J., Sobel, A., Galanaud, P., Crevon, M. C., and Colombani, J. Leukocyte migration inhibition with spleen extracts and other antigens in patients with renal allografts. Transplant. Proc., *4:*265, 1972.
33. Dossetor, J. B., MacKinnon, K. J., Gault, M. H., and McLean, L. D. Cadaver kidney transplants. Transplantation, *5:*844, 1967.
34. Dossetor, J. B., and Myburgh, J. A. Posttransplant immunologic monitoring summation. Transplant. Proc., *10:*1978, 661.
35. Ettenger, R. B., Opelz, G., Walker, J., Terasaki, P. I., Malekzadeh, M. K., Pennisi, A. J., Uittenbogaart, C. M., and Fine, R. N. Donor-specific preformed lymphocyte antibodies and mixed lymphocyte culture (MLC). Blocking in cadaver renal allograft recipients. Transplant. Proc., *10:*479, 1978.
36. Falk, R. E., Thorsby, E., Möller, E., and Möller, G. In vitro assay of cell-mediated immunity: The inhibition of migration of sensitized human lymphocytes by HL-A antigens. Clin. Exp. Immunol., *6:*445, 1970.
37. Fauchère, J. L., Berche, P., Kreis, H., Dandavino, R., and Crosnier, J. Accidents

infectieux au cours des transplantations rénales. Resultats et intérêt d'une surveillance bactériologique systématique. Nouv. Presse Med., *8:*1991, 1979.
38. Festenstein, H., Sachs, J. A., Paris, A. M. I., Pegrum, G. D., and Moorhead, J. E. Influence of HL-A matching and blood transfusion on outcome of 502 London transplant group renal-graft recipients. Lancet, *I:*157, 1976.
39. Fine, R. N. Renal transplantation in children. In *Advances in Nephrology*, edited by J. Hamburger, J. Crosnier and M. H. Maxwell, vol 5, p. 201. Year Book Medical Publishers, Chicago, 1975.
40. Friedman, E. A. Mithylpredenisolone therapy and allograft rejection. Comparison of daily and alternate day administration. Transplantation, *10:*552, 1970.
41. Fuller, T. C., Delmanico, T. L., Cosimi, A. B., Huggins, C. E., Kurg, M., and Russel, P. S. Effects of various types of RBC transfusions on HL-A alloimmunization and renal allograft survival. Transplant. Proc., *9:*117, 1977.
42. Gailiunas, P., Suthanthiran, M., Person, A., Strom, T. B., Carpenter, C. B., and Garovoy, M. R. Posttransplant immunologic monitoring of the renal allograft recipient. Transplant. Proc., *10:*609, 1978.
43. Garovoy, M. R., Suthanthiran, M., Gailiunas, P., Carpenter, C. B., Graves, M., Busch, G., and Tilney, N. L. Anti-Ia antibody eluted from rejected human renal allografts. Transplant. Proc., *10:*613, 1978.
44. Gluckman, J. C., Beaufils, H., Berger, J., Hinglais, N., Legrain, M., and Küss, R. Rapidly progressive glomerulonephritis with linear fluorescence in a kidney transplant. Clin. Nephrol., *1:*40, 1973.
45. Goodwin, W. E., Kaufman, J. J., Mims, M. M., Turner, R. D., Glassock, R., Goldman, R., and Maxwell, M. H. Human renal transplantation. I. Clinical experiences with six cases of renal homotransplantation. J. Urol., *89:*13, 1963.
46. Green, C. J., and Allison, A. C. Extensive prolongation of rabbit kidney allograft survival after short-term cyclosporin A treatment. Lancet, *I:*1182, 1978.
47. Grushkin, C. M., and Fine, R. N. Growth in children following renal transplantation. Am. J. Dis. Child., *125:*514, 1973.
48. Guttmann, R. D., Beaudoin, J. C., and Morehouse, D. D. Reduction of immunogenicity of human cadaver renal allografts by donor treatment. Transplant. Proc., *5:*663, 1973.
49. Gutmann, R. D., and Lindquist, R. R. Renal transplantation in the inbred rat. XI. Reduction of allograft immunogenicity by cytotoxic drug pretreatment of donors. Transplantation, *8:*490, 1969.
50. Hamburger, J. Immunologic follow up of renal allograft recipients. Transplant. Proc., *4:*669, 1972.
51. Hamburger, J. Recent advances in the understanding of rejection. In *Advances in Néphrology*, edited by J. Hamburger, J. Crosnier and M. H. Maxwell, vol. 5, p. 101. Year Book Medical Publishers, Chicago, 1975.
52. Hamburger, J., Crosnier, J., Dormont, J., and Bach, J. F. *Renal Transplantation: Theory and Practice*, p. 26. Williams & Wilkins, Baltimore, 1972.
53. Hamburger, J., Dimitriu, A., Bankir, L., Debray-Sachs, M., and Auvert, I. Collection of lymph from kidneys homotransplanted in man: cell transformation in vivo. Nature, *232:*633, 1971.
54. Hamburger, J., Vaysse, J., Crosnier, J., Auvert, J., and Dormont, J. Kidney homotransplantation in man. Ann. NY Acad. Sci., *99:*808, 1962.
55. Hamburger, J., Vaysse, J., Crosnier, J., Tubiana, M., Lalanne, C. M., Antoine, B., Auvert, J., Soulier, J., Dormont, J., Salomon, C., Maisonnet, M., and Amiel, J. L. Transplantation d'un rein entre jumeaux non monozigotes, après irradiation du receveur. Bon fonctionnement au quatrième mois. Presse Med., *67:*1771, 1959.
56. Hattler, B. G., and Miller, J. Changes in human mixed lymphocyte culture reactivity as an indicator of kidney rejection. Transplant. Proc., *4:*655, 1972.

57. Haxhe, J. J., Alexandre, G. P. J., and Kestens, P. J. The effect of Imuran and Azaserine on liver function tests in the dog. Arch. Int. Pharmacodyn. Ther., *168:*366, 1967.
58. Hersh, E. M., Butler, W. T., Rossen, R. D., and Morgan, R. O. Lymphocyte activation: a rapid test to predict allograft rejection. Nature, *226:*757, 1970.
59. Hersh, E. M., Butler, W. T., Rossen, R. D., Morgan, R. O., and Saki, W. In vitro studies of the human response to organ allografts: appearance and detection of circulating activation lymphocytes. J. Immunol., *107:*571, 1971.
60. Hume, D. M. Kidney transplantation. In *Human Transplantation*, edited by F. T. Rapaport and J. Dausset, p. 110. Grune and Stratton, New York, 1968.
61. Jamieson, S. W., Burton, N. A., Bieber, C. P., Reitz, B. A., Oyer, P. E., Stimson, E. B., and Shumway, N. E. Cardiac-allograft survival in primates treated with cyclosporin A. Lancet, *I:*545, 1979.
62. Jeffery, J. R., Downs, A., Grahame, J. W., Lye, C., Ramsey, E., and Thomson, A. E. Failure of blood transfusions to improve cadaveric renal allograft survival. Transplantation, *25:*344, 1978.
63. Kerman, R. H., and Geis, W. P. T-RFC monitoring of CMI events in renal allograft recipients. Transplant. Proc., *10:*633, 1978.
64. Kerman, R. H., Ing, T. S., Hano, J. F., and Geis, W. P. Predictive value of active T-RFC in renal allograft survival. Transplant. Proc., *10:*637, 1978.
65. Kostakis, A. J., White, D. J. G., and Calne, R. Prolongation of the rat heart allograft survival by cyclosporin A. IRCS Med. Sci. Surg. Transplant., *5:*280, 1977.
66. Kovithavongs, T., Schlaut, J., Pazderka, V., Lao, V., Pazderka, F., Bettcher, K. B., and Dossetor, J. B. Posttransplant immunologic monitoring with special consideration of technique and interpretation of LMC. Transplant. Proc., *10:*547, 1978.
67. Kreis, K. Procedure for performing renal transplantation. In *Nephrology*, edited by J. Hamburger, J. Crosnier and J. P. Grünfeld, p. 1311. John Wiley, New York, 1979.
68. Kreis, K., Mansouri, R., Descamps, J. M., Dandavino, R., N'Guyen, A. T., Bach, J. F., and Crosnier, J. Anti-thymocyte globulin in cadaver kidney transplantation. A randomized trial based on T-cell monitoring. Kidney Int., in press.
69. Kreis, H., Noel, L. H., Chailley, J., Lacombe, M., Descamps, J. M., and Crosnier, J. Kidney graft rejection: Has the need for steroids to be re-evaluated. Lancet, *II:*1169, 1978.
70. Küss, R., Legrain, M., Mathé, G., and Nedey, R. Epilogue d'une homotransplantation rénale de soeur à frère non jumeaux. Presse Med., *II:*1473, 1960.
71. Küss, R., Legrain, M., Poisson, J., and Guedon, J. Human renal transplantation: acute late rejection after complete withdrawal of steroid therapy. In Abstracts from the Fourth International Congress on Nephrology, p. 447, Stockholm, 1969.
72. Legrain, M., Jacobs, C., and Küss, R. Are there contraindications to renal transplantation. In *Advances in Nephrology*, edited by J. Hamburger, J. Crosnier, and M. H. Maxwell, vol. 4, p. 203. Year Book Medical Publishers, Chicago, 1974.
73. Leski, M., Kreis, H., Descamps, B., and Crosnier, J. Les complications extra-rénales des transplantations de rein. In *Actualités Nephrologiques de l'Hôpital Necker*, edited by J. Hamburger and J. Crosnier, p. 229. Med. Flammarion, Paris, 1969.
74. Liburd, E. M., Pazderka, V., Kovithavongs, T., and Dossetor, J. B. Evidence for suppressor cells and reduced CML induction by the donor in transplant patients. Transplant. Proc., *10:*557, 1978.
75. Lippman, M. E., Halterman, R. H., Leventhal, B. G., Perry, S., and Thompson, E. B. Glucocorticoid-binding proteins in human acute lymphoblastic leukemic blast cells. J. Clin. Invest., *52:*1973, 1715.
76. London, W. J., Drew, J. S., Blumberg, B. S., Grossman, R. A., and Lyons, P. J. Association of graft survival with host response to hepatitis B infection in patients with kidney transplant. N. Engl. J. Med., *296:*241, 1977.

77. Luciani, J., Frantz, P., Thibault, P., Shesquiere, F., Conseiller, C., Cousin, M. T., Glaser, P., Legrain, M., Viars, P., and Küss, R. Early anuria prevention in human kidney transplantation. Transplantation, *28:*308, 1979.
78. McConnachie, P. R., Finch, W. T., and Birtch, A. G. Monitoring and predicting rejection. Transplant. Proc., *10:*543, 1978.
79. Merrill, J. P. Medical management of the transplant patient. In *Human Transplantation*, edited by F. T. Rapaport and J. Dausset, p. 66. Grune and Stratton, New York, 1968.
80. Murray, J. E., Barno, B. A., and Athinson, J. Fifth report of the human kidney transplant registry. Transplantation, 5:752, 1967.
81. Myburgh, J. A., and Smit, J. A. B-cell antibodies and clinical kidney transplantation. Transplant. Proc., *10:*529, 1978.
82. Opelz, G., Sengar, D. P. S., Micket, M. R., and Terasaki, P. I. Effect of blood transfusions on subsequent kidney transplants. Transplant. Proc., *5:*253, 1973.
83. Opelz, G., Terasaki, P. I., Graver, B., Sasaki, N., Langston, M., Cohn, M., and Mickey, M. R. Correlation between number of pretransplant blood transfusions and kidney transplant survival. Transplant. Proc., *11:*145, 1979.
84. Parsons, F. M., Brunner, F. P., Burck, H. C., Graser, W., Gurland, H. J., Harlen, H., Scharer, K., and Spies, G. W. Condensed report including pediatrics on regular dialysis and transplantation in Europe, IV, 1973. Proc. Eur. Dial. Transplant. Assoc., *11:*3, 1974.
85. Paul, L., Van Es, L. A., Kalff, M. W., and De Graeff, J. Intrarenal distribution of endothelial antigens recognized by antibodies from renal allograft recipients. Transplant. Proc., *11:*427, 1979.
86. Pedersen, N., and Morris, B. The role of the lymphatic system in the rejection of homografts: a study of lymph from renal transplants. J. Exp. Med., *131:*936, 1970.
87. Persijn, G. G., Van Hoof, J. P., Kalff, M. W., Lansberger, Q., and Van Rood, J. Effect of blood transfusion and HLA matching on renal transplantation in the Netherlands. Transplant. Proc., *5:*503, 1977.
88. Sells, R. A., Brookes, L., Baser, P., and Whitemore, D. Methylprednisolone blood levels in cadaveric renal allograft recipients. Transplant. Proc., *10:*651, 1978.
89. Sengar, D. P. S., Rashid, A., and Jindal, S. L. Effect of blood transfusions on renal allograft survival. Transplant. Proc., *11:*179, 1979.
90. Soulillou, J. P., Peyrat, M. A., and Guenel, J. Studies of the antibodies against HLA, Ia-like, FC and/or C3 receptors present in retransplant sera: Anti B cell antibodies not associated with accelerated graft loss. Transplant. Proc., *10:*475, 1978.
91. Starzl, T. E. *Experience in Renal Transplantation*, p. 383. Saunders, Philadelphia, 1964.
92. Starzl, T. E., Porter, K. A., Iwasaki, Y., Marchioro, T. L., and Kashiwagro, N. The use of heterologous antilymphocyte globulin in human renal homotransplantation. *Antilymphocyte Serum, A Ciba Foundation Study Group* (No. 29), edited by G. E. W. Wolstenholme and M. O'Conner, p. 4. Churchill, London, 1967.
93. Stiller, C. R., Dossetor, J. B., and Sinclair, N. R. Stc. First international symposium on immunologic monitoring of the transplant patient. Part II. Transplant. Proc., *10:*525, 1978.
94. Stiller, C. R., and Sinclair, N. R. Stc. Monitoring of rejection. Transplant. Proc., *11:* 343, 1979.
95. Stiller, C. R., Sinclair, N. R. Stc., Abrahams, S., McGirr, D., Singh, H., Howson, W. T., and Ulan, R. A. Anti-donor immune responses in prediction of transplant rejection. N. Engl. J. Med., *294:*978, 1976.
96. Stiller, C. R., Sinclair, N. R. Stc., McGirr, D., Jevnikar, A., and Lkan, R. A. Diagnostic and prognostic value of donor specific posttransplant immune responses: Clinical

correlates and in vitro variables. Transplant. Proc., *10:*525, 1978.
97. Stinnett, J. D., Alexander, J. W., Ogle, C. K., McClellan, M. A., Brody, D., and First, R. Immune function of kidney transplant patients in relation to infection. Transplant. Proc., *10:*639, 1978.
98. Surmont, J., Dutreix, A., and Lalanne, C. M. Les irradiations toto pour greffe de tissu ou transplantation d'organe chez l'homme. J. Radiol. Electrol. Med. Nucl. *41:*679, 1960.
99. Suthanthiran, M., Gailiunas, P., Fagan, G., Strom, T. B., Carpenter, C. B., and Garovoy, M. R. Detection of anti-donor "Ia" antibodies: A strong correlate of rejection. Transplant. Proc., *10:*639, 1978.
100. Svejgaard, A., and Solheim, B. G. Blood transfusion and kidney transplantation. In *Proceedings of the Ninth Scandinavian Transplantation Meeting.* Scand. J. Urol. Nephrol. (Suppl.), *42:*79, 1977.
101. Terasaki, P. I., Mickey, M. R., and Krasler, M. Presensitization and kidney transplant failures. Postgrad. Med., *47:*89, 1971.
102. Thomas, F., Lee, H. M., Wolf, J. S., Mendez-Picon, G., and Thomas, J. Monitoring and modulation of immune reactivity in human transplant recipients. Surgery, *79:* 408, 1976.
103. Thomas, F., Mendez-Picon, G., Thomas, J., Lee, H. M., and Lower, R. Effective monitoring and modulation of recipient immune reactivity to prevent rejection in early posttransplant period. Transplant. Proc., *10:*537, 1978.
104. Thomas, F., Thomas, J., Mendez, G., Lee, H. M., and Lower, R. Individualization of recipient immunosuppression by use of in vitro monitoring parameters. Transplant. Proc., *10:*621, 1978.
105. Thomas, J., Thomas, F., Johns, C., and Lee, H. M. Considerations in immunologic monitoring of long-term transplant recipients. Transplant. Proc., *10:*569, 1978.
106. Tilney, N. L., and Murray, J. E. The thoracic duct fistula as an adjunct to immunosuppression in human renal transplantation. Transplantation, *5:*1204, 1967.
107. Tilney, N. L., Strom, T. B., Vineyard, G. C., and Merrill, J. P. Factors contributing to the declining mortality rate in renal transplantation. N. Engl. J. Med., *299:*1321, 1978.
108. Ting, A., and Morris, P. J. Pre- and posttransplant B-cell antibodies in renal transplantation. Transplant. Proc., *11:*393, 1979.
109. Torisu, M., Yokoyama, T., Amemiya, H., Hohler, F. F., Schoter, G., Martineau, G., Penn, I., Palmer, W., Halgrimson, C. G., Pietriam, C. W., and Starzl, T. E. Immunosuppression, liver injury, and hepatitis in renal, hepatic, and cardiac homograft recipients: With particular reference to the Australia antigen. Ann. Surg., *174:*621, 1971.
110. Traeger, J., Revillard, J. P., Fries, D., Brochier, J., Touraine, J. L., and Berthoux, F. Etude critique des tests d'immunosuppression chez les malades traités par des serums anti-lymphocytes. In *International Symposium on Antilymphocyte Serum; Symposium Series in Immunological Standardization*, edited by J. F. Bach, J. Dormont, A. Eyquem, M. Raynaud and R. N. Regamay, vol. 16, p. 207. Karger, Basel, 1971.
111. Tursz, T., Fournier, C., Kreis, H., Crosnier, J., and Bach, J. F. T-lymphocytes in kidney allograft recipients. Br. Med. J., *1:*799, 1976.
112. Van Hoof, J. P., Kalf, M. W., Van Poelgeest, A. E., Persijn, G. G., and Van Rood, J. J. Blood transfusion and kidney transplantation. Transplantation, *22:*306, 1976.
113. Veith, F. T., Luck, R. J., and Murray, J. E. The effects of splemectomy on immunosuppresive regimen in dog and man. Surg. Gynecol. Obstet., *212:*229, 1965.
114. Waksman, B. H., Arbowys, S., and Arnasson, B. G. The use of specific "lymphocyte" antisera to inhibit hypertensive reactions of the "delayed" type. J. Exp. Med., *114:*997, 1961.
115. Williams, K. A., Ting, A., Cullen, P. R., and Morris, P. J. Transfusions: Their influence on human renal graft survival. Transplant. Proc., *11:*175, 1979.

116. Wolf, J. S., and Hume, D. M. Prolongation of renal homograft survival by external radiation of renal arterial blood. Fed. Proc., *24:*573, 1965.
117. Wonigeit, K., and Pichlmayr, R. Posttransplant monitoring of donor-specific T-cell reactivity at the precursor cell level. Transplant. Proc., *10:*563, 1978.
118. Woodruff, M. F. A., and Anderson, N. F. Effect of lymphocyte depletion by thoracic duct fistula and administration of antilymphocytic serum on the survival of skin homografts in rats. Nature, *200:*702, 1963.
119. Woodruff, M. F. A., Forman, B., and Fraser, K. B. The effects of antilymphocyte serum on circulating antibody levels. J. Immunol., *67:*57, 1951.

CHAPTER SEVEN

Transplanted Kidney:Natural History

Henri Kreis

Uncomplicated outcome—Complications involving the transplanted kidney:renal failure, graft rejection, glomerulonephritis, spontaneous rupture of the transplanted kidney.

UNCOMPLICATED OUTCOME

Postoperative progress may be divided into two stages: the first stage, from the day of transplantation to the day the patient leaves the hospital, an average of 3 weeks; the second stage, that of progressive return to normal life after leaving the hospital.

Immediate Postoperative Period

Diuresis and Renal Function

In most cases of a living donor transplant or of a cadaver kidney without undue ischemia (see below), there is immediate satisfactory function of the grafted kidney. Urine begins to flow between 2 and 10 min after circulation is restored. It reaches 2 to 10 ml/min[74] during the first hours, then progressively diminishes to a normal volume between 24 and 48 hours.[69, 131, 140, 176]

This early urine has a high sodium content (80 to 125 mmol/liter) and contains a significant amount of potassium (14 to 27 mmol/liter). Urine creatinine concentration is usually low (about 2 to 3 mmol/liter), but its 24-hour output is high and can lower the plasma creatinine level within the 1st day. The postoperative polyuria represents an osmotic diuresis with diminished reabsorption in the proximal tubules. This is easily explained by the following factors: 1) at the time of transplantation the patients have hyperosmolar plasma because of elevated blood urea; 2) in many cases, despite regular dialysis treatment, they have some degree of water and salt retention; and 3) ischemia and cooling of the kidney may cause lesions which affect tubular reabsorption, especially when cadaver kidneys are used.

When the polyuria is marked, close attention must be paid to water and electrolyte balance in order to avoid complications due to dehydration or hypokalemia.[131] Rehydration of the recipient must take into account possible preoperative overhydration; it must be sufficient to prevent any serious dehydration but must not be so excessive as to perpetuate the polyuria. When urinary output is less than 200 ml/hour, it is our practice to give fluid in amounts equal to the urinary output. Half of this fluid is an isotonic glucose solution containing 1 g of potassium chloride/liter; the other half is an isotonic sodium chloride solution. When diuresis is 200 ml/hour or more, 2 volumes of saline solution are given for each volume of glucose solution, and it is advisable to keep the fluid intake slightly below the urine output. The difference, however, must not exceed a total of 1/30 of the patient's body weight. This rule must of course be adapted in each individual case to the results of urine and blood analysis performed 6 and then every 24 hours after transplantation.

Renal function in the first hours[94, 95, 112, 140] and in the first weeks[3, 12, 65, 118, 169] after transplantation has been studied by many workers. Kountz et al[95] found a mean glomerular filtration rate of 54 ml/min and a mean plasma flow of 672 ml/min, with a mean renal blood flow of 979 ml/min. These figures suggest considerable intrarenal vasodilation. The mean filtration fraction is 0.089. Para-aminohippuric acid extraction is diminished and ^{125}[I]Hippuran and ^{131}[I]Diodrast extraction are diminished even more. The crude clearance figures are normal for a single kidney, but they do not reflect the renal plasma flow, which is remarkably increased. Kountz et al[95] did not find the glycosuria which other authors have reported and have interpreted as the consequence of tubular damage from prolonged ischemia. The hyperchloremic acidosis with inability to lower urinary pH below 5.8 and a diminished tubular bicarbonate reabsorption previously described[65, 112] was not observed by Ladefoged[104] at 14 to 60 days after transplantation, although disturbances in acid-base balance are not infrequent.[182] All authors have noted inversion of the normal circadian urinary rhythm and increased output of sodium when the patient is recumbent.[4, 17, 158]

The immediate establishment of effective glomerular filtration and the polyuria are very often instrumental in restoring plasma urea and creatinine to near normal levels by the 3rd day, when live related kidneys are used. With cadaver kidneys, when the management of the donor and the harvesting procedure is careful, uncomplicated and as untraumatic as possible, the onset of diuresis and function is immediate in more than 80% of recipients when total ischemia time in cold Collins' solution is less than 36 to 48 hours.[100] A high percentage of immediate function is most likely to be observed in cadaver kidney recipients either when they are volume-overexpanded,[113] pre- or peroperatively, or if they receive a large dose of furosemide before release of the vascular clamps. However, when ischemia, and especially warm ischemia, is too long or when the donor kidney has been obtained under difficult circumstances from a cadaver that had poor circulation during the agonal period, there may be early anuria due to acute tubular necrosis. One or more hemodialyses may then be necessary.

Proteinuria

Relatively marked proteinuria occurs immediately after transplantation and may persist for some weeks.[36, 122, 164, 195] This proteinuria is not derived from the recipient's own kidneys. In our series preoperative bilateral nephrectomy did not alter proteinuria levels.[36] Neither does the proteinuria signify an immune phenomenon; it is found in all recipients, even in the absence of rejection crises, and we have seen it in grafts from identical twins. The proteinuria is probably due to ischemic damage to the renal tubules and is characterized by a significant excretion of both albumin and low molecular weight proteins.[164] Tubular damage is likely to be present when the electrophoretic pattern is that of a tubular proteinuria (triple globulinuria),[36, 122] just as in the recovery stage of acute tubular necrosis.[41, 43, 184] On the other hand, heavy excretion of albumin suggests some temporary glomerular damage, with increased glomerular permeability. It is usually observed only during the first days. Thereafter, the electrophoretic pattern becomes that of tubular proteinuria.[164] Immunoprecipitation in a gel medium of the urinary proteins by specific antikidney immune serum demonstrates the excretion of protein of tissue origin in the postoperative period.[8, 71]

In favorable cases, the proteinuria diminishes or disappears completely in the following days, and its later reappearance always indicates some complication.[97]

In this period, fibrinuria is also very commonly found.[9, 21, 195] It disappears 2 to 3 weeks after transplantation but may reappear during rejection episodes. It consists of fragments of fibrin, the amount of which bears no relation to the level of proteinuria. This is generally thought to be due to the elimination in the urine of the products of fibrinolysis of intrarenal microthrombi[9, 21] or to be evidence of increased intravascular fibrinogenolysis.[195]

Blood Pressure and Ocular Fundi

The remission of the hypertension which developed during end-stage kidney disease following renal allotransplantation in man has been well documented.[91, 92] However, the drop in blood pressure may occur somewhat more slowly, due to the use of large doses of corticosteroids, to the narrowing of the arterial lumen by edema of the anastomosis or to postoperative renal failure. Remission of hypertension is observed even when the patient's own diseased kidneys are not removed.[91]

Once restored to a physiologic level, the blood pressure remains normal as long as there is good function in the transplanted kidney. The recurrence (or the appearance) of permanent post-transplant hypertension is most often explained by arterial stenosis of the transplanted kidney, by chronic rejection with interstitial fibrosis and vascular lesions of the graft or by recurrent glomerulonephritis. In addition, hypertension may be related to the presence of the recipient's own diseased kidney(s)[33, 64, 83] (see p. 254).

Parallel to the relief of hypertension, there is a spectacular improvement in the appearance of the *ocular fundi* after transplantation.[50, 69, 147] The regression of retinal changes follows an identical pattern in all patients. The tension in the central artery of the retina returns rapidly to normal, reflecting the general reduction in blood pressure; after 2 weeks the edema of the optic disc disappears. After 3 months at the most, exudates and hemorrhages are resorbed. Visual acuity, often very diminished, is restored even when there are pigmented chorioretinal scars around the disc. The retinal arterioles may improve more slowly. The arteriolar caliber increases, even where vascular changes were pronounced, but nipping at the arteriovenous intersections may persist for a long time.

Postoperative Biopsy of the Transplanted Kidney

Kincaid-Smith et al[88] have taken biopsies of the graft 20 to 25 min after restoration of renal blood flow. They concluded that the presence of more than two polymorphonuclear cells per glomerulus was an indication of poor tolerance and repeated rejection crises. More than five polymorphonuclears per glomerulus indicated rapid rejection, as already reported by Williams et al,[189] and might be related to the presence of preformed antibodies. Millard et al,[135] in 75 cases with immediate postoperative biopsy, were unable to confirm the correlation between the number of polymorphonuclear cells and the subsequent course. They did find many cases of tubular damage due to ischemia. In fact, as pointed out by Porter,[151] immediate postoperative biopsy of the transplant gives little indication of the severity of the injury, as there has been insufficient time for morphologic changes to appear. Later it will become impossible to differentiate between changes secondary to nonimmunologic injury, such as ischemia, preservation methods or traumatic vascular injury, and changes caused by rejection.

Subsequent Progress After Transplantation

In the months after transplantation, there is rapid improvement in the general condition of the patient. Weight gain in the first 2 months is often 30 to 40% of the preoperative weight.

Renal function improves progressively because of compensatory hypertrophy; urea and creatinine clearances reach 75 to 100% of the values found with two normal kidneys. Maximal osmolar concentration and the response to induced acidification of the urine return to normal. Cardiovascular complications disappear, anemia is corrected and peripheral nerve disorders are cured; disturbances of calcium and phosphorus metabolism may clear more slowly. More or less rapidly, there is full rehabilitation in work and social life.

Improvement of Hematologic Disorders

Anemia. Despite the theoretically possible interference of immunosuppressive drugs, anemia disappears during the course of the first 3 months, particularly if the iron depletion frequently seen in patients on long-term hemodialysis is corrected. The red cell count returns to normal; hematocrit and hemoglobin may even rise above normal levels because of a macrocytic reaction. Erythropoietic activity in the serum, absent in chronic uremia, is normal after transplantation,[5, 117, 129] as is ^{59}Fe incorporation into the red blood cells.[129] In fact, erythropoietic activity during the first post-transplantation weeks or months is probably higher than in the normal individual.

In some patients a period of transitory polycythemia is even seen.[85] This rather frequent abnormality is usually observed during the 1st post-transplantation year and lasts for a few months. Among possible explanations, such as graft ischemia or renal vein thrombosis, none has been clearly proven to be the cause.

If anemia recurs, it is usually due either to overdosage of azathioprine (anemia associated with leukopenia and thrombocytopenia) or to diminished function of the transplanted kidney (anemia without leukopenia).

Leukocytes. When recipients are submitted to large doses of steroids in the post-transplantation period, a high increase in the white blood cell count may be seen. Subsequently the leukocyte count runs between 3500 and 5000 white cells/mm on a standard dose of 3 mg/kg body wt azathioprine.

Leukopenia due to azathioprine overdosage may be preceded, accompanied and followed by an increase in the eosinophil count; this is infrequent, however, and in general does not go beyond 10 to 15%.

Platelets. In patients treated with azathioprine but not receiving antilymphocyte serum, thrombocytopenia is rare except as part of a pancytopenia. High susceptibility to azathioprine in a previously splenectomized recipient, or simple azathioprine overdosage, may be responsible for thrombopenia. Among post-transplantation complications, infection, whether disseminated or not, as well as severe rejection, can induce a large drop in platelet count.

An increased platelet count is observed in a few cases during the post-transplantation period. It is sometimes associated with an increase in the steroid regimen, and especially with intravenous bolus of 1 g prednisolone. When the platelet count remains over 500,000/mm, it may be safer to prescribe antiaggregant agents.

Some preparations of antilymphocyte serum (see Ch. Five) may cause thrombocytopenia, but since such sera can now be recognized by in vitro tests, their use can be avoided.

Effects of Transplantation on Polyneuritis

The tremendous improvement in the methods used for regular dialysis treatment during the past years has made the occurrence of severe polyneuritis among chronic dialysis patients much less frequent.

Nevertheless, in the rare cases where uremic neuritis is still present at the time of transplantation, it usually resolves rapidly. Within a few weeks of transplantation, functional disorders (itching, burning, muscular weakness) improve.[138] Objective signs, such as disturbance of gait and nerve conduction velocity, improve much more slowly, requiring from 6 to 12 months to return to normal.[154] It is unlikely that a steppage gait will persist indefinitely, but it has been observed in a few patients.

Effects of Transplantation on Bones and on Phosphorus and Calcium Metabolism

Most patients with chronic uremia, whether treated or not by hemodialysis before transplantation, have secondary hyperparathyroidism with or without bone changes,[125, 193, 174] although the changes in blood calcium and phosphorus, normally so typical of hyperparathyroidism, may be masked by the fact that renal failure itself causes blood calcium to drop and phosphorus to rise. It has been said that in most cases soon after successful renal transplantation the calcium and phosphorus levels in the blood return to normal and the osteodystrophic bone undergoes repair.[6, 86] Parathyroidectomy is thus seldom considered to be required after renal transplantation. Today the situation appears more complex, and the major difficulties in the analysis of phosphorus and calcium metabolism in transplant recipients are technical. Measurement of parathyroid hormone is based on a difficult radioimmunoassay. Since several sites of the molecules are antigenic, there are important differences between the antisera used. Some of them may recognize large amounts of inactive hormone fragments, whereas others directed against the N terminal end of the molecule, for example, will give different results. Vitamin D metabolite measurement, as well as ionized calcium dosage, requires sophisticated chemical analysis.

Persistent hypercalcemia after transplantation has now been reported by many groups,[29, 58, 162] with an incidence of about 20%. In most cases hypercalcemia is mild and resolves spontaneously within 2 years after transplantation.[30]

The present discrepancy with previous works is probably related to the fact that the simple determination of total serum phosphorus and calcium concentrations is not adequate screening for diagnosis, whereas the ionized calcium level provides the decisive clue.[58, 111]

In some patients with normal renal function, the persistance or the reappearance of hypercalcemia many years after kidney transplantation raises the contentious question of "tertiary hyperparathyroidism."

Autonomous (Tertiary) Hyperparathyroidism. There have been many reports of autonomous secondary hyperparathyroidism (tertiary hyperparathyroidism)[58, 108, 115, 193] since the initial report of McPhaul et al.[119] In fact, the hyperplastic parathyroid glands take time to involute, and when serum parathormone levels are periodically determined, a progressive decrease is usually observed. Nevertheless, a persistently elevated serum parathormone level suggests the presence of autonomous hyperparathyroidism and may require parathyroidectomy.[58] So far, 13 of our patients have undergone parathyroidectomy. Nine had classical subtotal parathyroidectomy; in the other patient all the parathyroid tissue was excised, but a small piece of one gland was autografted under the skin of the forearm. In all cases but one, in which adenoma was found in the removed glands, hyperplastic changes of the parathyroid were demonstrated.

It cannot be assumed that these hyperplastic changes would have persisted indefinitely, but the insidious consequences of long-lasting hyperparathyroidism may be deleterious enough to justify surgery when serum calcium or parathormone levels do not reach normal values within a few months.

It is possible that a state of phosphate depletion may develop as a consequence of diminished tubular reabsorption of phosphorus,[75] frequently observed in transplanted kidneys, and may contribute to the development of hypercalcemia.

Effect of Steroids on Skeleton. High or prolonged steroid dosage causes persistence or even aggravation of bone disorders present before transplantation.[81] We have seen vertebral collapse, rib fractures and fracture of the pelvis[108] in patients with no evidence of hyperparathyroidism. The osteoporosis in these patients appeared to be explained by the prolonged use of prednisone in high doses. More severe bone complications may occur in association with steroid therapy. For example, bone aseptic necrosis, whose incidence in our series is over 20% in patients with a minimum 1-year follow-up, has not been observed in transplant recipients who have never received steroid therapy (see p. 252).

Effect of Transplantation on Sexual Function. It has been well established that females receiving chronic hemodialysis treatment still have impaired sexual function despite a clear amelioration related to improved dialysis membranes.[87] A similar situation is observed among male patients. After transplantation, no abnormality is seen in the spermogram of males, and in females menstruation returns in all cases.[1, 19, 130]

Since the early years of human kidney transplantation when it was thought that pregnancy should be avoided in graft recipients, there have been numerous reports of normal pregnancies carried successfully to term.[52, 79, 157, 163, 180] A recent international survey[156] reported 86 normal pregnancies in 76 allograft recipients. Our own group has observed 11 infants born to 10 allograft recipients. Complications of pregnancy were minimal, and no transplants were rejected because of pregnancy. In addition, 21 male recipients fathered normal children despite immunosuppressive therapy.

Based on our experience and that reported in the literature, we conclude that: 1) sexual function is restored by successful renal transplantation, and 2) pregnancy has a minimal adverse effect on allograft function.

Very few studies have so far been reported on the offspring of renal allograft recipients. In a very recent report on 10 infants born to eight allograft recipients (five female and three male), Korsch et al[93] found no physical or developmental abnormalities in the offspring. Today, one of the main reasons for performing renal transplantation in patients receiving chronic hemodialysis treatment is to offer the patient the possibility of fathering a child or bearing a child of her own.

Social and Professional Rehabilitation

In the absence of complications, patients are restored to full health within several weeks to 6 or 10 months after transplantation.

Usually the return to normal activity poses no problem; 73% of our patients either have resumed their normal work or, in the case of younger patients, have begun professional training within 6 months of transplantation.[155] This social and professional rehabilitation is more difficult to achieve when there has been a very long period of invalidism before transplantation.[59] Rehabilitation is easier when the patient is already skilled in some trade or profession.

Pathologic Changes

It is our custom to perform routine renal biopsy 6 months and 2 and 10 years after transplantation. These biopsies are studied by light and electron microscopy and by immunofluorescent techniques. (see Appendix III, p. 366).

The significant finding is that in clinically normal recipients without complications and with normal renal function tests, renal biopsy often reveals latent changes (Fig. 7.1). These changes are usually minor but

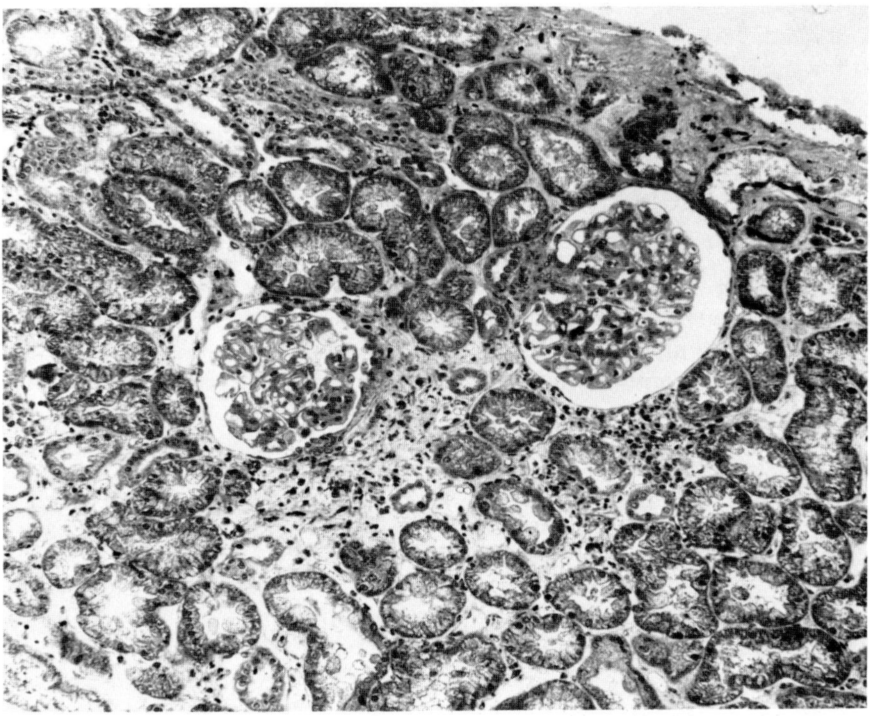

Fig. 7.1. Cadaver kidney transplantation. Renal biopsy specimen 4 years post-transplantation. Although transplant function was normal, a fibrotic area and focal cellular infiltration can be seen (original magnification × 350).

definite even on light microscopy. Biopsies at 6 months were normal in only 41% of our homotransplants with normal function. At 2 years, only 47% of homotransplants with normal function were histologically normal. Latent changes include edema, fibrosis, focal cellular infiltration into the interstitial tissue and glomerular or vascular alterations. Two or more changes can occur in association. Occasionally immunofluorescence reveals small subendothelial deposits of IgG in the glomeruli. Minor glomerular changes are found even more often, of course, if each glomerulus is examined by electron microscopy.

These pathologic changes are more frequently observed in patients who have had one or more rejection crises, even when these crises appeared fully reversible. In the 6-month biopsies, the patients with histologic changes had had an average of twice as many crises as those with histologically normal kidneys.

When 2-year biopsies were compared with those at 6 months, a similar picture was seen in 73%, disappearance of the lesions in 10% and the appearance of lesions in 17%.

Overall, these biopsies show that even where clinical tolerance of the graft is excellent, morphologic changes in the graft are common. When only cadaveric grafts are considered, almost every biopsy shows at least a few mild changes. Whether these changes reflect a latent immunologic process or are a later consequence of early nonimmunologic damage has not been determined (see below).

COMPLICATIONS INVOLVING THE TRANSPLANTED KIDNEY

Failure of the transplant to function, temporarily or definitively, is one of the most frequent of the complications threatening the allograft recipient. Renal damage and the subsequent impairment of renal function may result from various processes other than rejection. Nevertheless, whatever the origin of the complication, its main, constant and striking hallmark is a decline in renal function reflected by a rise in serum creatinine level.

Post-transplantation Renal Failure

Episodes of renal failure (RFE) frequently follow kidney transplantation. Most of them appear reversible with appropriate medical or surgical therapy, but in a relatively small number of cases the transplanted kidney will never function again, whatever the treatment. Early and accurate diagnosis of post-transplant RFE is probably the key to better long-term survival.

Immediate Renal Failure Episodes

Kidneys taken from living related donors do not suffer preoperative damage; the warm, and even the cold, ischemia times are always very short since removal and transplantation of the kidney are usually almost simultaneous. Postoperative RFE are therefore extremely uncommon in grafts from living related donors, whether or not the pair is HLA-identical (human leucocyte A),[73] and they probably need not be anticipated unless kidney removal or reimplantation complications led to prolonged ischemia.

A period of renal failure is much more likely with cadaver kidneys since premortem incidents in the donor can induce severe lesions of the kidney. Among these incidents, vascular collapse frequently occurs, as does short-term cardiac arrest, which can lead to severe tubular lesions or even to disseminated intravascular coagulation. Then follows the harvesting procedure, during which the kidney suffers surgical trauma, with the possiblity of definitive cardiac arrest. Finally, the kidney is stored for many hours or days, and the preservation method itself may induce various lesions.[31, 63, 76, 172] Because of ischemia and other stresses suffered by the kidney before transplantation, the majority of cadaver kidneys have at least mild tubular lesions, which can progress to tubular necrosis and result in acute renal failure.[90] In this regard, warm ischemia is much more prejudicial than cold ischemia (see Ch. Four).

The symptomology of immediate RFE varies according to the intensity and nature of the lesions. Minimal changes may involve only partial defects of tubular functions. Isolated hyperkalemia was observed by Defronzo et al[42] in 23 of 75 patients in the first 3 months following renal transplantation. This was attributed to a reversible defect in urinary potassium excretion. Hyperchloremic acidosis has been reported by numerous authors.[18, 65, 74, 192] Gyorgy et al[65] noted an acidification defect in 21 of 24 transplant recipients. It was frequently associated with increased phosphate clearance, hypercalcemia, concentrating defect and glycosuria. Acidifying, concentrating and diluting defects characteristic of distal tubular dysfunction were reported by Better et al.[18]

Generalized proximal tubular dysfunction referred to as a Fanconi-like syndrome (glycosuria, aminoaciduria, phosphaturia, uricosuria and bicarbonaturia) has been reported in rare instances.[106, 124] The pathophysiology of post-transplantation tubular dysfunction remains obscure. Ischemia of the transplant, as well as rejection episodes, may damage proximal tubular cells. Hyperparathyroidism, which is almost always present during the first weeks or months following surgery, has been shown to decrease bicarbonate and, of course, phosphate reabsorption. Steroid administration is often responsible for glycosuria. Therefore, the meaning of these initial and incomplete disturbances of graft function is not unequivocal. Nevertheless, nonimmunologic lesions are likely to play the major role in their occurrence.

Complete renal failure may occur under other circumstances in the postoperative period. Sometimes the patient still passes a certain amount of urine despite a creatinine clearance below 5 ml/min. However, the most frequent problem is that the kidney produces no or very little urine and that this anuria can last for several days, necessitating dialysis. Various groups have reported different incidences of immediate RFE,[15, 32, 100, 169] because various mechanisms may lead to RFE in the transplant recipient. For example, in our department, despite the use of kidneys that have been subjected to a long period of ischemia, the frequency of immediate postoperative renal insufficiency has been reduced from 54% to less than 20% by intravenous injection of 500 mg furosemide before completing anastomosis of the transplant vessels (Table 7.1).[100] Similar and even better results were attained in other groups either by infusing enough fluid to the recipient during surgery to avoid chronic fluid depletion, which is frequent in hemodialyzed recipients, or by careful selection of the donor and the elimination of 6 to 10% of kidneys because of poor perfusion characteristics during machine perfusion.[15] In other reports, the percentage of initial nonfunction varies from 28%[32] to 74%.[169]

In a recent study,[97] our group found that the clinical presentation and biochemical parameters of immediate RFE were those usually observed in acute tubular necrosis without regard to etiology. Fever was generally present, but its frequency varied according to the presence and the amount of corticosteroids. Anuria was usually seen, but diuresis was observed in 15 to 20% of cases. When a few milliliters of urine could be collected, the urine/plasma creatinine ratio was near 10 or lower in about half of the patients, whereas the urinary sodium concentrations were higher than 30 mEq/liter in more than 75% of patients.

Hypertension was less frequent in the postoperative period even in patients whose blood pressure was elevated before surgery. The use of large amounts of steroids did not significantly increase the number of

TABLE 7.1

Influence of furosemide recipient pretreatment on postoperative renal function

Pretreatment with Furosemide	No. of Cases	No. of Patients Needing Postoperative Dialysis	No. of Irreversible Immediate RFE
Yes	131	26 (19.8%)	13 (9.9%)
No	94	51 (54%)	10 (10.6%)
Total	225	77 (34.2%)	23 (10.2%)

hypertensive patients (10%) as compared to hypertensives among those not receiving steroids (29.5%).

In general, the postoperative anuric period lasts only a few days (Fig. 7.2). It may, however, be as long as 4 to 5 weeks. In a few patients, irreversible renal failure may be observed immediately after transplantation. For example, 8 such episodes occurred in 65 of our patients who developed immediate renal failure.

It is generally said that the length of time that elapsed between transplantation and the onset of renal function has no influence on the long-term survival of the transplant, provided the recipient has been maintained on dialysis until recovery.[90, 190] However, some workers[40, 166, 185] have suggested that delayed primary function was probably detrimental to long-term function. In a recent study of recipients 1 year or more after transplantation,[40] those with delayed primary function had only 70% of the functional capacity of patients with immediate function. It is not known whether this decreased function resulted from a continuous decline in renal function or whether it had already occurred by the time of recovery. In fact, it is highly probable that initial nonimmunologic lesions responsible for primary nonfunction of the kidney may progress to chronic renal failure.

When kidney biopsy is made during the early oliguric renal failure period, acute tubular necrosis appears to be the major histologic feature. Unfortunately, biopsy provides no evidence as to its precise cause. It is now well known that acute rejection is responsible for a severe reduction in kidney perfusion,[78] leading to necrosis of tubular cells; this necrosis can also be the result of antemortem blood pressure collapse in the donor or of any kind of surgical mishap. Vascular lesions are also frequent on kidney sections and/or on angiography of the transplant, regardless of the reason for transplant failure.

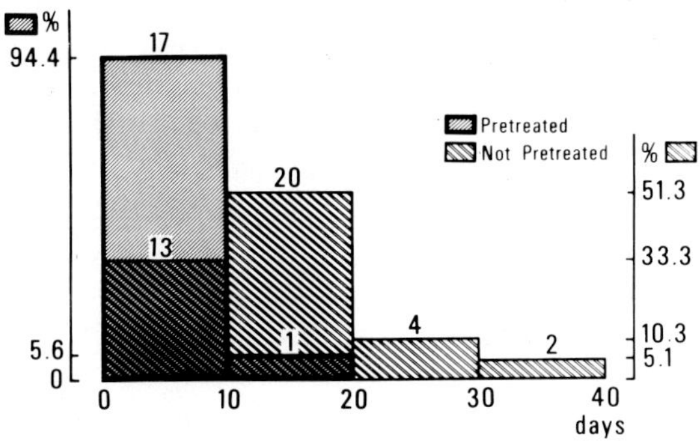

Fig. 7.2. Duration of immediate renal failure episodes according to corticosteroid regimen in cadaver kidney graft recipients.

Diagnosis of immediate RFE is not easy. The principal problem in the immediate postoperative phase is to differentiate between irreversible rejection and reversible acute tubular necrosis related to the status of the donor or to surgical problems. In this regard, it is important to weigh on the one hand the cumulative effects of antemortem events in the donor, harvesting difficulties, perservation methods, ischemic injury and the implantation procedure, and on the other hand, the immunologic status of the host, with special attention to possible anti-HLA antigen preimmunization.

Nonimmunologic factors responsible for primary nonfunction are usually reversible with appropriate treatment, except when the kidney has been severely harmed before transplantation. On the contrary, hyperacute rejection leading to immediate renal failure is not reversible but requires prompt removal of the transplant in order to avoid severe complications related to the presence of a necrosed organ in the recipient. It is thus clear that the etiology of early transplant nonfunction must be elucidated as quickly as possible. Generally, during the course of a rejection episode, urinary creatinine concentration is elevated and that of sodium is reduced; during the course of tubular necrosis, the exact opposite occurs. In practice, however, the simultaneous occurrence of the two complications often makes precise interpretation of the results difficult.

The following is the sequence of diagnostic steps taken by our group for management of allograft recipients developing immediate post-transplantation RFE. 1) Verify that there is no functional or organic bladder obstruction, which is not infrequent after anesthesia and bleeding inside the urinary tract. 2) Check that the recipient has normal, or better, even slight overhydration, with a pulmonary artery pressure of around 20 mmHg. 3) Assess the patency of the ureter and the absence of urinary leakage by ultrasound scan, which gives much better results than intravenous pyelography when the surgical wound is closed. 4) Ascertain patency of the transplant circulation with renal isotope scans with technetium and hippuric acid; if necessary, perform renal angiogram to visualize intrarenal vascular branches. When all the above procedures give normal results, the reversibility of renal failure is assured and a transplant biopsy is not necessary. A vascular defect on the isotope scan and/or vascular abnormalities on the angiogram (irregularities on arteriolar branches, infarction areas, severe slowing of the blood flow) make re-examination and biopsy of the graft necessary. Angiographic "dead tree" aspect or corticonecrosis demonstrated during the nephrogram phase of the angiogram indicates irreversible vascular damage and the necessity of removing the transplant.

Routine use of the above protocol provides the basis for diagnosis of the major causes of initial RFE. However, when it provides no data for diagnosis, possible undetectable trauma of the kidney must be considered and it is necessary to re-evaluate the preagonal status, the surgical procedures and the preservation methods in each case. In a recent work[97] we discovered in 41.5% of patients with initial nonfunction, one or more factors that could have caused or contributed to the occurrence of renal failure such as those shown in Table 7.2.

Immediate hyperacute rejection is frequently said to be responsible for irreversible immediate RFE[186] when severe vascular lesions are demonstrated. This rejection might be due to anti-HLA cytotoxic antibodies in the recipient that are directed against the donor and are thus injurious to the vascular endothelium.[20, 181] This interpretation appears less plausible, however, when the donor-recipient cross-match is negative, as is the general rule. However it is highly probable that antidonor sensitized T lymphocytes can be directly responsible for immediate graft destruction in the absence of circulating humoral antibodies.

Delayed Acute Renal Failure Episodes

Delayed RFE may be observed at any time post-transplantation, and even after many years, regardless of whether the transplant originally functioned well or not. They are, however, much more frequent during the first 6 months, and especially during the first weeks after surgery. In our series,[97] 85% of patients who received a cadaver kidney allograft developed delayed RFE during the 1st month, and only 9.3% of 156 patients never had an episode of renal failure. The overall incidence of delayed reversible renal failure is much higher in patients receiving cadaver kidneys than in those receiving transplants from living related donors.[46] This is the consequence of an increased number of rejection episodes due not only to the lack of complete identity between the cadaver donor and the receipient but also to a higher incidence of

TABLE 7.2
Major factors responsible for or contributing to the occurrence of immediate renal failure episodes

Infarcts	4
Frozen kidney	1
Rupture	3
Technical accident	14
Urinary tract fistula	3
Warm ischemia time (10–50 min)	5
Perirenal collection	1
Cortical necrosis	3
Miscellaneous	2

nonimmunologic complications such as infections, which are probably related to the higher dosage of immunosuppressive agents which cadaver kidney recipients receive.

It is common practice to consider most RFE occurring after kidney transplantation, and in particular those which do not occur immediately postsurgery, to be the result of rejection phenomena. In fact, many of them are not the consequence of a recipient immune response to the graft antigens but rather can be due to various causes.[120] Diagnosis of delayed RFE therefore poses a difficult challenge that is generally not resolved by conventional laboratory and clinical criteria. Sonography (or intravenous pyelography when ultrasound cannot be used), transplant angiography and renal biopsy must always be performed. Immunologic monitoring[179] has never given reliable results in individual clinical cases. When all above investigations have been done, it may still be necessary to surgically re-explore the transplant and perirenal area, although the routine use of sonography has drastically reduced the need for surgery. Thus, in 45% of our cases we demonstrated a factor responsible for, or at least contributing to the occurrence of renal failure.[98] Urinary tract fistula, rupture or infarcts of the kidney, local and systemic infection and pretransplantation mishaps were among the most frequent findings (Table 7.3). This does not mean that the remaining 55% of RFE were rejection episodes while all others were of nonimmunologic origin but simply that there is a better probability that unexplained RFE have an immunologic origin.

The protocol used in the management of transplant recipients certainly has a real influence on the frequency and the course of RFE. We have demonstrated[98] that steroids did not prevent the occurrence of RFE, even when the high doses used in the treatment of rejection episodes were given during the immediate postoperative period and thereafter (Table 7.4). On the contrary, antithymocyte globulin (ATG) significantly decreased the frequency of RFE as long as it was given (Fig. 7.3).[99] On the

TABLE 7.3

Major factors responsible for or contributing to the occurrence of delayed renal failures

Technical accident	8
Infections	
Urinary	3
Wound	9
Lung, Blood	4
Rupture	4
Infarcts	2
Ureter fistula	9
Miscellaneous	4

TABLE 7.4
Incidence of renal failure episodes in patients receiving high doses of steroids from the day of transplantation (pretreated) and in those receiving no steroids until the occurrence of RFE (not pretreated)

	Patient Pretreated ($N = 53$)	Patient Not Pretreated ($N = 54$)
Reversible RFE	39 (73%)	45 (83%)
Irreversible RFE	3 (6%)	4 (7%)
RFE improved by day 6	28 (53%)	34 (63%)
RFE improved by day 10	43 (82%)	45 (83%)
Functional graft at 6/12	42 (79%)	41 (76%)

other hand, the presence of large amounts of steroids delayed the onset of renal failure, which took place 1 to 5 days after transplantation when azathioprine was given alone, while renal failure occurred after day 5 in patients already receiving steroids. ATG has also been said to be able to modify the onset of RFE because some authors observed a rebound in the frequency of RFE after the withdrawal of ATG.

After the beginning of renal failure, urinary concentrations of creatinine and sodium were also found to be slightly different in patients submitted to steroid therapy. These recipients almost always had a high urine/plasma creatinine ratio and low urinary sodium concentration, whereas in those already treated by steroids a low urine/plasma concentration

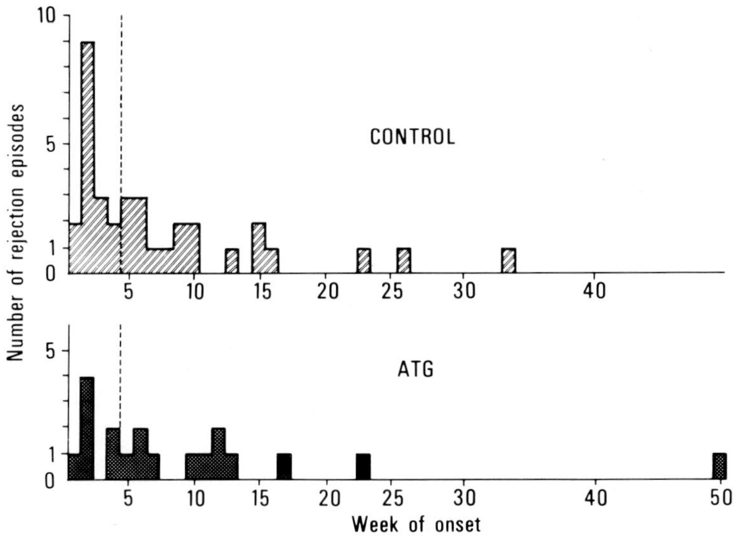

Fig. 7.3. Incidence and date of onset of renal failure episodes in patients treated with antithymocyte globulin (ATG) and in those receiving only conventional therapy (azathioprine + steroids).

and a high urinary sodium concentration may also be observed in some cases (Fig. 7.4).

These observations probably reflect two varieties of delayed renal failure: one which responds to steroids and is prevented by high doses of steroids immediately after transplantation, and the other which does not respond to steroids but still has a spontaneously favorable course in the majority of cases.

Thus, the clinical appearance of renal failure in the post-transplantation course is deeply affected by the quality, amount and timing of the administration of immunosuppressive drugs. The pathologic aspect of kidney sections taken during RFE is also modified. For example, when patients do not receive steroids, infiltration of large cells and edema are generally observed in the interstitium of a cadaver transplant during the first days or weeks after surgery in addition to vascular lesions.[160] With

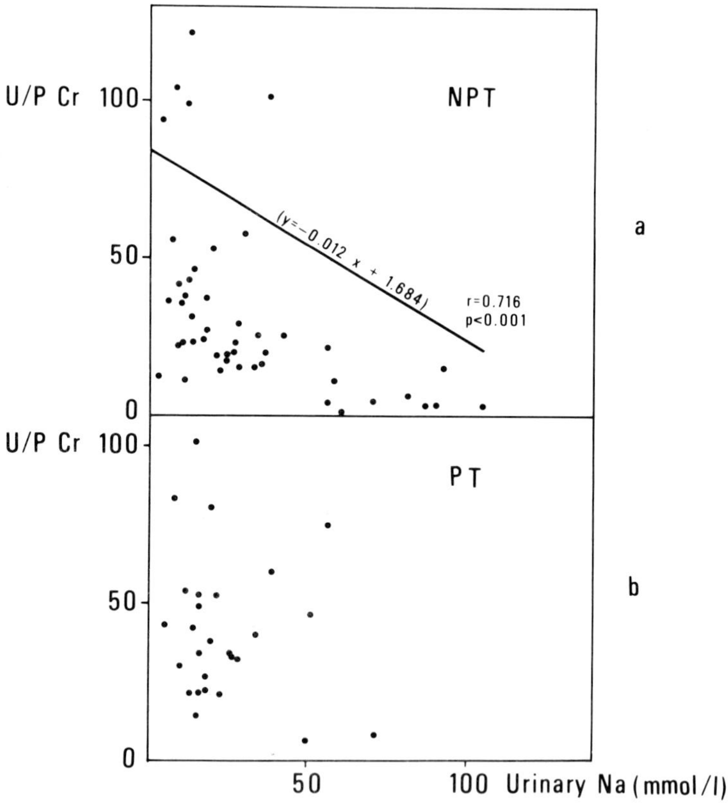

Fig. 7.4. Urine/plasma creatinine ratio and urine sodium at the onset of renal failure episodes in 1) patients pretreated with steroids (PT) and 2) patients not pretreated with steroids (NPT).

high doses of steroids, we did not detect significant cell infiltration and edema in the interstitium. Only vascular lesions were present and were similar to those observed in nonsteroid treated allograft recipients.[98]

On the contrary, once renal failure has occurred, its duration is not altered according to whether patients received steroids, ATG, azathioprine or a combination of drugs. Usually, when no extrarenal complications were detected, renal function began to improve in less than 6 days in the majority of patients. Recovery took more than 10 days in only 18% of our cases regardless of the type of treatment.[97] The severity of each RFE differs. Sometimes there is only a mild decline in renal function, attested by a slight increase in plasma creatinine level. On the other hand, oliguria or even anuria lasting for 1 to 3 days can also be observed; usually oliguria is followed by a rapid stepwise increment in urine volume and renal function, and the overall duration of the RFE is not longer than that in clinically minor episodes. In a few cases, however, severe vascular damage in the transplanted kidney can induce irreversible RFE, necessitating graftectomy. Similar episodes of irreversible renal failure occurring after the transplanted kidney has functioned for several days have been described in various reports.[54, 120, 160] It appears very difficult to assume that these episodes result from immunologic insult to the transplanted kidney, especially when they occur just a few days after surgery. In addition, it has also sometimes been observed that, when the two kidneys of a cadaver donor are transplanted by two different groups into recipients having different immunologic status, both recipients developed delayed irreversible renal failure. This is evidence for a nonimmunologic origin of this accident. On the other hand, it is clear that most of these accidents are likely to stem from an immunologic process, particularly when they occur around 8 to 10 days after grafting and when they are correlated with the appearance in the recipient serum of cytotoxic HLA antibodies specifically directed toward the donor antigens.[45]

Acute irreversible renal failure episodes are almost always the result of severe vascular lesions, whatever their origin. Diagnosis of these episodes is particularly difficult when the patient already has acute tubular necrosis. However, this type of RFE is best defined either by technetium scintiscans demonstrating the lack of the initial peak of radioactivity or by an angiographic "dead tree" image, the latter being almost reliable evidence.

The longer the time since grafting, the more unusual is the occurrence of acute RFE. Nevertheless, a few patients after a number of years of successful graft function do undergo either reversible or acute irreversible RFE. Because of their insidiousness, diagnosis of these accidents is possible only if patients are regularly checked for proteinuria, plasma creatinine, creatinine clearance and blood pressure. Treatment might still be effective, but in most instances complete recovery cannot be achieved and renal function will drop to a lower level. The slow development of RFE usually delays diagnosis and the institution of therapy, allowing the appearance of irreversible lesions.

Why late RFE can be severe enough to induce irreversible lesions is not well understood. Violent immunologic assault toward graft antigens by recipient immune systems is unlikely so long after transplantation. Non-HLA immune response, such as that to viral antigens cross reacting with graft antigens, is more likely. In many instances, RFE subsequent to infection is indistinguishable from those of graft rejection, even on kidney sections, where similar interstitial infiltrates of acute or chronic inflammatory cells may be associated with vascular lesions.

Chronic Renal Failure

A slowly progressing rise in serum creatinine level with a concomitant decrease in glomerular filtration rate can be observed in allograft recipients over a number of years. This is usually said to result from chronic graft rejection (see p. 210), despite the lack of any in vitro immunologic evidence of a permanent attack of the kidney target by a continuously developing immune process. The course of chronic renal failure is usually slow and its related complications appear progressively. Hypertension, anemia and hyperparathyroidism are among the most frequent and the earliest. Hypertension is often severe and difficult to control despite large amounts of antihypertensive drugs.

Since the transplanted kidney cannot generate a painful response to urinary pathway obstruction, it is of the utmost importance to detect the presence of any ureteral stone and/or stenosis in these cases.

The appearance of chronic renal failure always raises the question of its cause. Is it invariably the result of chronic rejection, or is it possible for initial nonimmunologic lesions of the kidney such as severe tubular necrosis and traumatic or ischemic vascular and glomerular changes to progress chronically toward interstitial fibrosis and fibrous endarteritis? An indirect positive response to this question can be found in many reports,[31, 142, 165] demonstrating that the mode of preservation has an important influence on graft survival (see Ch. Four) and that kidneys preserved by certain methods may give worse long-term graft survival than others. No valid evidence supporting or disproving this possibility can be furnished by comparing cadaver and living-donor grafts, since in the latter both histocompatibility and quality are better. However, the question remains important because in many cases chronic renal failure may be considered to be caused by rejection, leading to the maintenance or reintroduction of high amounts of immunosuppressive drugs. In our experience, as in that of others,[167] the withdrawal of azathioprine, when required by a complication related to this drug, is far from being harmful to the graft, even though its function was already chronically altered.[39]

It should be emphasized that biologic or immunologic studies performed in the recipient developing chronic renal failure unfortunately do not permit distinction of renal failure due to rejection from other disease processes. Even pathologic examination of kidney biopsies show only nonspecific lesions. Many nonimmunologic disorders of the kidney are marked by varying degrees of acute and chronic inflammation involving both vessels and interstitium, changes that can be seen in graft rejection as well.[160]

In conclusion, three major types of RFE can be described, according to their course:

1. *Irreversible renal failure,* which is almost always the consequence of severe vascular changes. It can occur immediately after surgery but is often delayed by a few days. It is the result either of rejection or of nonimmunologic trauma of the kidney. So far, no treatment has proved efficient and the transplant must be removed rapidly in order to avoid toxic complications.

2. *Reversible renal failure,* which, when it occurs in the *immediate postoperative phase,* usually is caused by acute tubular necrosis of nonimmunologic origin. This type of renal failure can be prevented and its course shortened by various types of routine preoperative treatment such as the use of high doses of furosemide and/or fluid loading of the recipient. Constant care in the management of the donor and in kidney removal are also necessary.

3. *Delayed reversible renal failure* is sometimes related to a specific nonimmunologic cause, even if not evident, but it is frequently idiopathic. Nevertheless, even in the latter case it is usually not possible to prove that this delayed failure is caused by an immunologic rejection process. This probably explains the confusing discrepancies reported by various authors in their attempts at immunologic monitoring of the transplant recipient.

One variety of idiopathic reversible renal failure is steroid-sensitive and occurs, in the absence of steroid therapy, within the first 5 days following transplantation. It can be prevented by the institution of high doses of steroids immediately after transplantation.

Another variety is steroid-independent, which occurs during the 2nd week following transplantation and has a spontaneously reversible course. It is highly probable that this type often represents the clinical expression of a rejection episode.

Graft Rejection

Until 1959, earlier attempts in that decade to transplant a cadaver kidney all led to more or less rapid destruction of the graft.[84, 101, 105] The impairment of renal function that occurred was considered to be the clinical feature of the rejection phenomenon. It is not surprising that thereafter all reversible renal failure episodes were labeled "rejection." Our group first proposed the term "rejection crisis" [72] to designate an acute alteration in transplant function which rapidly returned to the previous level, usually in response to the association of some therapy with the basic immunosuppressive treatment. In fact, any significant episode of rejection is associated with a measurable change in renal function, but this does not imply that every impairment in renal function originates in a rejection process. As discussed above, impaired renal function can be the result of a number of factors.

Transplant teams are thus faced with a major, still unsolved problem: to discriminate between rejection and other factors causing impairment of renal function. A large number of immunologic parameters have been assayed in vitro during renal failure episodes (see Ch. Six), but discrepancies are observed in the results from different centers using the same assay.[179] This lack of correlation is probably related to the heterogeneity of causes responsible for so-called "rejection episodes."

The description and classification of true rejection episodes is hindered by the fact that there are no pathognomonic data for rejection, whether clinical, biologic, immunologic, or even pathologic.

Another still unsolved question concerns the precise mechanisms by which the allograft is destroyed. Early work on graft rejection primarily concentrated on the cellular mechanisms. The initial reports of Medawar[127, 128] in the mid-40s emphasized the inflammatory cellular infiltration of the graft. It was believed that this represented the basic immune response of the host directed toward graft antigens. Graft rejection was consequently considered as a form of cellular immunity similar to delayed hypersensitivity, and cells found in the interstitium were thought to be the cause of graft rejection.

Later it was generally accepted that humoral immunity also plays an important role in allograft injury.[25, 150, 159, 178] Many reports have suggested that hyperacute or accelerated destruction of the kidney were more frequently observed in previously immunized recipients having developed circulating antidonor antibodies.[89, 144, 145] As vascular damage was predominant in this type of rejection,[24, 160] a correlation was made between the presence of antibodies and of vascular lesions.

Thus, a qualitative concept of transplant rejection, differentiating between cellular (tubulointerstitial) and humoral (vascular) rejection mechanisms was soon accepted. The first is responsible for the cellular infiltration of the kidney and the subsequent occurrence of fibrosis, whereas the second, involving the presence of antibodies directed against graft antigens, is responsible for hyperacute necrosis of the kidney.

Present Concept of Allograft Rejection

There is no doubt that the rejection reaction in an individual receiving an allograft is far from totaly suppressed by chemical immunosuppression. It is more intense when compatibility between donor and recipient is poor. Pre-existence of a sensitivity to some of the histocompatibility antigens of the donor exacerbates this reaction and occasionally renders it irreversible. On the other hand, in some patients it seems that the longer the recipient keeps his graft the more tolerance is shown with less and less evidence of rejection.

The classical description of human kidney allograft rejection usually comprises three main clinical types: 1) hyperacute and delayed hyperacute (or accelerated) rejection, 2) acute reversible rejection and 3) chronic rejection.[24, 35, 160, 186]

Hyperacute Rejection. The renal allotransplant can undergo hyperacute rejection within minutes of revascularization.[89] It becomes blue and flaccid rather than taking on the firm, pink aspect normally observed when the graft is revascularized. Because of this intraoperative decrease in blood flow through the graft, no urine appears and the kidney must be rapidly removed.

Today hyperacute-like rejection episodes are usually not observed until several days or weeks after the kidney has begun to function. This accident, described as the delayed hyperacute or accelerated rejection episode,[186] generally occurs between the 5th and 10th postsurgical day. Diuresis suddenly stops, the patient's temperature rises and there is localized pain at the site of the graft; total anuria ensues, accompanied by weight gain. If the kidney is not removed, a toxic syndrome occurs. It is first marked by a drop in WBC or platelet count and subsequently by marrow aplasia and can lead rapidly to death. Tardy removal of the transplant may fail to allow reversal of the toxic complications and may lead to a fatal outcome. Early diagnosis of hyperacute rejection is thus of the utmost importance; however, this type of rejection is difficult to distinguish from the course of a kidney that suffered a long agonal period in the donor, mishaps during removal or faulty preservation techniques. In these last two cases, renal failure is often reversible after several days or weeks of anuria. In fact, when the cross-match reaction between donor cells and recipient serum is clearly negative, as is now an imperative requirement for organ transplantation, immediate hyperacute rejection is quite rare and the "soft blue kidney" is likely to be the result of nonimmunologic injury.[13, 55, 102]

Arteriography is the method best suited to defining this type of rejection, or at least to differentiating between irreversible and reversible rejection.[25, 133] Early it may show slowing of the renal flow, demonstrated by the persistence of the contrast dye within the branches of the transplant arteries, although more distal peripheral arteries are already filled with the contrast dye or have even already disappeared. Early and explosive appearance of renal veins[78] is frequently seen on arteriograms performed during hyperacute rejection, but a similar image can also be observed during the course of fully reversible renal failure episodes. Their meaning remains unclear.[194] After a few days, patchy filling defects are present, mainly in the outer cortex; arterioles demonstrate irregularities and cut-off of distal branches, arcuate, interlobular or intralobular, giving rise to the end-stage image of a dead tree (Fig. 7.5). The nephrogram phase is pale, showing a corticonecrosis or, in some cases, multiple infarcts responsible for a fleecy aspect of the nephrogram.

Renal scintiscan and renogram, using both hippuric acid and technetium,[7, 103, 121, 173] have proved to be useful. The initial so-called vascular or perfusion phase, which follows the injection of the radiolabeled bolus, is particularly valuable.[187] The rapid appearance of the radioactive bolus in the kidney gives rise to a sharp peak on the activity curve. If this peak disappears, serious perfusion problems are certainly present and an arteriogram should be performed. It is thus usually possible to avoid repeating the angiogram.

The pathologic lesions (Fig. 7.5) are characteristic but certainly not pathognomonic of hyperacute rejection.[25, 26, 160] They are the consequence of circulating antibody binding to endothelial cell membrane bound HLA antigens, with prompt fixation of complement. This results in necrosis and lysis of endothelial cells (Fig. 7.6). Platelet and fibrin thrombi develop in close contact with either the basement membrane, as in peritubular capillaries, or in the media in larger vessels. Large numbers of polymorphonuclear leukocytes are seen in the injured area, infiltrating the vascular walls. This process progresses rapidly to thrombosis of the vessel lumen, leading to partial or total cortical necrosis (Fig. 7.7). In the interstitium, an intense congestion of the peritubular capillaries is generally seen during the early stage, often accompanied by multiple flame hemorrhages. In some situations there may well be neither edema nor cellular infiltration, in particular when thrombosis occurs rapidly and obstructs large vessels, or in patients who have received massive doses of corticosteroids.

Since the first lesions appear at the vascular endothelium in this type of rejection,[189] the term "vascular rejection" is sometimes used rather

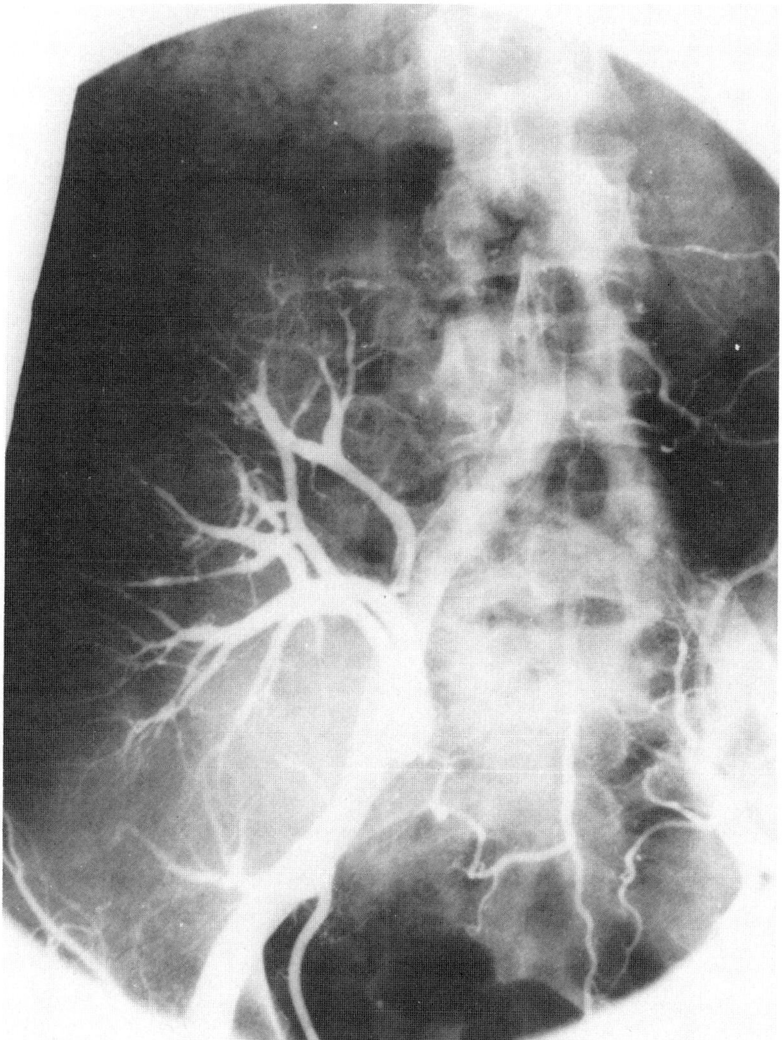

Fig. 7.5. Angiographic aspect of irreversible rejection. The "dead tree" image.

than hyperacute rejection. This vascular type of irreversible rejection with the same clinical, arteriographic and pathologic pictures occasionally occurs several weeks or even several months after transplantation.

The mechanism of hyperacute rejection is thought to be well established.[20, 160] It occurs when the recipient is preimmunized against HLA antigens of the donor,[149] as demonstrated by the presence of circulating antibodies in the serum of the recipient. Routine performance of cross-

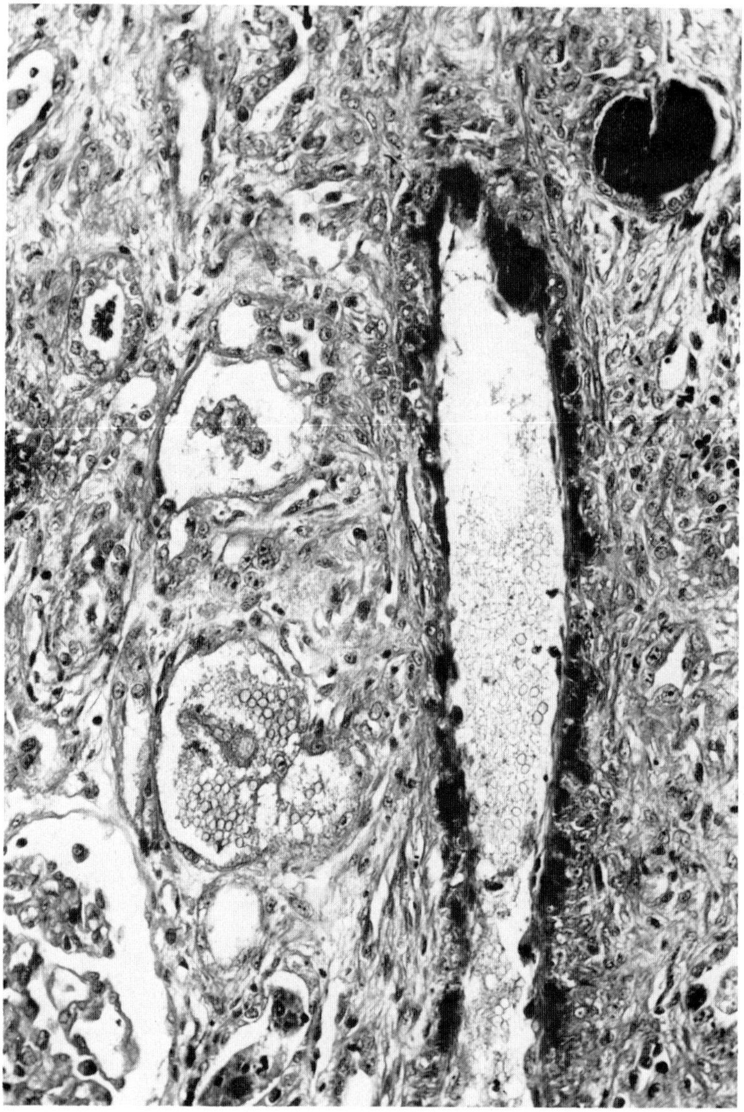

Fig. 7.6. Transplant biopsy 11 days after grafting. Fibrinoid necrosis of the entire muscle wall of an interlobular artery, interstitial oedema, tubular necrosis. Histologic appearance of severe rejection (original magnification × 300).

match between periodically collected recipient sera and donor lymphocytes will avoid most cases of this type of rejection, which is usually due to preimmunization by blood transfusions, pregnancy or previous grafts.

The interpretation of vascular rejection is much more difficult when

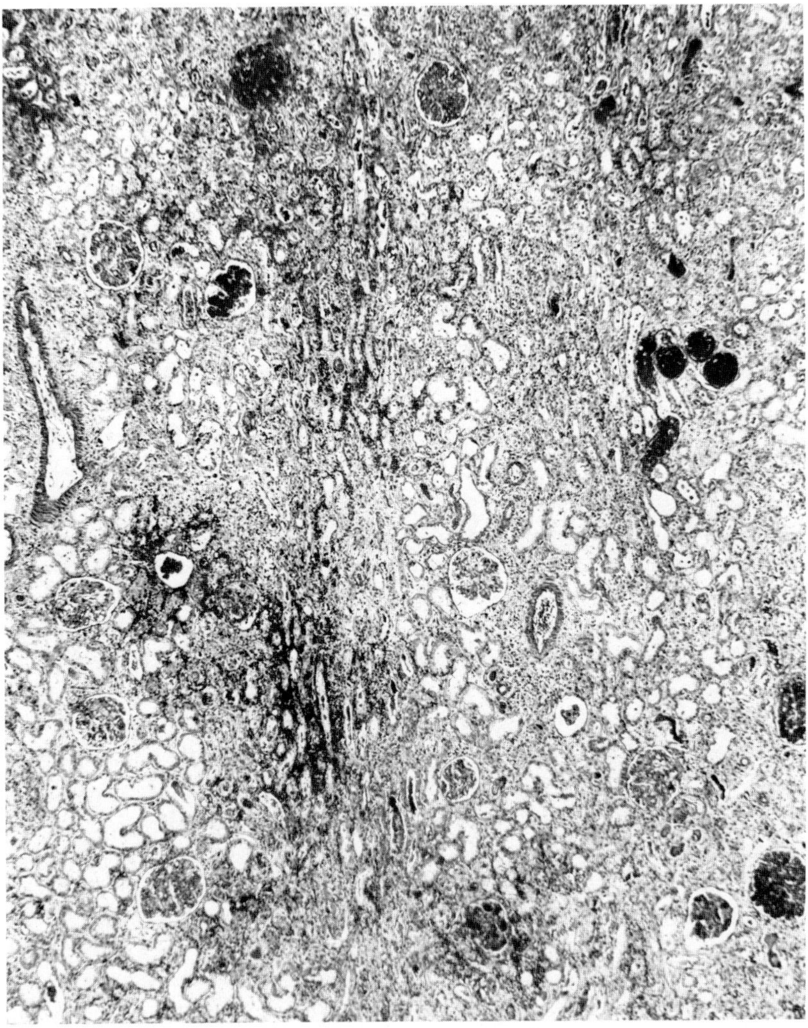

Fig. 7.7. Cadaver kidney transplantation. Hyperacute rejection episode. Ischemic and hemorrhagic necrosis of all the constituents of the renal parenchyma. Total necrosis of the transplant (original magnification × 130).

there is no antibody detectable in the recipient. In recipients who have been previously sensitized, it is possible to suggest that the cross-match test was not sensitive enough. However, presensitization can persist for several years despite the disappearance of circulating cytotoxic antibodies. In these cases transplantation produces a reactivation and a secondary immune response. This phenomenon could explain the finding by Terasaki et al[181] that the incidence of hyperacute rejection was much higher in those recipients who had preformed cytotoxic antibodies against a panel even though antibodies could not be detected against their specific donors.

When presensitization can definitely be excluded, it is difficult to explain how a primary immune response in an immunosuppressed individual would be sufficiently strong to produce immediate graft destruction. Thus, it may be suggested that nonimmunologic mechanisms may be involved. In fact, similar injury to vessels may be mediated by factors other than antibody directed at donor HLA antigens. Prolonged vascular collapse in the donor might be responsible for local clotting; multiple areas of necrosis, vascular necrosis, thrombosis and cortical necrosis may be the consequence of a variety of bacterial or viral infections. Some authors have suggested that the observed lesions might be due to a Schwartzman phenomenon.[175] The length of ischemia or the method of graft preservation have also been incriminated.[32, 76] Furthermore, renal lesions analogous to those found in hyperacute rejection have been observed in experimental rabbit autotransplantation.[114]

Finally, it is impossible to distinguish between these two hypotheses without clear evidence that preformed antibodies against the donor were not present in the recipient. Nor are the two necessarily exclusive, because pre-existing lesions in the kidney as a result of ischemia or other nonimmunologic factors could contribute to or even increase the harmful effect of cytotoxic antibodies. Delayed hyperacute rejection is more likely to be the result of the immunologic process of rejection as they are often correlated with the appearance in recipient serum of cytotoxic HLA antibodies directed against HLA-A and B[45] or DR(D-related)[171] antigens present in the donor, which were not present prior to transplantation. Thus, we think that so-called "immediate" hyperacute rejection is, at least in cross-match negative transplantation, almost always delayed. They might give the impression of being immediate when they occur in patients who already had acute tubular necrosis.

Acute Rejection. The existence of post-transplantation rejection episodes which are reversible, either by appropriate therapy or even spontaneously, is accepted by all authors. Described for the first time in 1959[72] as "crise du transplant," they have since been commonly labeled "acute rejection episode'" denoting an episode of reversible rejection in the patient's clinical course.[28, 160, 186] These episodes, which are by far the most common form of rejection, can occur at any time after grafting. However, they are most frequent during the first 2 weeks following surgery. Their inception and their manifestations can vary[97] depending on the immunosuppressive protocol. They can sometimes be triggered by a too rapid withdrawal of or even a decrease in steroids.

It is during the course of these early acute rejection episodes that clinical manifestations are most clearly seen.[10] This is particularly true in either living related or cadaver kidney recipients who had not been started on corticoid therapy. In a few hours or days, diuresis stops, the volume of the transplant increases and the patient's temperature and arterial blood pressure rise. Renal function diminishes, as attested by a rise in serum creatinine level. Most often, although previous values were already low because of sodium restriction, urinary sodium excretion decreases still further. This drop is more clearly observed at the very beginning of rejection, and sometimes even before the serum creatinine rises. It probably reflects a decreased renal blood flow, which is the first consequence of rejection. Later, tubular cell alteration or necrosis will modify sodium excretion. The patient's initial weight gain is probably the consequence both of renal failure and of exaggerated sodium reabsorption. Proteinuria usually reappears if it had already disappeared. In the absence of proteinuria, the diagnosis of an acute rejection episode should be made only with the utmost caution.

None of these clinical manifestations are pathognomonic for rejection, and despite a multitude of procedures monitoring renal injury (see below) and attempting to monitor the immunologic processes (see Ch. Six), the daily determination of serum urea and creatinine concentrations remains the best indicator.[186]

The symptomatology of reversible late rejection episodes develops much more slowly and is much less marked. The most important sign is the reappearance of proteinuria, even very slight, and a mild increase in the level of serum creatinine. But several diseases of the transplant, other than rejection, can lead to similar disorders.

More important is the fact that these rejection episodes can be totally latent and only discovered fortuitously by routine renal biopsy in patients with normal and stable renal function. On a routine 6-month biopsy (Fig. 7.8), we were surprised to find in many of our patients histologic changes very suggestive of rejection, with interstitial edema and heavy cellular infiltration, although routine clinical and laboratory studies were completely normal. Whether this pathologic aspect is the hallmark of latent rejection episodes requiring treatment or is merely an inflammatory process developing in the transplanted kidney remains an unresolved but important question. In some instances where patients were then submitted to the classical steroid treatment used for rejection, subsequent biopsy showed an improved aspect, but this is not proof that the long-term outcome was modified in any way. Furthermore, it is highly probable that steroids act more by an anti-inflammatory effect than by creating a high degree of immunodepression.

Pathology of Acute Reversible Rejection. The traditional description of transplant biopsies performed during acute reversible episodes empha-

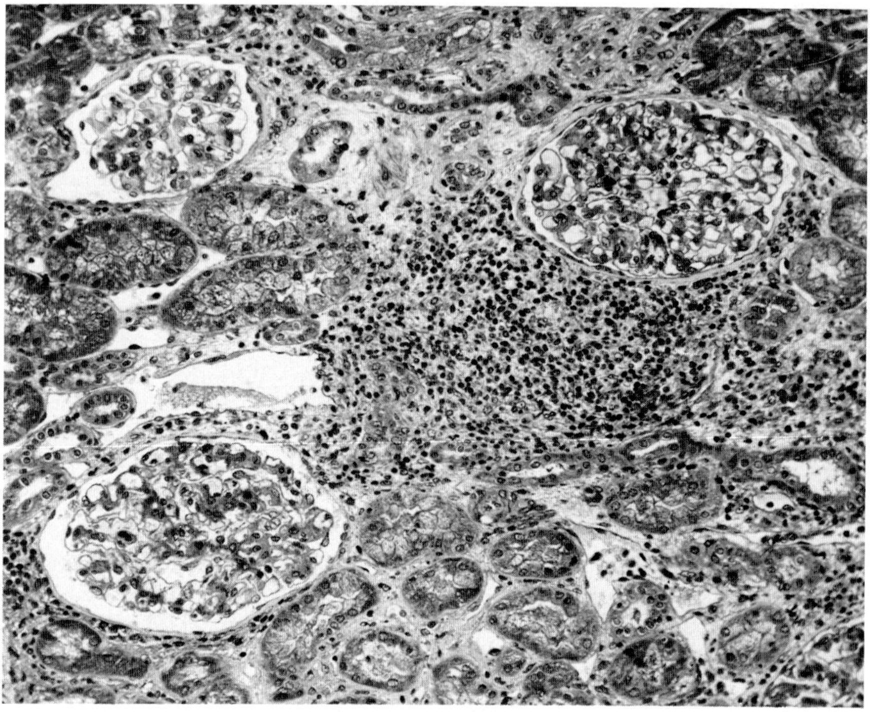

Fig. 7.8. Transplant biopsy 6 months after grafting. Localized infiltration of lymphoid and plasma cells. The interstitial tissue, glomeruli and tubules are normal (original magnification × 210).

sizes the prevalance of interstitial lesions, which are generally considered characteristic.[35, 38, 44, 69, 77, 110, 177] The interstitial tissue is considerably altered by marked and diffuse edema, with diffuse infiltration of small round cells (Fig. 7.9), particularly marked in foci which are generally perivascular. The peritubular capillaries are dilated and contain the same round cells.

Study of these cells by electron microscopy[57, 137] shows that they consist of lymphocytes, plasma cells, macrophages, polymorphs with occasional basophils and blast cells which are similar to transformed lymphocytes found in mixed lymphocyte cultures. It has been emphasized by Rowlands et al[160] that, contrary to what its name might suggest in terms of the concepts of general pathology, acute rejection is not marked by any significant number of granulocytes. Although the cellular exudate felt to represent cell-mediated injury dominates the changes seen in these patients, it has more recently been demonstrated that vascular lesions are quite frequently if not always, observed.[151, 160, 188] They consist in necrosis of only isolated smooth muscles in some cases, or in various

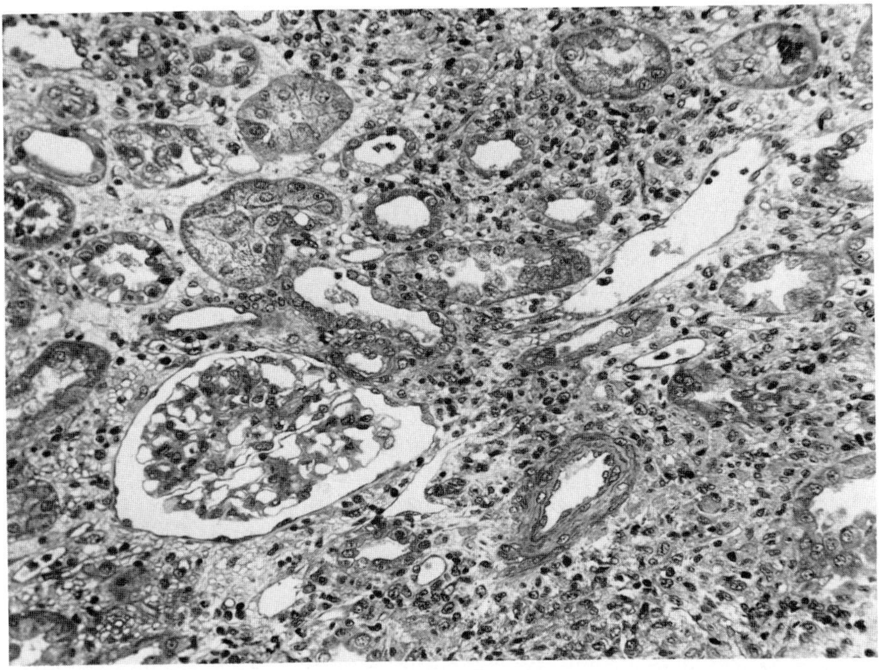

Fig. 7.9. Histologic appearance of reversible acute rejection episode. Diffuse interstitial edema and extensive infiltration by lymphoids and plasma cells. Normal glomeruli, tubules and blood vessels (original magnification × 250).

endothelial cell lesions in others (lysis, fibrinoid necrosis, hyperplasia).[160] The internal elastic lamina may focally disappear, with fibrinoid necrosis in the media. Microthrombosis is probably the late consequence of vascular injury.

Glomerular and tubular lesions may also occasionally be seen, the latter probably being the result of kidney ischemia subsequent to vascular lesions.

IgG, IgA, C_3 or IgG, IgM, C_3 and fibrinogen are more frequently found in the kidney during the course of rejection episodes than in biopsies taken when function is stable.[116]

Immunofluorescent studies performed by Berger et al[16] on biopsy material taken from our patients during acute rejection episodes showed deposits of IgG, IgM and C_3, either confined to the glomeruli or in the arterioles and vessels, in nearly 50% of cases undergoing acute rejection and in only 27% of biopsies taken outside of these episodes.

Mechanisms of Acute Reversible Rejection. Host immune responses, stimulated by allotransplantation, are responsible for acute attack of the kidney target because such episodes do not occur during transplantation between monozygous twins. The exact nature of the phenomenon, however, remains uncertain. It is now well established that the antiallograft reaction depends both on cell-mediated and on antibody-mediated responses of the host.[150, 160] Blast transformation of the host lymphocytes and the presence of specifically cytotoxic lymphocytes inside the graft has been well established, even if these phenomena are not reflected in the circulating blood and can thus not be used as a routine test by the clinician. Moreover, lymphocytes may be assisted by the nonspecific effect of "activated" macrophages (see p. 6), as suggested in man by the presence of numerous macrophages in graft biopsies.[137]

Parameters Used in the Assessment of Acute Rejection. Clinical evaluation of the post-transplant patient is important in diagnosing rejection, but renal failure due to rejection still cannot be distinguished from other disease processes, either by clinical and biological study of the graft or by the various assays for monitoring the immunologic response of the recipient (see p. 163). The various nonimmunologic parameters used to assess rejection all reflect tissue damage, whether tubular, interstitial, glomerular or vascular, but none is well correlated with a precise cause of kidney lesions. The main parameters are the following:

1. The Level of Renal Function. The most universally accepted marker for kidney transplant rejection is a rise in serum creatine level, reflecting a drop in renal function. Renal clearance determinations, as well as a variety of other assays of renal function, are also available. Their performance is much more complicated and more expensive, and they are less reliable than the daily determination of serum creatinine concentrations[28, 120, 186] when patients are followed serially in the same laboratory. Patients having a rise in serum creatinine concentration can only be classified as having impaired renal function, however, and this, of course, has many causes.

2. Urinary Parameters. a. Proteinuria, especially when it is nonselective and recurs after initial disappearance, strongly suggests rejection but is also commonly seen during glomerulonephritis (recurrent or de novo), pyelonephritis, obstructive uropathy, and so on.

b. The presence of a clump of lymphocytes, of red cell casts or of fibrin fragments is far from diagnostic.

c. The presence of lactate dehydrogenase (LDH) or lysozymuria has not been of substantial value in diagnosing rejection and probably represents only tubular damage, whatever its origin, and inflammatory lesions of the kidney.[120]

d. Low concentration of urinary sodium[28,, 186] is only the expression of decreased renal blood flow. Furthermore, since some degree of tubular damage often exists as a result of ischemia at the time of transplantation, or rapidly occurs after rejection when there is a large reduction in renal blood flow, the significance of urinary sodium concentration can be ambiguous.

3. Clinical Parameters. a. Fever, tenderness and increased size of the kidney and a rise in blood pressure may be present in complications other than rejection and may be considerably modified by the amount of steroids received by the patient at the onset of rejection.

b. Oliguria and subsequent weight gain is characteristic only of altered renal function and may be the consequence of obstruction, ureteric leak, infection, decreased renal blood flow, etc. Moreover, diuresis can persist from the patient's own kidneys and mask oliguria.

c. Leukocytosis may also occur but is certainly not a reliable monitor of rejection.[37]

d. ^{131}I Hippuric acid or technetium renogram and scintiscan[7, 123, 161] can be informative as to renal blood flow and tubular function but are in no way a reliable index of rejection. It is sometimes an early parameter indicating improvement in renal function in an oliguric patient.

e. Intravenous pyelography is helpful for excluding a nonimmunologic cause of renal failure such as urinary leak or obstructive uropathy, but it may result in further transient deterioration of renal function. Ultrasound scans are therefore much more useful and more reliable, particularly since they can also assess the absence of perirenal collections such as hematoma, abscess or lymphocele. They are also noninvasive and can be performed as often as necessary.

f. *Transplant biopsy* performed during a clinically assumed rejection episode cannot alone provide pathognomonic evidence for rejection. Interstitial edema and infiltration of polymorphs, lymphocytes or plasma cells are evidence only of inflammation. Vascular lesions are more likely to be the result of rejection, but various other diseases may also result in similar vascular changes. In our group renal biopsy is routinely performed during renal failure episodes, but it provides only support to other evidence. Some groups[143] have stressed the value of fine needle aspiration biopsy, which is said to give reliable data. As it is less invasive than ordinary percutaneous or open biopsy, it can be performed as often as necessary. Biopsy can provide an idea, however, as to the long-term prognosis of the graft. If vascular lesions (endothelial cell proliferation or vascular necrosis) associated with congestive blood-filled capillaries or interstitial hemorrhage are present, the prognosis is poor, whatever the origin of the lesion. Similarly, when large areas of fibrosis are seen throughout the biopsy sections, it can be assumed that treatment will be ineffective. Finally, none of the pathologic lesions observed during rejection episodes can be considered specific to rejection because pathological aspects similar to all of them have also been described in experimental kidney allotransplantation.[114]

g. *Angiography* will give information as to the extent of vascular changes, the presence of cortical infarct and the rate of blood flow through the renal artery. It will elucidate the declining renal function, but again it will be inadequate evidence of rejection.

Treatment of Acute Rejection. The diagnosis of an acute rejection episode not only has theoretical importance but it usually also represents an event considered to require modification of the baseline immunosuppressive therapy. Acute rejection is treated in much the same manner by most transplant groups. Glucocorticoids are either increased or instituted, and high doses are always used (see p. 103). Azathioprine is generally unaltered, and adjunctive therapy (local irradiation, antilymphocyte serum or heparin) is seldom used. Since steroid related complications are still the major cause of death and morbidity after transplantation, the question of its necessity can reasonably be raised. We have already shown[98] that steroids are probably effective only in treating inflammatory lesions and thus cannot drastically modify the appearance and course of rejection. On the other hand, the rejection process certainly begins long before serum creatinine levels rise, and ideally it should be halted before changes occur in the kidney. We found that a potent antithymocyte globulin prevented the occurrence of most rejection episodes as long as it was administered.[99] It thus appears that: 1) immunosuppressive drugs are more efficient in preventing the occurrence of rejection than in its treatment once it is clinically established; and 2) corticosteroids probably have a mild immunosuppressive effect but a high anti-inflammatory effect.

Chronic Rejection. Independent of acute rejection episodes, whose frequency diminishes with time, there is a constant immunologic conflict between host and transplant, which results from imperfect immunosuppression and defective donor-recipient histocompatibility. This clinically and biologically latent conflict is detectable on repeat biopsy specimens, which show progressive destruction of the transplant. During the course of this destruction, the lesions can be vascular, interstitial and/or glomerular.[150, 160]

Arterial Lesions (Fig. 7.10). The severity of the arterial lesions plays the most important role in determining the survival of the transplant. Narrowing of the arterial and arteriolar lumen by hyperplasia of intimal cells or frank proliferation and then by fibrosis of the media is the most striking morphologic lesion. Disruption and thickening of the lamina elastica interna, which may even disappear, may also be seen as the residue of fibrinoid necrosis. It is frequently associated with the progressive destruction of the transplant. Immunofluorescence microscopy usually shows a positive fluorescence for fibrin.[25, 160] There may also be staining for C_3 or for C_3 and IgM.

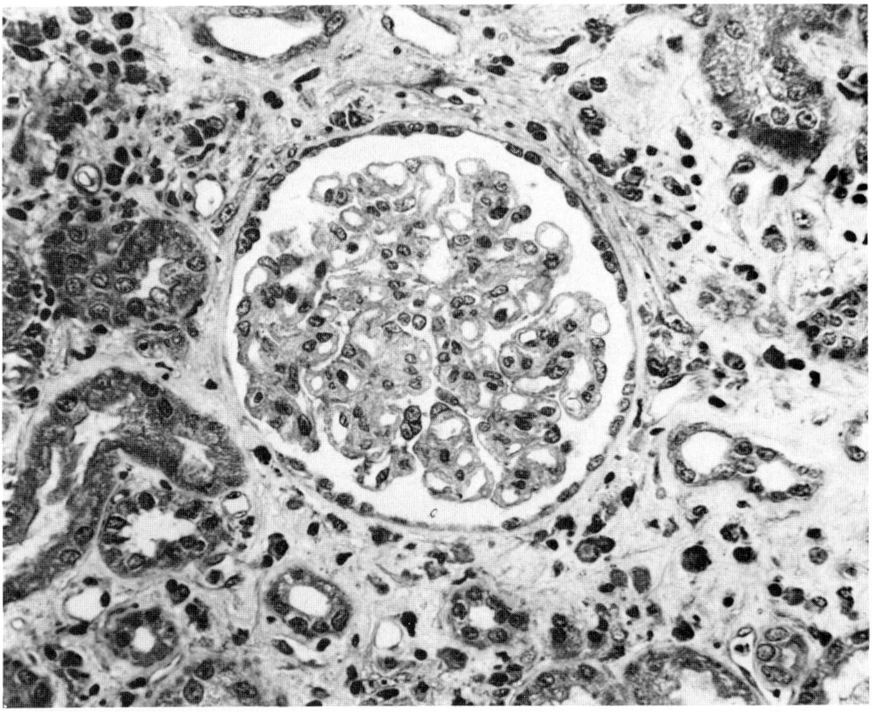

Fig. 7.12. Transplant biopsy specimen 4 years after grafting. Glomerular changes related to chronic rejection. Diffuse thickening of the glomerular basement membranes and enlargement of the intercapillary regions (original magnification × 570).

basement membrane is often irregular and the foot processes of the epithelial cells are often fused. Subendothelial deposits, intercapillary proliferation and glomerular fibrosis can also be observed. The immunoglobulin and complement deposits found in a transplanted kidney are not always associated with proliferative glomerulonephritis and can occasionally disappear after several years. These observations must be taken into consideration when interpreting the relationships that might exist between the deposits and lesions occurring in spontaneous glomerulonephritis.

Their significance is still unknown. Because of the immunoglobulin deposits, it has been suggested that circulating immune complexes could be induced by the antigraft response of the host. However, the relationship between immune deposits and glomerular lesions has not been completely elucidated in these cases. On the one hand, immunoglobulin and complement deposits may be found in transplanted kidneys with no glomerular lesions, inducing no glomerular cell proliferation at any time. Conversely, little or no immunoglobulin or complement deposition may be found, despite glomerular cell proliferation and other alterations in the glomerulus.[70]

In our experience, "rejection" glomerulonephritis is not incompatible with normal and stable renal function for several years. The only abnormality detected is marked proteinuria, which occasionally may lead to a nephrotic syndrome and, occasionally also, to microscopic hematuria.

Toward a New Concept of Graft Rejection

In recent years evidence has accumulated that vascular changes are common in many, if not in all, renal allografts. First to be observed were thickened vascular walls in long-standing renal allografts. It was soon demonstrated, however, that acute vascular alterations were frequent in human renal allografts undergoing acute rejection, even in the absence of patent preimmunization of the recipient.[25, 160, 186] Whether the vascular injury comes about solely as the result of direct antigen-antibody interaction is still uncertain. Accumulating evidence strongly suggests that some of the vascular lesions induced by rejection may be produced not only by antibodies or various mediators (lymphotoxins, chemotactic factors, platelet activating factors, histamine, etc.) but also by lymphocytes, and in particular by primed lymphocytes.[151, 186]

The vascular endothelial cells of the graft are in fact the first target for any type of "killer agent" directed toward the graft antigens. It is now well known that endothelial cells demonstrate many antigenic determinants, among which are the ABO blood group antigens, the HLA-A, B and DR antigens, and some recently described non-HLA endothelial antigens also present on monocytes.[136, 146] Thus, there is binding of circulating antibodies and complement, as well as cytotoxic cells, to endothelial or muscle cell membrane bound antigens. The subsequent cell membrane injury will result in altered permeability and surface properties of vascular cells, with two further possibilities:

1. Vascular cell changes are irreversible, leading to cell death. In the areas of injured endothelium, platelets aggregate, releasing platelet factors and activating fibrinogen. This can result in vascular thrombosis and infarction of the supplied area, or in complete cortical necrosis when endothelial damage extends throughout vascular branches. This type of rejection corresponds to what is generally described as hyperacute or accelerated rejection, but here circulating antibodies are not the only factor involved.

2. Endothelial changes are less severe and less disseminated. The capillary and arteriolar lumen is focally narrowed, giving rise to increased vascular resistance and decreased renal blood flow, resulting in kidney ischemia. Endothelial damage secondary to both immunologic killer

agents and ischemia may lead to disruption of the capillary walls and/or to increased permeability with leakage of fluid and cells into the interstitium. Tubular necrosis may also be the consequence of decreased blood supply to the tubular cells. The clinical appearance will be that of acute renal failure because of the decreased renal blood flow and possible tubular changes. Within a few days, endothelial swelling will decrease, and organization of thrombus and fibrinolysis occurs. The vascular lumen reopens, leading to improved renal blood flow. Renal function improves and serum creatinine concentration returns to the previous level. When ischemia was severe enough to induce acute tubular necrosis, recovery will take a few more days. The interstitial inflammatory reaction to vascular wall damage probably acts as an amplifier of rejection by increasing intraparenchymal resistance and thus resulting in a further drop in renal blood flow.

Corticosteroids, which are a potent anti-inflammatory agent, can abolish the interstitial reaction or prevent its appearance if they are instituted before the inception of the rejection process. In the former case, renal function will improve after the institution of steroid therapy, more especially as vascular lesions are mild and inflammatory reaction severe. In the latter case, only the vascular component will be reponsible for renal failure and will not be modified by any alterations in the steroid regimen. On the other hand, a potent immunosuppressive agent should be able to prevent some rejection episodes when given before the appearance of lesions, whereas after their appearance it will be ineffective.

When a patient developing a rejection episode is not treated by either steroids or any kind of potent nonsteroid anti-inflammatory drug, the course of the vascular lesion will probably not be modified. Instead, interstitial lesions will progress to fibrosis and chronic renal failure.

In this hypothesis,[96] rejection appears a unique phenomenon, more or less severe, and with more or less acute destruction of transplant vascular walls, resulting in various secondary lesions (interstitial inflammatory reaction, vascular thrombosis with infarction, cortical necrosis, or fibrous endarteritis). Chronic rejection represents the association of permanent uncontrolled and latent aggression of the transplant vessels and the progressing sequelae of the early acute attacks.

If this concept is correct, steroids should be: 1) unable to prevent the occurrence of rejection; 2) unnecessary in the treatment of the major and primary lesion subsequent to rejection, i.e., the vascular lesion; and 3) replaced by a nonsteroid anti-inflammatory agent. We have recently shown[98] that when high doses of steroids (5 mg/kg body wt/day po) are given to allograft recipients as of the day of surgery, the incidence of renal failure episodes is not significantly different from that observed in a control group of recipients receiving no steroids at all. These accidents spontaneously resolved even though steroid dosage was reduced during the course of the episode. We have also shown that ATG prevented the occurrence of most reversible acute RFE and that steroids failed to do so. In a new study we are now using a nonsteroid anti-inflammatory agent in addition to ATG as a substitute for steroids.

The first results are encouraging, as illustrated by the course of one patient who received no steroids, had an episode of spontaneously reversible renal failure and now has normal function, 5 months later (Fig. 7.13). On the other hand, we have reversed the course of acute delayed renal RFE without altering the maintenance steroid regimen, although very severe vascular lesions were seen by angiography, through the continuous infusion of dopamine for 10 days at a dose of 2 μg/kg/min. We feel that dopamine, acting as a vasodilator, both increased renal blood flow, thus improving renal function, and prevented the appearance of arteriolar thrombosis.

In fact, injury to vessels may be mediated by factors other than immunologically generated "killer agents" directed against transplantation antigens. Prolonged ischemic time of the donor kidney or infectious complications in the recipient, for example, might produce sufficient vascular injury to promote vascular necrosis, local clotting, patchy infarction or cortical necrosis. Finally, we are still faced with the same problem: the lack of specific criteria to differentiate between rejection and nonimmunologic lesions in the transplant.

Glomerulonephritis of the Transplanted Kidney

Since 1963[62] several authors have reported recurrence in a transplanted kidney of the glomerulonephritis (GN) which was responsible for the destruction of the recipient's own kidneys.[48, 56, 61, 82, 153] The report by Glassock et al[61] of recurrence of the original GN in a series of renal transplantations between identical twins was strong evidence that the glomerular disease of the transplant was actually a recurrence of the patient's initial GN and not a feature of rejection. The very high incidence of GN recurrence (61%) and its severity in Glassock's series was not found, however, in subsequent series and in allografts, raising the possibility that immunosuppressive drugs may exert some protective effect.

In 1969 our group[68] described another type of glomerular lesion in renal allografts when the patient's own kidneys had been destroyed by a dissimilar disease (e.g. hereditary GN, pyelonephritis or congenital abnormalities). We suggested that this could be a form of rejection. This "rejection glomerular disease" was confirmed by Porter[153] and many others (see p. 212).

In addition to these two main causes of glomerular damage in renal grafts, other possibilities include "de novo" GN.[22, 23, 170]

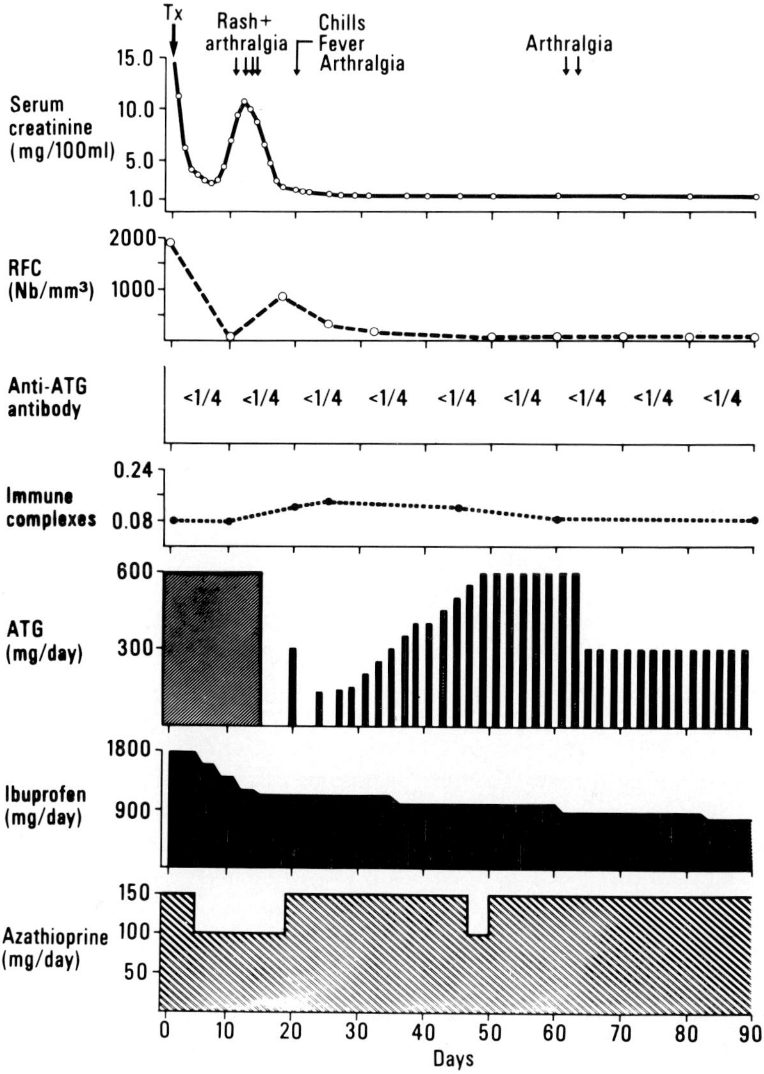

Fig. 7.13. First 3 months post-transplantation course of a patient treated with antithymocyte globulin (ATG) and ibuprofen rather than steroids.

Transmission of the Patient's Original Glomerulonephritis to the Graft

The main types of chronic GN subject to recurrence in the graft are the nephrotic syndrome with focal glomerular sclerosis, membranous GN, membranoproliferative GN, rapidly progressive GN and Immunoglobulin A (IgA) mesangial deposits. In a recent study of our first 500 allograft recipients,[70] recurrence was observed in 17.5% of 166 patients whose own kidneys had been destroyed by GN (Table 7.5). The subsequent course, however, was far from severe in all these cases.

Recurrence of the Nephrotic Syndrome with Focal and Segmental Glomerulosclerosis. Recurrence was observed in 4 out of 14 allografted patients in our series. Similar results have been reported by Hoyer et al,[80] Habib[66] and many others.[27] Special features usually characterize recurrence in these cases. Massive proteinuria, often seen in the hours immediately following transplantation, may be followed rapidly by a nephrotic syndrome, which is often uninfluenced by corticosteroids. Biopsy shows only minimal changes during this initial stage. Some months later segmental and focal sclerosis of the graft glomeruli may appear, with focal deposits of IgM, C_3 and rarely IgG. Loss of the graft due to recurrence is far from constant. In two patients receiving a second transplant, immediate recurrence was seen in the second as well as in the first graft. In this form of GN, recurrence seems more frequent and severe the shorter was the course of the primary disease toward renal failure.

Focal and segmental glomerulosclerosis with the nephrotic syndrome has sometimes, however, been observed in failing allografts of patients whose original renal disease was not focal glomerulosclerosis;[51] it has then been considered the result of chronic rejection with associated nephrotic syndrome.

Recurrence of Membranous Glomerulonephritis. Recurrence has very rarely been reported in GN with extramembranous deposits. According to Cameron and Turner,[27] evidence of recurrence is firmly established in only two published cases.[27] It may seem surprising that recurrence appears rare in a type of GN considered a result of circulating immune complexes, whose formation may continue for a long time. But

TABLE 7.5
Incidence of recurrent glomerulonephritis (GN) *in the series of Necker Hospital*

Type of GN	No. of Patients	No. of Cases With Recurrence
Focal and segmental glomerulosclerosis	14	4
Membranous GN	2	0
Membranoproliferative GN with sub-endothelial deposits	23	2
Membranoproliferative GN with isolated C_3 deposits	4	3
Membranoproliferative GN, lobular form	13	2
Dense deposits disease	11	8
Rapidly progressive GN	1	0
IgA mesangial deposits	20	9
Shönlein-Henoch purpura	6	1
Unclassified GN	72	—
Total	166	29

it must be pointed out that membranous GN often has a benign or slow course so that a limited number of cases require transplantation.

Recurrence of Membranoproliferative Glomerulonephritis. In the common form of membranoproliferative GN with subendothelial deposits, the study of recurrence is difficult because clinical and pathologic findings are similar to those of the "rejection glomerular disease" described above. In our series, only 2 of 23 cases were classified as certain recurrences. More frequent, or perhaps more easily demonstrated, was recurrence in the three special forms which follow.

Membranoproliferative GN with C_3 deposits (no immunoglobulin deposit) is prone to recur with the same immunofluorescent pattern and persistently low level of C_3 in the serum. In our cases, clinical manifestations were limited and the course was benign.

In the *"lobular" type of proliferative nephritis*, an identical lesion can appear on the allograft. This was observed in 2 of 13 transplanted patients (Fig. 7.14). One of these cases was studied with serial biopsies. There first appeared mesangial deposits of IgG and C_3, then subepithelial deposits, and only thereafter endocapillary proliferation and formation of lobular nodules. This observation of the development of a nephritis in a normal kidney is of course important for the understanding of spontaneous GN.[67]

Finally, the "*dense deposits disease*" described by Galle and Berger in 1963, associating endocapillary proliferation with intramembranous, electron-dense deposits of a still unknown substance, recurs in a large number of cases: 8 patients of 11 in our series and at least 18 others in the literature.[77, 183] The recurrent lesion can remain latent, but nevertheless these cases are evidence that the lesion depends upon some systemic factors. The serum C_3 level, which is almost constantly low in this disease, may either remain low or return to normal after transplantation, even when biopsy shows development of the membrane lesion. In addition, C_3 nephritic factor (NF) serum activity, commonly detected in this type of GN, often disappears soon after transplantation.[49]

Recurrence of Rapidly Progressive (Malignant) Glomerulonephritis. Most studies concern cases of crescentic GN with linear IgG deposits along the glomerular capillary wall, with or without anti-glomerular basement membrane (GBM) antibodies detectable in the serum or in kidney eluates.[14, 47, 49, 107, 191] In such cases, a similar linear IgG fixation has been reported in the transplanted kidney, with or without crescent formation. This has been seen even in patients with no circulating anti-GBM antibodies, although they were found in transplant eluates.[34] These patients may show clinical manifestations, but several cases of recurrent linear deposits without kidney damage have been reported.[14] Dixon and Wilson[47, 191] report that in 15 patients with anti-GBM disease (excluding Goodpasture's syndrome), 6 showed clinical or

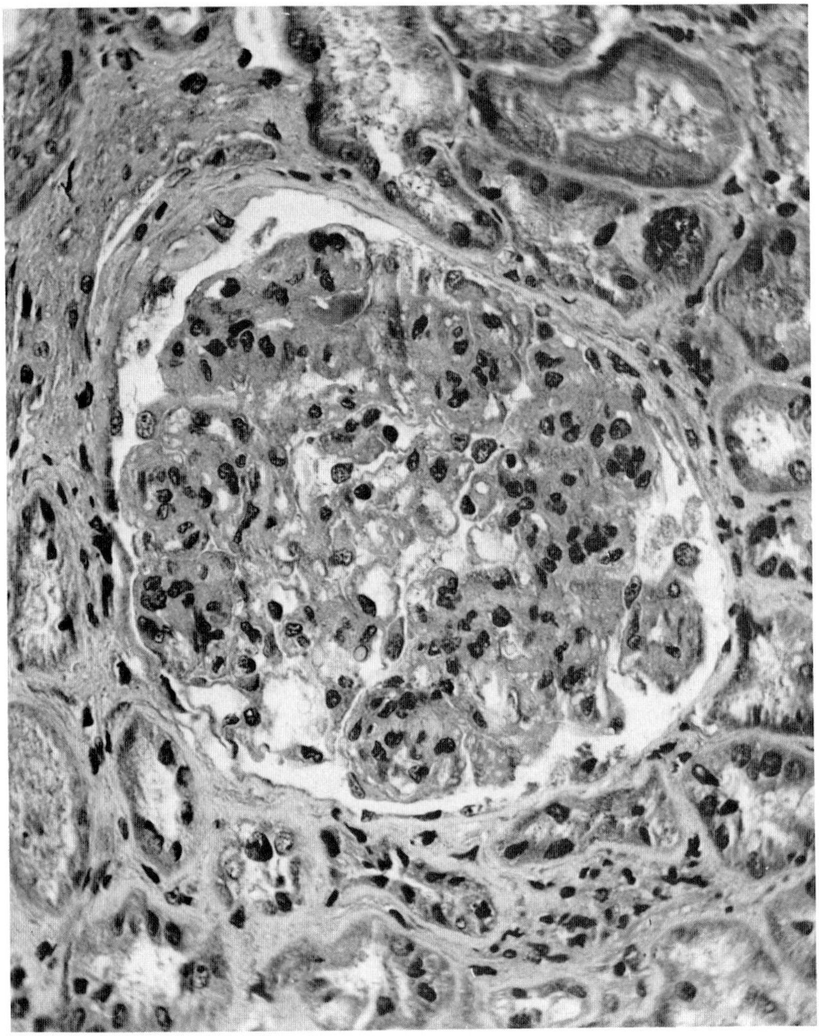

Fig. 7.14. Kidney biopsy 18 months after transplantation. Recurrent glomerulitis, marked proliferation of endothelial cells. The tuft has a lobulated appearance. Many early centrolobular nodules. The original disease in the recipient was a lobular glomerulonephritis (original magnification × 870).

immunofluorescent evidence of recurrence and graft failure ensued in at least 3. Anti-GBM antibodies may fix on the graft within minutes after transplantation[107] but when no linear IgG fixation is found on the first biopsy, it never appears subsequently.

Goodpasture's syndrome may also be mentioned in this regard. The 1971 Human Renal Transplant Registry reported 12 patients with this syndrome having undergone transplantation: in 8 of them the graft was unaltered after 3 months to 5 years.

Recurrence of IgA Mesangial Deposits. Also seen to recur in the transplant is the special form of glomerulonephritis described by Berger in 1969, associating diffuse mesangial deposits of IgA and IgG with usually segmental and focal glomerular lesions. Early IgA mesangial deposits were seen in 9 of 20 patients in our series[16] and in two patients reported by Mathew et al.[126] The diffuse IgA deposits often remain latent with excellent allograft function for as long as 8 years after transplantation.

Recurrence of Glomerulonephritis Associated with a Systemic Disease. Interestingly enough, some types of secondary GN associated with a systemic disease may have a low incidence of recurrence, if any. We have already mentioned Goodpasture's syndrome. The 1975 Renal Transplant Registry[2] reports 56 patients with systemic lupus receiving renal transplants and never showing recurrence either on biopsy specimens or autopsy material. The concept that circulating immune complexes explain most cases of GN is not supported by observations on transplanted kidneys. In the GN of Schönlein-Henoch purpura, only three cases of recurrence have been reported (see references in Levy et al[109]). Of six patients in our series, only one showed histologic evidence of recurrence.

The fact that a potential recipient has a type of GN that can recur is not a contraindication to transplantation. It has been established that in those types with a high incidence of recurrence (such as GN with dense deposits) the overall prognosis is not modified, and that in the other types recurrence is neither constant nor always severe. One can, however, suggest that only cadaver kidneys be transplanted to patients having rapidly progressive focal glomerusclerosis.

De Novo Glomerulonephritis

When GN develops following hepatitis B,[170] glomerular alterations provoked by the administration of antilymphocyte serum[23] or transplantation of kidneys already altered by latent GN,[22] there is no serious doubt about the origin of the GN, especially when the recipient's original disease was not a GN and when there is no evidence of graft rejection. More difficult to interpret are the few cases in which the occurrence of GN cannot be related either to graft rejection or to the transmission of the patient's original disease.[134, 148] We have observed three patients who developed membranous GN after transplantation. None of them had membranous GN in their own diseased kidneys, and all have normal function of the transplant. Only one of the three had had hepatitis, more than 1 year before the occurrence of the nephrotic syndrome. In two cases, circulating immune complexes were found together with the glomerular lesions.

Spontaneous Rupture of the Transplanted Kidney

Several authors[11, 60] have reported spontaneous rupture of the transplant, and in our own series it occurred in 4% of cases. It is usually seen during the first 15 postoperative days, sometimes insidiously and only discovered by chance during surgical exploration. However, most of these patients complain of local pain, and increased volume of the kidney and sudden anuria are also observed. Hemorrhage may cause circulatory collapse that may be sufficiently severe to require emergency surgery. The kidney may usually be saved by careful local hemostasis. Postoperatively, the function returns to normal in a few hours or days. The precise cause of the rupture is not clear. It is probably the combined result of post-transplantation interstitial edema and of small cortical infarctions. We have never found any correlation with a rejection episode, with the duration of ischemia or with pathological evidence of tubular necrosis. Similar ruptures have also been observed after experimental autotransplantation.

REFERENCES

1. Abramovici, H., Brandes, J. M., Better, O. S., Peretz, A., and Paldi, E. Menstrual cycle and reproductive potential after kidney transplantation. Report of two patients. Obstet. Gynecol., *37:*121, 1971.
2. ACS/NIH Organ Transplant Registry. The 12th Report of the Human Renal Transplant Registry, JAMA, *233:*787, 1975.
3. Advisory Committee of the Transplant Registry. Description of kidney transplant function during first year. Transplantation, *8:*728, 1969.
4. Albertsen, K., and Posborg-Petersen, V. Urinary rhythm after renal transplantation. Lancet, *2:*636, 1968.
5. Albrecht, P. H., and Greene, J. A., Jr. Serum erythropoietin after renal homotransplantation. Ann. Intern. Med., *65:*908, 1966.
6. Alfrey, A. C., Jenkins, D., Groth, C. G., Schorr, W. S., Gecelter, L., and Ogden, A. Resolution of hyperparathyroidism after renal homotransplantation. N. Engl. J. Med., *279:*1349, 1968.
7. Anderson, E. A., and Wilson, R. E. Radioisotope renography and radioscintillation scanning in the diagnosis of homograft rejection. Surg. Gynecol. Obstet., *122:*1273, 1966.
8. Antoine, B., Neveu, T., Leski, M., and Bach, J. F. Histuria during renal transplantation. Transplantation, *8:*110, 1969.
9. Antoine B., Neveu, T., and Ward, P. D. Fibrinuria during renal transplantation. Transplantation, *8:*98, 1969.
10. Bach, J. F., and Leski, M. The rejection crisis in human renal transplantation. Rev. Fr. Etud. Clin. Biol., *15:*1048, 1970.
11. Barbanel, C., Lacombe, M., and Descamps, B. Spontaneous rupture of the kidney in

human transplantation and experimental autotransplantation. Abstract of the Fifth International Congress of the Transplantation Society, p. 178, Jerusalem, 1974.

12. Barnes, B. A., Murray, J. E., and Atkinson, J. Data from the kidney transplant registry: Survival of secondary renal transplants and an analysis of early renal function. In *Advance in Transplantation*, edited by J. Dausset, J. Hamburger and G. Mathe, p. 351. Munksgaard, Copenhagen, 1968.
13. Beachley, M. C., Pierce, J. C., Boykin, J. V., and Lee H. M. The angiographic evaluation of human renal allotransplants. Arch. Surg., *111:*134, 1976.
14. Beleil, O. M., Coburn, J. W., Shinaberger, J. H., and Glassock, R. J. Recurrent glomerulonephritis due to anti-glomerular basement membrane antibodies in two successive allografts. Clin. Nephrol., *1:*377, 1973.
15. Belzer, F. O., Schweizer, R. T., Hoffman, R., and Kountz, S. L. Preservation and transplantation of human cadaver kidneys. Transplantation, *14:*363, 1972.
16. Berger, J., Yaneva, H., Nabarra, B., and Barbanel, C. Recurrence of mesangial deposition of IgA after renal transplantation. Kidney Int., *7:*232, 1975.
17. Berlyne, G. M., Mallick, N. P., Scedat, Y. K., Edwards, E. C., Harris, R., and McOrr, W. N. Abnormal urinary rhythm after renal transplantation in man. Lancet, *2:*435, 1968.
18. Better, O. S., Chaimovitz, C., Niveth, Y., Stein, A., Nahir, A. M., Barzilai, and Erlik, D. Syndrome of incomplete renal tubular acidosis after cadaver kidney transplantation. Ann. Intern. Med., *71:*39, 1969.
19. Bierman, M., and Nolan, G. H., Menstrual function and renal transplantation. Obstet. Gynecol., *49:*186, 1977.
20. Boehmig, H. J., Giles, G. R., Amemiya, H., Wilson, C. B., Coburg, A. J., Genton, E., Bunch, D. L., Dixon, F., and Starzl, T. E. Hyperacute rejection of renal homografts with particular reference to coagulation changes, humoral antibodies and formed blood elements. Transplant. Proc., *3:*1105, 1971.
21. Braun, W. E., and Merrill, J. P. Urine fibrinogen fragments in human renal allografts. N. Engl. J. Med., *278:*1366, 1968.
22. Brutel de la Riviere, G., and Van de Putte, L. B. A. Pre-existing glomerulonephritis in allografted kidneys. Arch. Pathol., *100:*196, 1976.
23. Busch, G. J., Birtch, A. G., Luke, P., Jr., Kobayashi, K., Galvanek, E. G., and Carpenter, C. B. Human renal allografts. Glomerular deposits of horse immunoglobulin G and nephritis following administration of antilymphocyte globulin. Hum. Pathol., *2:*299, 1971.
24. Busch, G. J., Martins, A. C. P., Hollenberg, N. K., Wilson, R. E., Colman, R. W. A primate model of hyperacute renal allograft rejection. Am. J. Pathol., *79:*31, 1975.
25. Busch, G. J., Reynolds, E. S., Galvanek, E. G., Braun, W. E., and Dammin, G. J. Human renal allografts. The role of vascular injury in early graft failure. Medicine, *50:* 29, 1971.
26. Callard, P., Bedrossian, J., Idatte, J. M., Belair, M. F., Grossetete, J., Mandet, C., and Bariety, J. The arterial lesions in the course of renal allograft rejection phenomena. In *Advances in Nephrology*, edited by J. Hamburger, J. Crosnier and M. H. Maxwell, vol. 5, p. 333. Year Book Medical Publishers, Chicago, 1975.
27. Cameron, J. S., and Turner, D. R. Recurrent glomerulonephritis in allografted kidneys. Clin. Nephrol., *7:*47, 1977.
28. Carpenter, C. B. The early diagnosis of renal allograft rejection in man. In *Advances in Nephrology*, edited by J. Hamburger, J. Crosnier and M. H. Maxwell, vol. 5, p. 229. Year Book Medical Publishers, Chicago, 1975.
29. Chatterjee, S. N., Friedler, R. M., Berne, T. V., Oldham, S. B., Singer, F. R., and Massry, S. G. Persistent hypercalcemia after successful renal transplantation. Nephron, *17:*1, 1976.

30. Christensen, M. S., Nielsen, H. E., and Torring, S. Hypercalcemia and parathyroid function after renal transplantation. Acta Med. Scand., *201:*35, 1977.
31. Clark, E. A., Mickey, M. R., Opelz, G., and Terasaki, P. I. Evaluation of Belzer and Collins kidney preservation methods. Lancet, *1:*361, 1973.
32. Clark, E. A., Terasaki, P. I., Opelz, G., and Mickey, M. R. Cadaver kidney transplant failures at one month. N. Engl. J. Med., *291:*1099, 1974.
33. Coles, G. A., Crosby, D. L., Jones, G. R., Jones, J. H., and McVeigh, S. Hypertension following cadaveric renal transplantation. Postgrad. Med. J., *48:*399, 1972.
34. Couser, W. G., Wallace, A., Monaco, A. P., and Lewis, E. J. Successful renal transplantation in patients with circulating antibody to glomerular basement membrane: Report of two cases. Clin. Nephrol., *1:*381, 1973.
35. Crosnier, J. The transplanted kidney. In *Kidney in Systemic Diseases,* edited by S. G. Massry. Karger, Basel, 1977.
36. Crosnier, J., Antoine, B., Dormont, J., Debray-Sachs, M., Leski, M., and Bach, J. F. La protéinurie des reins transplantés. Bull. Mem. Soc. Méd. Hôp. Paris, *118:*233, 1967.
37. Daar, A. S., Morris, P. J., and Oliver, D. O. Leucocytosis is not a manifestation of rejection. Br. Med. J., *2:*1570, 1977.
38. Damin, G. J. The pathology of human renal transplantation. In *Human Transplantation,* edited by F. T. Rapaport and J. Dausset, p. 170. Grune and Stratton, New York, 1968.
39. Dandavino, R., Trunet, P., Descamps, B., and Kreis, H. Prolonged withdrawal of Azathioprine in kidney transplantation. Transplant. Proc., *9:*655, 1978.
40. Davison, J. M., Uldall, P. R., and Ross-Taylor, R. M. Relation of immediate post-transplant renal function to long term function in cadaver kidney recipients. Transplantation, *23:*310, 1977.
41. Debray-Sachs, M., and Sachs, C. Proteinuria in patients with homotransplanted kidneys. Nature, *212:*209, 1966.
42. De-Fronzo, R. A., Goldberg, M., Cooke, C. R., Barker, C., Grossman, R. A., and Agus, Z. S. Investigation into the mechanisms of hyperkalemia following renal transplantation. Kidney Int., *11:*357, 1977.
43. Dempster, W. J. Renal function after transplantation. Lancet, *i:*243, 1970.
44. Dempster, W. J., and Williams, M. A. Cellular infiltration in homotransplanted kidneys. Br. Med. J., *1:*18, 1963.
45. Descamps, B., Gagnon, R., Barbanel, C., Debray-Sachs, M., and Crosnier, J. Complement dependent and lymphocyte dependent antibodies in human allograft recipients. Transplant. Proc., *7:*1, 1975.
46. Descamps, B., Hinglais, N., and Crosnier, J. Renal transplantation between 33 HLA identical siblings. Transplant. Proc., *5:*231, 1973.
47. Dixon, F. J., McPhaul, J. J., and Lerner, R. A. The contribution of kidney transplantation to the study of glomerulonephritis. The recurrence of glomerulonephritis in renal transplants. Transplant. Proc., *1:*194, 1969.
48. Dixon, F. J., McPhaul, J. J., Jr., and Lerner, R. A. Recurrence of glomerulonephritis in the transplanted kidney. Arch. Intern. Med., *123:*554, 1969.
49. Droz, D., Zanetti, M., Noel, L. H., and Leibowitch, J. Dense deposits disease. Nephron, *19:*1, 1977.
50. Ducrot, H., Jungers, P., Funck-Brentano, J. L., Perrin, D., Crosnier, J., and Hamburger, J. La correction de l'hypertension artérielle par la transplantation rénale chez l'homme. Pathol. Biol. (Paris), *13:*1070, 1965.
51. Ettenger, R. B., Heuser, E. T., Malekzadeh, M. H., Pennisi, A. J., Uittenbogaart, C. H., and Fine, R. N. Focal glomerulosclerosis in renal allografts. Association with the nephrotic syndrome and chronic rejection. Am. J. Dis. Child, *131:*1347, 1977.

52. Farber, M., Kennison, R. D., Jackson, H. T., and Sbarra, A. J. Obstet. Gynecol. (Suppl.), *48:*25, 1976.
53. Fine, R. N. Renal transplantation in children. In *Advances in Nephrology*, edited by J. Hamburger, J. Crosnier and M. H. Maxwell, vol. 5, p. 201. Year Book Medical Publishers, Chicago, 1975.
54. Flanigan, W. J., Aron, L. F., Brewer, T. E., and Caldwell, F. T. Etiology and diagnosis of early post transplantation oliguria. Am. J. Surg., *132:*808, 1976.
55. Foley, W. D., Bookstein, J. J., Tweist, M., Gikas, P. W., Mayor, G. H., and Turcotte, J. G. Arteriography of renal transplants. Radiology, *116:*271, 1975.
56. Galle, P., Hinglais, N., and Crosnier, J. Recurrence of an original glomerular lesion in three renal allografts. Transplant. Proc., *3:*368, 1971.
57. Galle, P., and Montera, H. de. Examen au microscope électronique des cellules infiltrant le tissu interstitiel d'un homotransplant rénal humain. Rev. Fr. Etud. Clin. Biol., *7:*40, 1962.
58. Geiss, W. P., Popovtzer, M. M., Gorman, J. L., Halgrimson, C. G., Groth, C. G., and Starzl, T. P. The diagnosis and treatment of hyperparathyroidism after renal homotransplantation. Surg. Gynecol. Obstet., *137:*997, 1973.
59. George, C. R. P., Tiller, D. J., Burrows, S. M., and Perceval, L. M. Life with a transplanted kidney. Med. J. Aust., *57:*461, 1970.
60. Ghose, M. K., Kest, L. M., Cohen, S. M., Roza, O., Berman, L. B., Lidsky, I., Tertelbaum, S., and Galvin, J. B. Spontaneous rupture of renal allotransplants. J. Urol (Baltimore), *109:*790, 1973.
61. Glassock, R. J., Feldman, D., Reynolds, E. S., Dammin, G. J., and Merrill, J. P. Human renal isografts: A clinical and pathologic analysis. Medicine, *47:*411, 1968.
62. Goodwin, W. E., Kaufman, J. J., Mims, M. M., Turher, R. D., Glassock, R., Goldman, R., and Maxwell, M. H. Human renal transplantation. I. Clinical experiences with 6 cases of renal homotransplantation. J. Urol. (Baltimore), *89:*13, 1963.
63. Grundmann, R., Strümper, R., Eichmann, J., and Pichlmayer, H. The immediate function of the kidney after 24 to 72 hr preservation. Transplantation, *23:*437, 1977.
64. Grünfeld, J. P., Kleinknecht, D., Moreau, J. F., Kamoun, K., Sabto, J., Garcia-Torres, R., Ossorio, M., Kreis, H. Permanent hypertension after renal homotransplantation in man. Clin. Sci., *48:*391, 1975.
65. Gyorgy, A. Z., Stewart, J. H., George, C. R. P., Tiller, D. J., and Edwards, K. D. G. Renal tubular acidosis, acidosis due to hyperkalemia, hypercalcemia, disordered citrate metabolism and other tubular dysfunctions following human renal transplantation. Q. J. Med., *38:*231, 1969.
66. Habib, R. Focal glomerular sclerosis. Kidney Int., *4:*355, 1973.
67. Hamburger, J., Berger, J., Hinglais, N., Descamps, B. New insights into the pathogenesis of glomerulonephritis afforded by the study of renal allografts. Clin. Nephrol., *1:*3, 1973.
68. Hamburger, J., Crosnier, J., and Dormont, J. Observations in patients with a well tolerated homotransplanted kidney. Ann. NY Acad. Sci., *120:*558, 1964.
69. Hamburger, J., Crosnier, J., Dormont, J., Reveillaud, R. J., Hors, J. H., and Alsina, J. Homotransplantation rénale humaine. Résultats personnels chez 52 malades. II. Histoire naturelle du greffon dans les cas de tolérance prolongée. Presse Méd., *73:*2873, 1965.
70. Hamburger, J., Crosnier, J., and Noel, L. H. Recurrent glomerulonephritis after renal transplantation. Annu. Rev. Med., *29:*67, 1978.
71. Hamburger, J., Vaysse, J., Crosnier, J., Auvert, J., and Dormont, J. Résultats de quatorze transplantations rénales chez l'homme. Bull. Mem. Soc. Med. Hôp. Paris, *114:*225, 1963.

72. Hamburger, J., Vaysse, J., Crosnier, J., Tubiana, M., Lalanne, C. M., Antoine, B., Auvert, J., Soulier, J. P., Dormont, J., Salmon, Ch., Maisonnet, M., and Amiel, J. L. Transplantation d'un rein entre jumeaux non monozygotes après irradiation du receveur. Bon fonctionnement au quatrième mois. Presse Méd., *67:*1771, 1959.
73. Hansen, H. E., and Skov, P. E. The functional pattern of the transplanted living donor kidney during the early posttransplant period. Acta. Med. Scand., *196:*507, 1974.
74. Henderson, L. W., Nolph, K. D., Puschett, J. B., and Goldberg, M. Proximal tubular malfunction as a mechanism for diuresis after renal homotransplantation. N. Engl. J. Med., *278:*467, 1968.
75. Herdman, R. C., Michael, A. F., Vernier, R. L., Kelly, W. D., and Good, R. A. Renal function and phosphorus excretion after human transplantation. Lancet, *1:*121, 1966.
76. Hills, G. S., Light, J. A., and Perloff, L. J. Perfusion related injury in renal transplantation. Surgery, *79:*440, 1976.
77. Hinglais, N., and Leski, M. Pathologie des crises aigües du transplant. In *Cours Internat. Transpl. Lyon 1971*, p. 201, Simep, 1971.
78. Hollenberg, N. K., Birtch, A., Rashid, A., Mangel, R., Briggs, W., Epstein, M., Murray, J. E., and Merrill, J. P. Relationships between intrarenal perfusion and function serial hemodynamic studies in the transplanted human kidney. Medicine, *51:*95, 1972.
79. Horbach, J., Van Liebergen, T., Mastboom, J., and Wijdeveld, F. Pregnancy in a patient after cadaveric renal transplantation. Acta. Med. Scand., *194:*237, 1973.
80. Hoyer, J. R., Raij, L., Vernier, R. L., Simmons, R. L., Najarian, J. S., and Michael, A. F. Recurrence of idiopathic nephrotic syndrome after renal transplantation. Lancet, *2:* 343, 1972.
81. Hume, D. M. Kidney transplantation. In *Human Transplantation*, edited by F. T. Rapaport and J. Dausset, p. 110. Grune and Stratton, New York, 1968.
82. Hume, D. M., and Bryan, C. P. The development of recurrent glomerulonephritis. Transplant. Proc., *4:*673, 1972.
83. Hume, D. M., Magee, J. H., Kauffman, H. M., Rittenbury, M. S., and Prout, G. R. Renal homotransplantation in man in modified recipients. Ann. Surg., *158:*608, 1963.
84. Hume, D. M., Merrill, J. P., Miller, B. F., and Thorn, G. W. Experiences with renal homotransplantation in the human. Report of nine cases. J. Clin. Invest., *67:*1771, 1955.
85. Jepson, J. H., Leeuw, N. K. M. de, Gault, M. H., Dossetor, J. B., and Manay, B. Characteristics of erythropoiesis following human renal homotransplantation. Transplant. Proc., *3:*353, 1971.
86. Johnson, J. W., Hattner, R. S., Hampers, C. L., Bernstein, D. S., Merrill, J. P., and Sherwood, L. M. Secondary hyperparathyroidism in chronic renal failure, effects of renal transplantation. JAMA, *215:*418, 1971.
87. Jungers, P., Lambert-Netter, A., Pelissier, C., Zingraff, J., and Crosnier, J. Etude des troubles de la fonction gonadique chez les urémiques hémodialysés. Gynecology, *27:* 525, 1976.
88. Kincaid-Smith, P., Morris, P. J., Saker, B. M., Ting, A., and Marshall, V. C. Immediate renal-graft biopsy and subsequent rejection. Lancet, *ii:*748, 1968.
89. Kissmeyer-Nielsen, F., Olsen, S., Petersen, V. P., Fjeldborg, O. Hyperacute rejection of kidney allografts associated with pre-existing humoral antibodies against donor cells. Lancet, *2:*662, 1966.
90. Kjellstrand, C. M., Casali, R. E., Shideman, J., Simmons, R. L., Buselmeir, T., and Najarian, J. S. The etiology and prognosis in acute post-transplant renal failure. Am. J. Med., *61:*190, 1976.
91. Kleinknecht, D., Jungers, P., Ducrot, H., Auvert, J., Leski, M., Kreis, H., Zingraff, J., Xerri, A., Man, N. K., Crosnier, J., and Hamburger, J. Transplantation nephrectomy and hypertension. In Die Niere in Kreislauf, 9th Int. Symp. Deutsch. Gesellschaft für

fortschritte aufdem gebiete der inneren medizin, Würzburg 1970, p. 218. Thieme, Stuttgart, 1971.

92. Kolff, W. J., Nakamoto, S., Poutasse, E. F., Straffon, R., and Figueroa, J. E. Effects of bilateral nephrectomy and kidney transplantation on hypertension in man. Circulation (Suppl.), *30:*23, 1964.

93. Korsch, B. M., Klein, J. D., Negrete, V. F., Henderson, D. J., and Fine, R. N. Physical and psychologic follow-up on offspring of renal allograft recipients. Pediatrics, in press.

94. Kountz, S. L., and Cohn, R. The pathophysiology of renal allotransplants in subjects on immunosuppressive therapy. In *Advance in Transplantation*, edited by J. Dausset, J. Hamburger and G. Mathe, p. 617. Munksgaard, Copenhagen, 1968.

95. Kountz, S. L., Truex, G., Earley, L. E., and Belzer, F. O. Serial hemodynamics after allotransplantation in man. Circulation, *41:*217, 1970.

96. Kreis, H. Insufisances rénales aigües et rejet des reins transplantés, Nouv. Presse Méd., *8:*2943, 1979.

97. Kreis, H., Finch, T. W., Moreau, J. F., Noel, L. H., Lacombe, M., Crosnier, J. Early renal failure after cadaver kidney transplantation. In *Advances in Nephrology*, edited by J. Hamburger, J. Crosnier, J. P. Grünfeld and M. H. Maxwell, vol. 8, p. 209. Year Book Medical Publishers, Chicago, 1979.

98. Kreis, H., Lacombe, M., Noel, L. H., Descamps, J. M., Chailley, J., and Crosnier, J. Kidney graft rejection: Has the need for steroids to be reevaluated? Lancet, *2:*1169, 1978.

99. Kreis, H., Mansouri, R. Descamps, J. M., Dandavino, R., N'Guyen, A. T., Bach, J. F., and Crosnier, J. Antithymocyte globulin in cadaver kidney transplantation. A randomized trial based on T cell monitoring. Kidney Int., to be published.

100. Kreis, H., Noel, L. H., Moreau, J. F., Barbanel, C., and Crosnier, J. Biologic, pathologic and radiologic studies of cadaver kidneys preserved in Collins' solutions. Transplant. Proc., *9:*1611, 1977.

101. Küss, R., Teinturier, J., and Milliez, P. Quelques essais de greffe de rein chez l'homme. Bull. Mem. Acad. Chir., *77:*755, 1951.

102. Laasonen, L., Edgren, J., and Wattson, T. Magnification angiography in the evaluation of transplanted kidneys. Acta Radiol., *17:*200, 1976.

103. Laasonen, L., and Kock, B. Angiography and isotope renography in active rejection of renal transplants. Scand. J. Urol. Nephrol., *12:*79, 1978.

104. Ladefoged, J. Tubular reabsorption of bicarbonate in transplanted cadaver kidneys. Nephron, *8:*216, 1973.

105. Lawler, R. H., West, J.W., McNuity, P. H., Clancy, E. J., and Murphy, R. P. Homotransplantation of the kidney in the human. JAMA, *144:*844, 1950.

106. Leonard, L., Vertuno, M. C., Preuss, H. G., Pargy, W., Jr., and Schreiner, E. G. Fanconi syndrome following homotransplantation. Arch. Intern. Med., *133:*302, 1974.

107. Lerner, R. A., Glassock, R. J., and Dixon, F. J. The role of antiglomerular basement membrane antibody in the pathogenesis of human glomerulonephritis. J. Exp. Med., *126:*989, 1967.

108. Leski, M., Kreis, H., Descamps, B., and Crosnier, J. Les complications extra-rénales des transplantations de rein. *Actualités Néphrologiques de l'Hôpital Necker*, p. 229. Med. Flammarion, Paris, 1969.

109. Levy, M., Broyer, M., Arsan, A., Levy-Bentolila, A., and Habib, R. Anaphylactoid purpura nephritis in childhood: natural history and immunopathology. Adv. Nephrol. *6:*183, 1976.

110. Lindquist, R. R., Guttmann, R. D., Merrill, J. P., and Dammin, G. J. Human renal allografts. Interpretation of morphologic and immunohistochemical observations. Am. J. Pathol., *53:*851, 1968.

111. Low, J. C., Schaaf, M., Earll, J. M., Piechocki, J. T., and Li, T. K. Ionic calcium determination in primary hyperparathyroidism, JAMA, *223:*152, 1973.
112. Lozada, E., Soberman, R., Gleedman, M., and Veith, R. Hydrogen ion excretion of transplanted kidneys. Bull. N. Y. Acad. Med., *45:*997, 1969.
113. Luciani, J., Frantz, Ph., Thibault, Ph., Ghesquiere, F., Conseiller, C., Cousin, M. T., Glaser, P., Legrain, M., Viars, P., and Küss, P. Early anuria prevention in human kidney transplantation. Transplantation, *28:*308, 1979.
114. Lund, B. *Renal Transplantation in Rabbits.* Munksgaard, Copenhagen, 1973.
115. McIntosh, D. A., Peterson, E. D., and McPhaul, J. J., Jr. Autonomy of parathyroid function after renal homotransplantation. Ann. Intern. Med., *65:*900, 1966.
116. McKenzie, I. F. C., and Wittingham, S. Deposits of immunoglobulins and fibrin in human allografted kidneys. Lancet, *2:*1313, 1968.
117. McMain, P. B., Hoffman, G. C., Nakamoto, S., and Kolff, W. J. Erythropoiesis and renal homotransplantation, Can. Med. Assoc. J., *93:*241, 1975.
118. McMillan, R., Evans, D. B., and Lines, J. G. Reversed rhythm of kidney transplants. N. Engl. J. Med., *280:*166, 1969.
119. McPhaul, J. J., Jr., McIntosh, D. A., Hammond, W. S., and Park, O. K. Autonomous secondary (renal) parathyroid hyperplasia. N. Engl. J. Med., *271:*1342, 1964.
120. Maher, J. F. A logical approach to the diagnosis of renal transplant rejection. Immunologic, ischemic and inflammatory impairement of renal function. Am. J. Med., *56:* 275, 1974.
121. Mandel, S. R., Mattern, W. D., Staab, E., and Johnson, G. Use of radionuclide imaging in the early diagnosis and treatment of renal allograft rejection. Ann. Surg., *181:*596, 1975.
122. Manuel, Y., Pali, S., Bernhardt, J. R., Revillard, J. P., Claudey, D., and Traeger, J. Proteinuria in human renal allografts. Helv. Med. Acta, *35:*3, 1969.
123. Martin, D. C., Hunter, J. L., Lawton, M. B., Berke, R. A., and Morton, M. E. Serial radionuclide quantitative function studies for evaluation of renal transplants. J. Urol., *112:*2, 1974.
124. Massry, S. G., Coburn, J. W., Popovtzer, M. M., Schinaberger, J. H., Maxwell, M. H., and Kleeman, C. R. Secondary hyperparathyroidism in chronic renal hemodialysis and after renal transplantation. Arch. Intern. Med., *124:*431, 1969.
125. Massry, S. G., Preuss, H. G., Maher, J. F., and Schreiner, G. E. Renal tubular acidosis after cadaver kidney transplantation. Am. J. Med., *42:*284, 1967.
126. Mathew, T. H., Mathews, D. C., Hobbs, J. B., and Kincaid-Smith, P. Glomerular lesions after renal transplantation. Am. J. Med., *59:*177, 1975.
127. Medawar, P. B. The behavior and fate of skin allografts and skin homografts in rabbits. J. Anat., *78:*176, 1944.
128. Medawar, P. B. A second study of the behavior and fate of skin homografts in rabbits. J. Anat., *79:*157, 1945.
129. Merans, E. A., Johnston, C. S., Huser, J. H., and Murphy, G. P. Renal transplantation in the Rhesus monkey. V. Alterations in erythropoietin activity. Invest. Urol., *2:*574, 1965.
130. Merkatz, I. R., Schwartz, G. H., David, S. H., Stenzel, K. H., Riggio, R. R., and Whistsell, J. C. Resumption of female reproductive function following renal transplantation. JAMA, *216:*1749, 1971.
131. Merrill, J. P. Medical management of the transplant patient. In *Human Transplantation*, edited by F. T. Rapaport and J. Dausset, p. 66. Grune and Stratton, New York, 1968.
132. Merrill, J. P. Glomerulonephritis in renal transplants. Transplant. Proc., *1:*994, 1969.
133. Michel, J. R., Moreau, J. F., and Japhet, Y. L'artériographie dans la transplantation rénale. Ann. Radiol., *16:*361, 1973.

134. Milgrom, F., Klassen, J., and Fujih, E. Immunologic injury of renal homografts. J. Ex. Med., *134:*1935, 1971.
135. Millard, P. R., Hebertson, B. M., and Evans, D. B. Renal biopsy in clinical management of renal transplantation. Lancet, *i:*113, 1970.
136. Moraes, J. R., and Stastny, P. A new antigenic system expressed in human endothelial cells. J. Clin. Invest., *60:*449, 1977.
137. Nabarra, B., Descamps, B., and Hamburger, J. Cell infiltration in human renal allografts: an ultrastructural study. Transplant. Proc. (Suppl.), *7:*645, 1975.
138. Nielsen, K. The peripheral nerve function in chronic renal failure. IX. Recovery after renal transplantation. Electrophysiological aspects (sensitory and motor nerve conduction). Acta Med. Scand., *195:*171, 1974.
139. O'Brien, J. P., and Hume, D. M. Membranous glomerulonephritis in two human renal homotransplants. Ann. Intern. Med., *65:*504, 1966.
140. Ogden, D. A., Sitprija, V., and Holmes, J. H. Function of the renal homograft in man immediately after transplantation. Am. J. Med., *38:*873, 1965.
141. Olsen, S., Bohman, S. O., and Petersen, V. D. Ultrastructure of the glomerular basement membrane in long term renal allograft with transplant glomerular disease. Lab. Invest., *30:*176, 1974.
142. Opelz, G., and Terasaki, P. L. Kidney preservation: perfusion versus cold storage. Transplant. Proc., *8:*121, 1976.
143. Pasternack, A., Virolainen, M., and Häyry, P. Fine needle aspiration biopsy in the diagnosis of human renal allograft rejection. J. Urol., *109:*167, 1973.
144. Patel, R., and Terasaki, P. I. Significance of the positive cross-match test in kidney transplantation. N. Engl. J. Med., *280:*735, 1969.
145. Patel, R., Wilson, R. E., Birtch, A.G., Merrill, J. P., Murray, J. E., and Vusch, G. Cadaveric kidney transplantation in a patient with donor specific antileukocyte cytotoxic antibodies: report of a case. Transplantation, *12:*88, 1971.
146. Paul, L. C. Antibodies directed against donor antigens in human renal allograft. Thesis, Drukkerij J. H. Pasmans, 'S. Gravenhage, 1976.
147. Perrin, D. Oeil et tranplantation rénale. Vie Med., *50:*1204, 1969.
148. Petersen, V. P., Olsen, T. S., Kissmeyer-Nielsen, F., Bohman, S. O., Hansen, H. E., Hansen, E. S., Skov, P. E., and Solling, K. Late failure of human renal tranplants. Medicine (Baltimore), *54:*45, 1975.
149. Pierce, J. C., Cobb, G. W., and Hume, D. M. Relevance of HLA antigens to acute humoral rejection of multiple renal allotransplants. N. Engl. J. Med., *285:*142, 1971.
150. Porter, K. A. Renal transplantation. In *Pathology of the Kidney*, edited by R. H. Heptinstall, ed. 2, vol. 2, p. 977. Little, Brown, Waltham, MA, 1974.
151. Porter, K. A. Histopathology in clinical renal transplantation. Transplant. Proc., *6:*79, 1974.
152. Porter, K. A., Dossetor, J. B., Marchioro, T. L., Peart, W. S., Rendall, J. M., Starzl, T. C., and Terasaki, P. I. Human renal transplants. I. Glomerular changes. Lab. Invest., *16:*153, 1967.
153. Porter, K. A., Rendall, J. M., Stolinski, C., Terasaki, P. I., Marchioro, T. L., and Starzl, T. E. Light and miroscopic study of biopsies from 33 human renal allografts and an isograft 1¾ to 2 years after transplantation. Ann. NY Acad. Sci., *129:*615, 1966.
154. Raskin, N. H., and Fishman, R. A. Neurologic disorders in renal failure (second of two parts). N. Engl. J. Med., *294:*204, 1976.
155. Reveillaud, R. J., Leski, M., and Crosnier, J. Indications et résultats de la transplantation rénale. Presse Méd., *78:*795, 1970.
156. Riffle, G., and Traeger, J. Pregnancy after renal transplantation: an international survey. Transplant. Proc. (Suppl. 1), *7:*723, 1975.

157. Robertson, J. G., Cockburn, F., and Woodruff, M. Successful pregnancy after cadaveric renal transplantation. J. Obstet. Gynecol. Br. Commonw., *81:*777, 1974.
158. Rossmann, P., and Jirka, J. *Rejection Nephropathy*, vol. 1, p. 368. Academia Praha, Prague, 1979.
159. Rowlands, D. T., Jr., and Bossen, E. H. Immunological mechanisms of allograft rejection. Arch. Intern. Med., *123:*491, 1969.
160. Rowlands, D. T., Hill, G. S., and Zmijewski, C. M. The pathology of renal homograft rejection. A review. Am. J. Pathol., *85:*774, 1976.
161. Salvatierra, O., Jr., Powell, M. R., Price, D. C., Kountz, S. L., and Belzer, F. O. The advantages of ^{131}I-orthoiodohippurate scintiphotography in the management of patients after renal transplantation. Ann. Surg., *180:*336, 1974.
162. Schwartz, G. H., David, D. S., Riggio, R. R., Saville, P. D., Whitsell, J. C., Stenzel, K. H., and Rubin, A. L. Hypercalcemia after renal transplantation. Am. J. Med., *49:*42, 1970.
163. Sciarra, J. J., Toledo-Pereyra, L. H., Bendel, R. P., and Simmons, R. L. Pregnancy following renal transplantation. Am. J. Obstet. Gynecol., *123:*411, 1975.
164. Sethi, K., First, M. R., Pesce, A. J., Fidler, J. P., and Pollack, V. E. Proteinuria following renal transplantation. Nephron, *18:*49, 1977.
165. Shell, A. G. R., Boulas, J., Drummond, J. M., May, J., Rogers, J. H., and Storey, B. G. Controlled clinical trial of machine perfusions of cadaveric donor renal allografts. Lancet, *2:*287, 1975.
166. Sheil, A. G. R., Stewart, J. H., Johnson, J. R., May, J., Charlesworth, J., Kalowski, S., Shard, A. M., and Bashir, H. Evaluation of cadaver donor renal transplantation. Transplant. Proc., *3:*347, 1971.
167. Sheriff, M. H. R., Yaha, T., and Lee, H. A. Is azathioprine necessary in renal transplantation. Lancet, *1:*118, 1978.
168. Shimamura, T., Gyorkey, F., Morgen, R. O., and Debakey, M. E. The fine structural observations in human kidney homografts. Invest. Urol., *3:*590, 1966.
169. Skov, P. E., and Hansen, H. E. The functional pattern of the cadaveric kidney in early post transplant period. Acta Med. Scand., *196:*285, 1974.
170. Sonnabend, W., Kistler, G. S., Thiel, G., Zollinger, H. U., Bianchi, L., Enderlin, F., Gudat, F., and Krech, U. Chronische herd-glomerulitis und chronisch-persistierende hepatitis nach nierentransplantation: Nachweis von hepatitis B und Epstein Barr-virus antigen. Schweiz. Med. Wochenschr., *104:*205, 1974.
171. Soulillou, J. P., Peyrat, M. A., and Guenel, J. Association between treatment-resistant kidney-allograft rejection and post-transplant appearance of antibodies to donor B-lymphocyte alloantigens. Lancet, *1:*354, 1978.
172. Spector, D., Limas, C., Frost, J. S., Zachary, J. B., Sterioff, S., Williams, G. M., Rolley, R. T., and Sadler, J. H. Perfusion nephropathy in human transplants. N. Engl. J. Med., *295:*1217, 1976.
173. Staab, E. V., Whittier, F., Patton, D. D., Ginn, E. H., and Acherman, J. R. Early evaluation of cadaver renal allotransplant by means of radionuclide imaging. Nuclear Med., *106:*147, 1973.
174. Stanbury, S. W. Bone disease in uremia. Am. J. Med., *44:*714, 1968.
175. Starzl, T. E., Lerner, R. A., Dixon, F. J., Groth, C. G., Brettschneider, L., and Terasaki, P. I. Schwartzman reaction after human renal homotransplantation. N. Engl. J. Med., *278:*642, 1968.
176. Starzl, T. E., Marchioro, T. L., Holmes, J. H., and Waddell, W. R. The incidence, cause and significance of immediate and delayed oliguria or anuria after renal human transplantation. Surg. Gynecol. Obstet., *118:*819, 1964.
177. Starzl, T. E., Marchioro, T. L., and Waddell, W. R. The reversal of rejection in human

renal homografts with subsequent development of homograft tolerance. Surg. Gynecol. Obstet., *117:*385, 1963.

178. Stetson, C. A., and Jensen, E. Humoral aspects of the immune response to homografts. Ann. NY Acad. Sci., *87:*249, 1960.
179. Stiller, C. R., Sinclair, N. R., McGirr, D., Jevnikar, A., and Ulan, R. A. Humoral and cellular presensitization and graft outcome. Transplant. Proc., *10:*525, 1978.
180. Tagatz, G. E., and Simmons, R. L. Pregnancy after renal transplantation. Ann. Med. Int., *82:*113, 1975.
181. Terasaki, P. I., Kreisler, M., and Mickey, R. M. Presensitization and kidney transplant failures. Postgrad. Med. J., *47:*89, 1971.
182. Thier, S. O., Henderson, L. W., and Root, R. K. Renal transplantation: Medical management of the transplant recipient. In *The Kidney*, edited by B. M. Brenner and F. C. Rector, vol. 2, p. 1819. Saunders, Philadelphia, 1976.
183. Turner, D. R., Cameron, J. S., Rewick, M., Sharpstone, P., Melcher, D., Ogg, C. S., Evans, D. I., Trafford, A. J. P., and Leibowitz, S. Transplantation in mesangiocapillary glomerulonephritis with intramembranous dense "deposits." Recurrence of Disease. Kidney Int., *9:*439, 1976.
184. Waldman, T., Strober, W., and Mogielnicki, P. The renal handling of low molecular weight proteinuria. II. Disorders of serum protein catabolism in patients with tubular proteinuria, the nephrotic syndrome or uremia. J. Clin. Invest., *51:*2162, 1972.
185. Whittaker, J. R., Veith, F. J., Soberman, R., Lalezari, P., Tellis, I., Freed, S. Z., and Gliedman, M. L. The fate of the renal transplant with delayed function. Surg. Gynecol. Obstet., *136:*919, 1973.
186. Williams, G. M. Clinical aspects of allograft rejection. Transplant. Proc., *6:*71, 1974.
187. Williams, G. M. Clinical course following renal transplantation. In *Kidney Transplantation. Principles and Practice*, edited by P. J. Morris, p. 203. Academic Press, London, 1979.
188. Williams, G. M., Haar, A., Parks, L. C., and Krajewski, C. A. Endothelial changes associated with hyperacute, acute and chronic renal allograft rejection in man. Transplant. Proc., *5:*819, 1973.
189. Williams, G. M., Hume, D. M., Hudson, R. P., Jr., Morris, P. J., Kano, K., and Milgrom, F. "Hyperacute" renal homograft rejection in man. N. Engl. J. Med., *279:*611, 1968.
190. Williams, G. M., White, H. J. O., and Hume, D. M. Factors influencing the long term functional success rate of human renal allograft. Transplantation, *5:*837, 1967.
191. Wilson, C. B., and Dixon, F. J. Antiglomerular basement membrane antibody induced glomerulonephritis. Kidney Int., *3:*74, 1973.
192. Wilson, D. R., and Siddiqui, A. A. Renal tubular acidosis after kidney transplantation. Ann. Intern. Med., *79:*352, 1973.
193. Wilson, R. E., Hampers, C. L., Katz, A. I., Bernstein, D. S., Wackman, A., Merrill, J. P., and Murray, J. E. Management of secondary hyperparathyroidism in renal allograft recipients. Transplant. Proc., *1:*206, 1969.
194. Zimmerman, R., and Sprayregen, S. Arterio-venous shunting in renal transplant rejection. Angiology, *29:*40, 1978.
195. Zuhlke, V., and Hermann, G. Immunological studies of proteinuria following human kidney allotransplantation. Transplant. Proc., *3:*361, 1971.

CHAPTER EIGHT

Extrarenal Complications

Jean Crosnier

Surgical complications—Infectious complications—Pulmonary complications—Hepatic complications—Bone complications—Arterial hypertension—Hematologic complications—Malignant tumors—Other complications.

The 13th Transplant Registry published in 1977[2] reports a global mortality of 31.58% among transplant recipients, with death occurring in patients having normal renal function in 64% of these cases.

Thus, mortality still bedevils transplantation statistics. However, death should be avoidable after transplantation because in the case of graft failure it is always possible to return the patient to hemodialysis.

In a study of patients transplanted at Necker Hospital between 1959 and 1968,[25] we found that 85% of deaths were due to extrarenal complications. This means that nearly always, death is secondary to surgery or due to the effects of immunosuppressive drugs, particularly corticosteroids.

The following study of extrarenal complications reflects our own experience with 471 renal transplantations performed in 437 patients at Necker Hospital between June 1959 and June 1977.

SURGICAL COMPLICATIONS

Wound Complications

Delayed healing and disruption of the wound occurred in 27% of our patients and at times posed difficult surgical problems. This complication is frequently observed in association with urinary fistulae or after repeated surgical intervention through the same wound.

Wound complications contributed to death in 7% of our cases (9 deaths in 128 complications) and to graftectomy in 25%.

Perirenal Collection

Hemorrhage and Perirenal Abscess

Hematoma are frequently due to surgery and should be avoided by careful surgical hemostasis.

This complication is often observed when nephrectomy of the patient's own kidney is performed at the same time as transplantation. This is one of the disadvantages of uretero-ureteral anastomosis when the patient's homolateral kidney has to be removed.

Hematoma may also be secondary to renal biopsy and to spontaneous rupture of the kidney.

The major risk of hematomas is in their tendency to become infected. They cause the majority of perirenal abscesses, but abscesses can also occur after bacterial contamination of the graft during its removal or preservation, and in these circumstances the course is often severe.

Clinical signs of infection or hemorrhage are often sparse. A swelling at the transplant site is diagnostic when it occurs, but usually only a reduction in renal function is observed, sometimes associated with fever.

Urinary Collection

Urinary collection always indicates a leakage secondary to a fistula of the excretory apparatus (see p. 239). When this complication results in the formation of an abscess, it becomes practically impossible to close the fistula surgically.

Lymphocele

A lymphocele, first described after renal transplantation by Hume,[54] occurs with variable frequency, from 1.2 to 14% in various series[14] and 3% in our own series, hence, much less frequently than after lymphadenectomy.

It is generally an early postsurgical complication, although first signs have been observed as late as 15 months post-transplantation in one of Starzl's[118] patients and 4 years in one of our cases. Symptomatology[83] depends on whether there is compression and whether it is venous or ureteric. Lymphocele can be latent and discovered only during surgical exploration for other complications. Conversely, it can provoke a unilateral edema on the side of the transplant, very rarely an obvious swelling below the graft. More often the first sign is a sudden reduction in renal function. Intravenous urography demonstrates ureteric compression (Fig. 8.1), and lymphography (Fig. 8.2) of the lower limb on the side of the

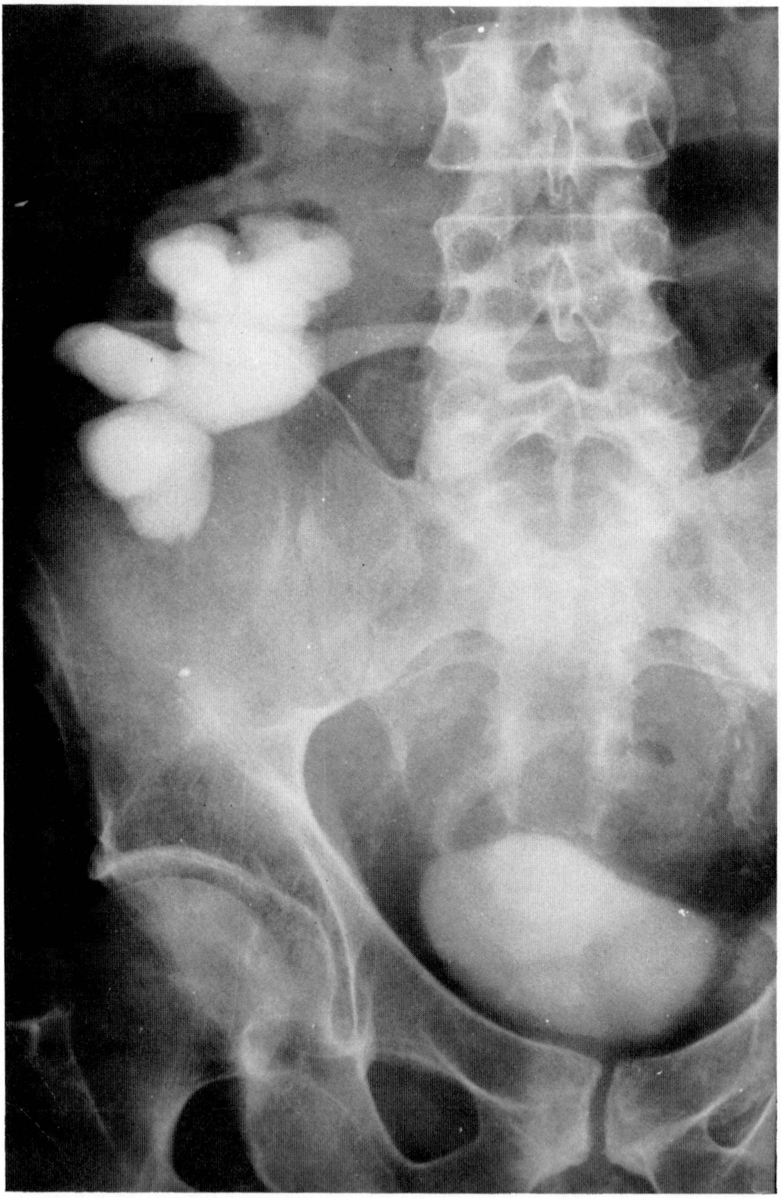

Fig. 8.1. Intravenous pyelography of a recently transplanted kidney. Enlargement of urinary tract is the consequence of ureteric compression by a lymphocele.

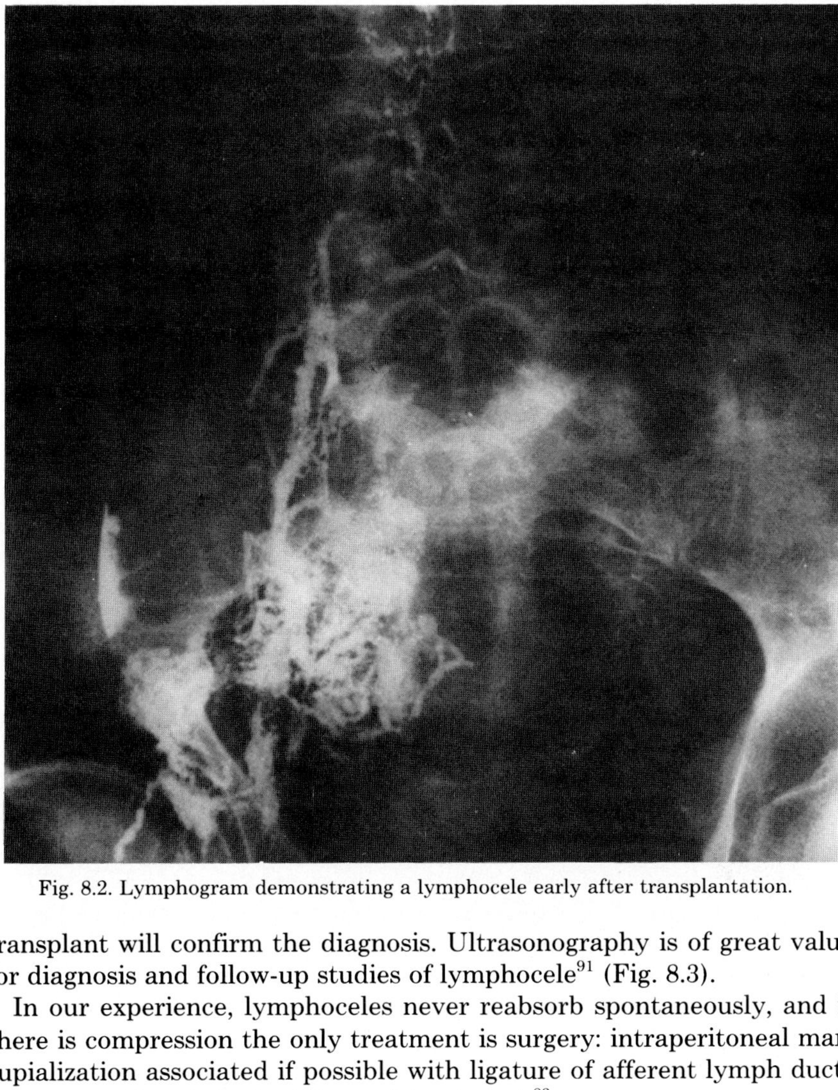

Fig. 8.2. Lymphogram demonstrating a lymphocele early after transplantation.

transplant will confirm the diagnosis. Ultrasonography is of great value for diagnosis and follow-up studies of lymphocele[91] (Fig. 8.3).

In our experience, lymphoceles never reabsorb spontaneously, and if there is compression the only treatment is surgery: intraperitoneal marsupialization associated if possible with ligature of afferent lymph ducts is now considered the best form of treatment.[83]

Complications Involving the Renal Vessels

Arterial stenosis is the most frequent vascular complication. Surveying our results in 1975,[66] we found 38 arterial stenoses in 306 renal transplants performed in 287 patients from June 1959 through December 1973 (12.4%), of which 8 occurred among 137 transplants from related living donors (5.8%) and 30 among 137 transplants from cadaver donors (17.7%).

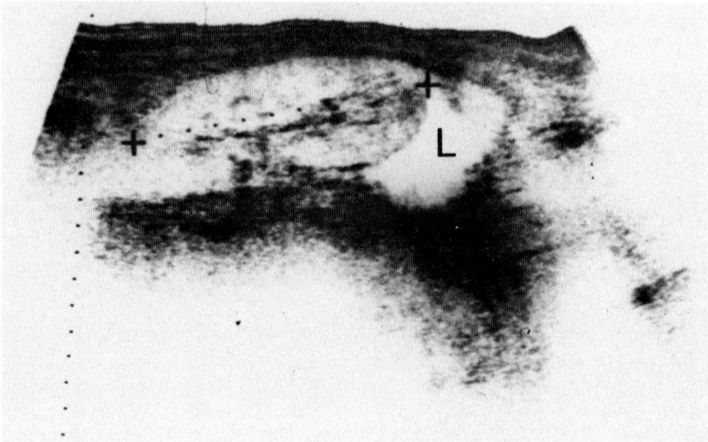

Fig. 8.3. Ultrasound scan demonstrating a nonechogenic area (L) between the lower pole of the transplant and the bladder. Transcutaneous needle puncture revealed the presence of lymph collection.

This high incidence in our series is probably explained by the fact that routine arteriography is performed in all our transplant recipients during the first 2 years after transplantation. In fact, arterial stenosis can be the cause of arterial hypertension but can remain latent, as was the case in 12 of our 38 patients who were normotensive and in whom the stenosis was discovered by routine arteriography (Fig. 8.4). We disagree with the view expressed by Hume[111] that it is unnecessary to perform post-transplantation arteriograms for the investigation of hypertension unless an arterial bruit is audible over the transplant; in our experience, such bruits have not consistently accompanied arterial stenosis.

Stenosis occurs at different sites and can be due to various causes. It can be preanastomotic, located on the hypogastric artery, usually due to an atheromatous plug. It can sometimes be found at the actual site of the anastomosis, probably due to faulty suture techniques. More frequently it is postanastomotic, due to intimal damage caused by trauma during removal of the kidney or during cannulation of the renal artery. An immune factor has been advanced as a cause of stenosis by Kincaid-Smith[60] and Porter.[100]

When the stenosis is very narrow and associated with hypertension and/or renal failure, surgical repair is necessary, but it is difficult to predict the cases in which correction of the stenosis will cure the hypertension.[47] In our series stenosis was surgically corrected in 14 patients. We observed 1 death, and in 10 of the other 13 patients blood pressure has remained normal since surgery; 5 of the 6 patients in the group having impaired renal function showed postsurgical improvement in function.

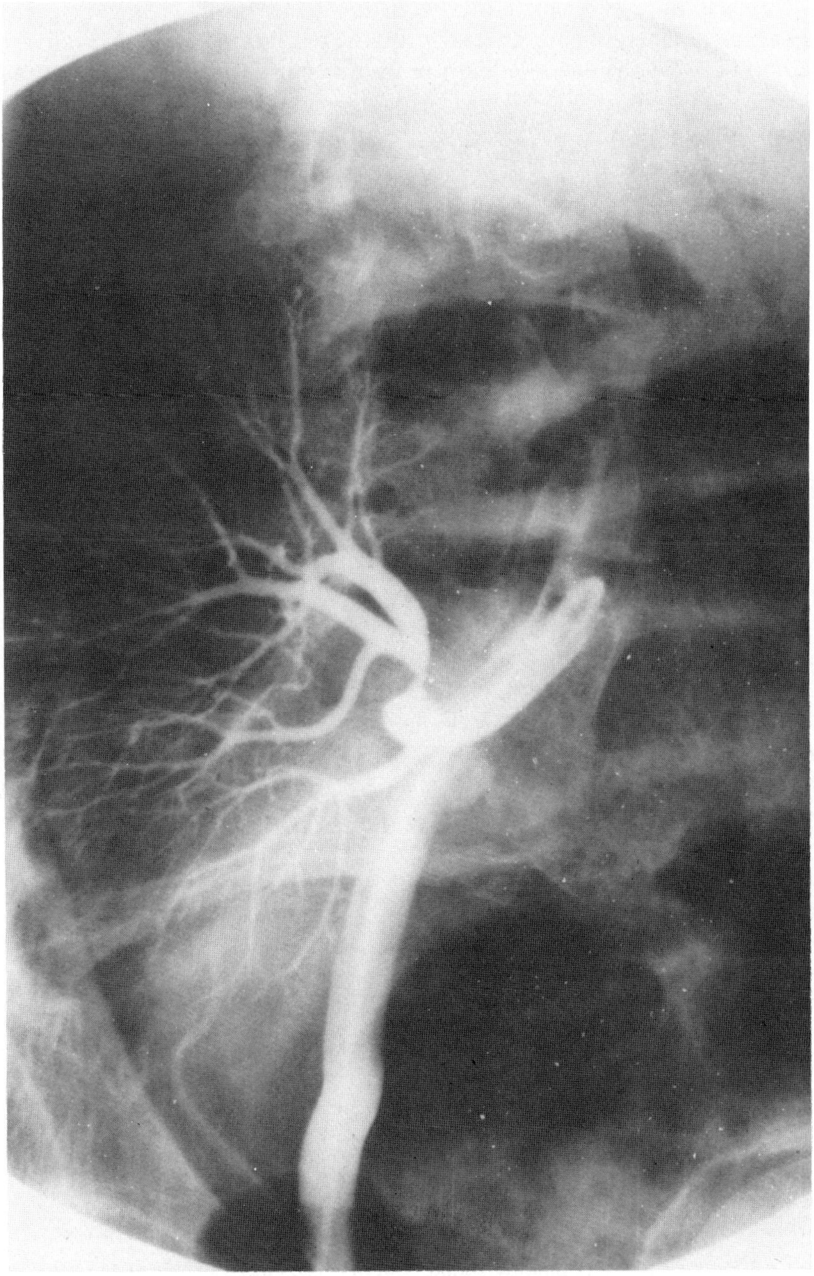

Fig. 8.4. Distal renal artery stenosis discovered 6 months after transplantation.

Rupture of the renal artery occurs at the site of anastomosis and in our series is always a consequence of local infection. It is very sudden and severe and often leads to death. In our own series, we observed seven cases: in two the patients died within minutes; in three emergency surgery was successful in (Fig. 8.5) restoring the blood flow; and in two the transplant was removed. When the arterial anastomosis has been made end-to-side, ligature of the iliac artery may be necessary to control hemorrhage.

Renal artery thrombosis usually occurs very early, during the 1st week after transplantation. It may be caused by surgical error or difficulties or provoked by intimal lesions caused by the catheter used to perfuse the kidney. When the main trunk of the artery is involved, there is massive infarction of the transplant, and graftectomy must be performed. Thrombosis of a small polar artery, after separate anastomosis, is much more frequent; it produces limited infarction, which can be the origin of a

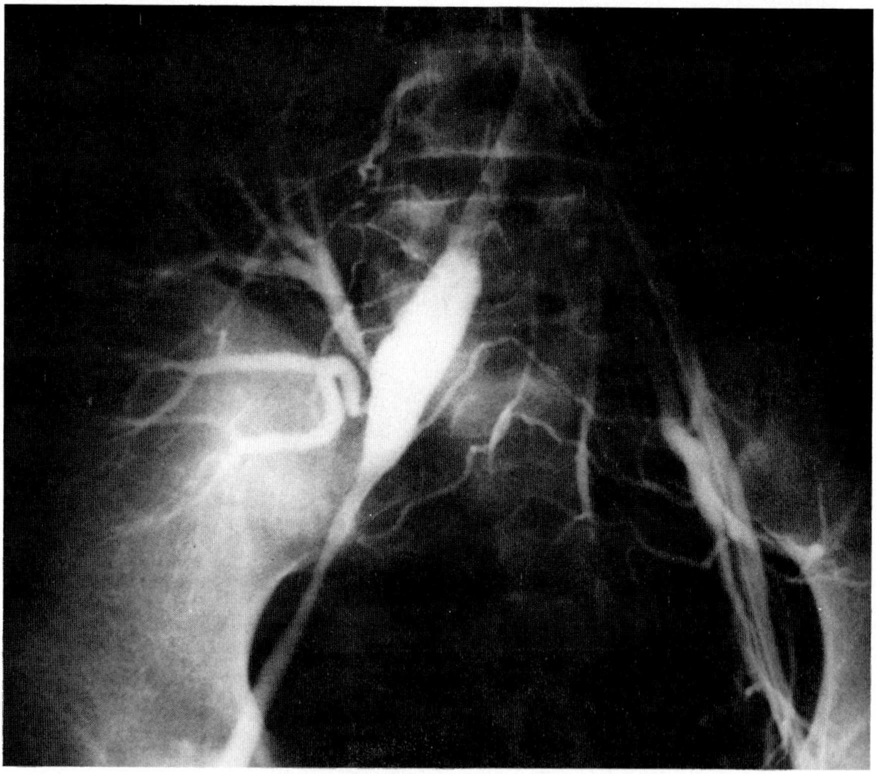

Fig. 8.5. Vein autograft repair after sudden rupture, 1 month after transplantation, of an aneurysm surrounding the renal artery of the graft and the internal and external iliac arteries.

sudden reduction in renal function and subsequently of arterial hypertension.

In some other cases thrombosis occurs later, several weeks or months after transplantation, and can be due to a number of factors: it may be associated with extensive thrombosis of the intrarenal arteries and arterioles, or it may be secondary to renal artery stenosis; an "immunocausative" factor has been suggested[60]; in his series of 13 vascular complications, Kountz[124] found occlusion of the renal artery at graftectomy in four rejected kidneys, due to a delay in nephrectomy; finally, thrombosis may be secondary to endarcteriectomy performed in the recipient at the time of transplantation.[124]

Renal vein thrombosis has been reported by Starzl[117] in a patient who died of pulmonary embolism and in whom autopsy revealed complete thrombosis of the renal vein of the graft. In our experience, it is very uncommon, despite the frequency of thromboembolic complications in transplant patients[25] (cf. p. 248). In one of our patients the graft had to be removed 8 days after transplantation because of massive infarction due to compression of the vena cava at the origin of the renal vein by a huge, tense, encysted hematoma.

Complications Involving the Urinary Tract

Urinary complications are found in 4 to 25% of cases.[98] They include reflux, stenosis, urinary fistula and ureteric obstructions.

Reflux, which occurs only when the ureter is anastomosed to the bladder as advocated by most authors, is uncommon if a suitable antireflux technique is used (cf. p. 319), with the ureter lying in a long submucous tunnel.

Stenosis is not rare with either uretero-ureteral or uretero-vesical anastomosis. It may cause progressive hydronephrosis with or without urinary infection; surgical repair may be necessary, but neither the patient nor his graft is at risk, since surgical cure is possible in most cases.

Urinary fistula is the most serious complication, with a mortality rate of between 14 and 60%.[106, 127] It generally occurs within the first 6 weeks after transplantation. A fistula may develop on the ureter, the bladder or a calyx.

Urinary ureteral extravasation is characterized by a decreased urinary output, pain, impaired renal function and frequently fever and swelling at the operative site. Diagnosis is confirmed by intravenous pyelography (Fig. 8.6) or ultrasonography. According to some authors, fistulae are less common after uretero-vesical[127] or pyelopelvic anastomosis[44] than after uretero-ureteral anastomosis. But whatever technique is adopted, a certain number of fistulae continue to occur, with an incidence of 4 to 25%,[98]

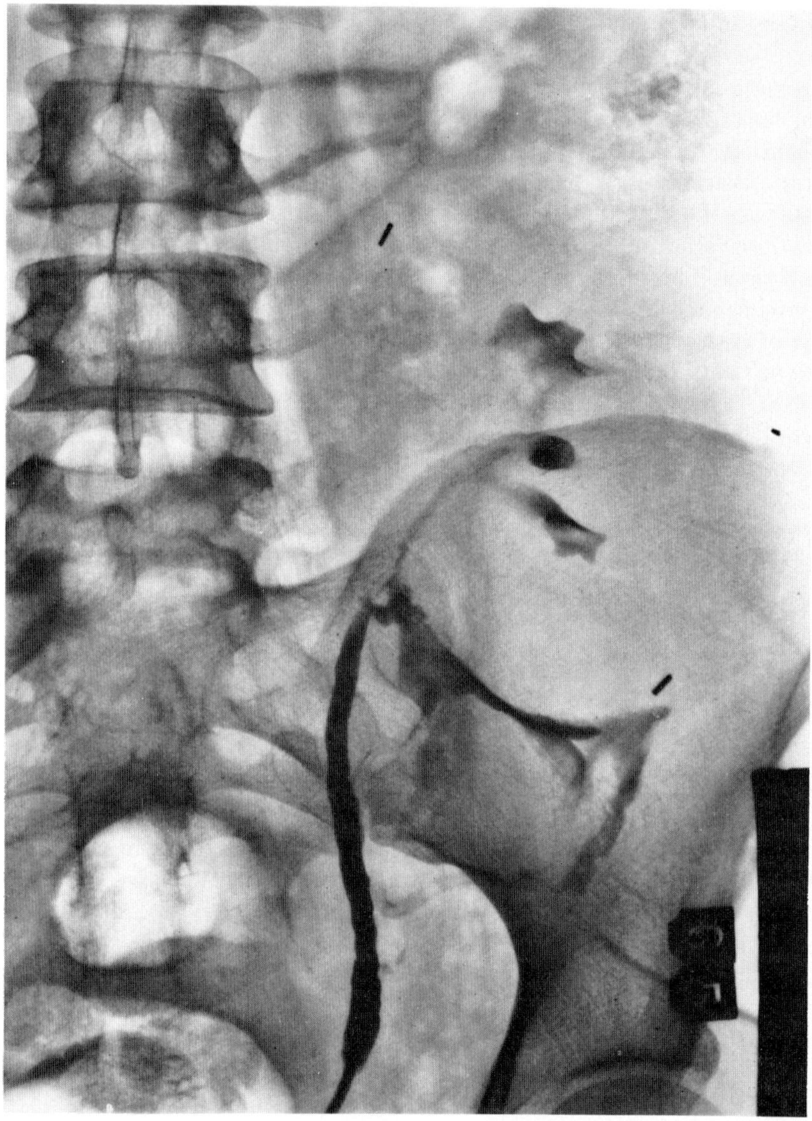

Fig. 8.6. Retrograde pyelogram 2 days after transplantation showing a ureteral fistula and a pocket surrounding the lower pole of the grafted kidney.

and 15% in our own series. This complication is generally accepted as due to the high doses of corticosteroids used during the early postoperative period. It may also be a manifestation of the rejection process directed against the ureter, as some authors[48] and we have found pathologic evidence of rejection in the wall of the grafted ureter and of its small arteries. Sometimes it is a technical complication due to trauma of the ureteric vessel during removal or during the anastomosis of the ureter to the bladder, particularly if the ureter is too short.[105] This is particularly the case when the fistula is due to focal ureteral necrosis at a distance from the site of anastomosis.

The symptoms of urinary leakage from bladder fistulae are very similar to those of ureteral extravasation. The diagnosis is confirmed by retrograde cystography. Bladder fistulae generally arise from the anterior bladder suture and are not always avoided despite a meticulous three-layer closure.[106] Bladder fistulae appear to be associated frequently with previous surgery of the bladder and are observed more frequently after second or third transplantations than in primary transplantation. If the fistula is small it may be managed solely by an indwelling catheter for at least 3 weeks. Cystography must be performed prior to catheter removal to confirm closure of the fistula. If the fistula is large or if ureteral catheter drainage fails to control urinary leakage, the bladder must be surgically repaired.[98]

Calyceal fistulae are usually related to segmental renal infarction due to difficulty in the removal of cadaveric kidneys or reanastomosis of an accessory renal artery.

Finally, urinary fistula is a very serious complication, often responsible for wound complication (cf. p. 292), perirenal abscess (cf. p. 233), septicemia (cf. p. 243) and/or progressive and irreversible deterioration of renal function. In our own series, 2.7% of patients died but 41% lost the graft and have returned to dialysis, fistulae having probably contributed to the failure of transplantation. However, fistulae involving the bladder had a significantly better prognosis than did ureteric fistulae.[98]

Ureteral obstruction may be due to several factors. The diagnosis can be very difficult, as the obstruction causes no pain in the transplant but does cause oliguria and deterioration of renal function.

In some cases obstruction was the result of compression by a large lymphocele. During the first few days after transplantation a blood clot may be responsible.

But more frequent are ureteral obstruction by calculi, particularly in patients who continue to have hyperparathyroidism after transplantation.[16, 69] Among the 19 cases we have observed, 9 were the subject of a detailed clinical and radiologic study that was reported in 1978.[3] Lithiasis is generally discovered late after transplantation because it is totally latent and inducing no pain, and the only symptoms are usually microscopic hematuria or pyuria.

INFECTIOUS COMPLICATIONS

It is not surprising that bacterial, viral and fungal infections should be common in patients treated with a combination of steroids and immunosuppressive drugs.[5] These complications play a major role in mortality after renal transplantation.[1, 25, 37, 67, 103]

Azathioprine is involved not only by its action on the immune response but also by its effect on the bone marrow, inducing leukopenia; however, it seems possible that in some cases leukopenia is not the cause of infection but is associated with it or is its consequence.[37]

Steroids, in addition to their immunosuppressive effect, also reduce the local inflammatory response, stabilize lysosomal membranes and increase the level of blood sugar, all factors which facilitate infection. Since the incidence of bacterial and fungal infections is higher during the first 4 months after transplantation, when doses of corticosteroids are particularly high, these infections are probably due to steroids. On the other hand, the daily doses of azathioprine remain consistent after transplantation, and this drug may therefore be responsible for viral infections and possibly also for tuberculosis.[63] We established, however, that an immunodepressive state obtained in mice by cyclophosphamide could in certain conditions decrease gentamicin activity against *Klebsiella pneumoniae* inoculated intraperitoneally.[38]

The risk of infection is increased in recipients over the age of 40,[51] in patients undergoing graft failure[25, 80] and in those with hypogammaglobulinemia.[103]

Bacterial Infections

We recently published a study of 80 infectious episodes occurring in the first six post-transplantation months in 51 kidney transplant recipients who underwent routine bacteriologic follow-up.[37] Table 8.1 shows the type of organisms implicated and the sites of infection in these 80 infectious episodes and the mortality in 21 cases of septicemia.

Clinical signs of bacterial infections are often reduced or even suppressed by corticosteroids, making diagnosis difficult. Fever remains the most reliable indicator, but in our study,[37] 40% of infectious episodes were nonfebrile.

The most frequently encountered bacteria are the gram-negative bacilli, but it is often difficult to isolate the responsible agents; blood cultures and cultures of samples from all potential sites should be repeated at regular intervals. When signs of severity, particularly neutropenia, occur,[37] antibiotic treatment must frequently be initiated before obtaining the results of bacterial investigations.

We must insist on the severity of infections due to *K. pneumoniae*, since in four of six cases of septicemia due to this organism, the infection was an important contributing factor to death. This severity is perhaps

TABLE 8.1
Organisms implicated in 80 bacterial infections observed in 51 allograft recipients[32]

Organisms Implicated	Site or Nature of Infectious Episode				Total
	Septicemia	Urinary Tract	Wound Abscess	Pneumonia	
Staphylococcus aureus	11 (3 deaths)	7	8	2	28
Staphylococcus epidermidis	1	10	0	0	11
Streptococcus species	1	12	1	0	14
Escherichia coli	0	9	0	0	9
Klebsiella pneumoniae	6 (4 deaths)	2	0	1	9
Salmonella typhi	0	1	0	0	1
Enterobacter cloacae	1	3	0	0	4
Proteus mirabilis	0	2	0	0	2
Serratia marcescens	0	1	0	0	1
Pseudomonas aeruginosa	1	0	0	0	1
Total	21	47	9	3	80

due to the tendency of septicemia caused by *Klebsiella* to be associated with neutropenia (three of the six cases).[37]

The most frequent bacterial infections involve the *urinary tract* and are often asymptomatic.[25, 37, 67] Often cured by the first course of antibiotics, they may become chronic if they are due to a lesion in the excretory tract and then may lead to acute pyelonephritis and septicemia.

Wound abscess, most often due to *Staphylococcus aureus,* requires surgical intervention. It is a serious complication that should be avoided by a high degree of asepsis during the course of the operation. For this reason, some authors believe that the nephrectomy of the patient's own kidney and the transplantation should be performed in two separate steps so that the nephrectomy site will be well healed and not provide a septic focus when immunosuppressive therapy is administered.[84]

Septicemia is reputed to have a very severe prognosis[25, 53, 84] with about 70% mortality. In the first edition of this book we reported a mortality of 52% in septicemia, but most of these deaths occurred during the period when total body irradiation was used. In our recent series we have had a less unsatisfactory outcome, with a mortality of 33.3%.[37]

Each group must carefully consider the precautions required for reducing the incidence of infections:[84] eliminate infection prior to transplantation; avoid, if possible, the use of catheters; avoid leukopenia and discontinue azathioprine if the white blood cell count is low; reduce, and in severe infections, discontinue the steroid dose, even though this may lead to sacrificing the kidney in order to control the infection; develop regular post-transplantation bacteriologic check-up procedures for detecting infectious complications.[38]

Viral Infections

In our own series we have observed 72 cases of proven viral infections. Viral hepatitis and viral pneumonia will be discussed with hepatic complications (p. 249) and pulmonary complications (p. 247). See also malignant tumors (p. 257).

In fact, the incidence of viral infections in allograft recipients is particularly difficult to determine. Isolation of the virus from the blood, urine or other samples is often difficult, and in many episodes of unexplained fever it is not possible to obtain positive proof for a viral origin although it is strongly suspected. Conversely, many viruses, such as of the herpes group, can exist in a latent state, and their detection in a renal graft recipient or the observation of antibody rises may be related to activation of a "latent virus" or to immunological dysfunction rather than to viral infection.[31]

In our experience ordinary viral infections such as herpes zoster, herpes simplex, chicken pox, mumps, influenza etc., are not particularly severe and resolve normally without any reduction in the dose of immunosuppressive drugs or steroids.

Apart from producing clinical disease, viral infections can modulate the immune system. Moreover, virus may be involved in oncogenesis, leading to the high incidence of malignant tumors in renal allograft recipients.[79]

Finally, some viruses, in particular cytomegaloviruses, can cause very severe infection in immunosuppressed individuals.[22, 71, 72] Some of these infections are reactivation of a latent virus and some are primary infections in initially seronegative patients transmitted by a kidney from a seropositive donor.[19] Contrary to the conclusions of some groups,[116] it seems that fever, arthralgia, pneumonitis, hepatitis and deterioration of renal function with histologic evidence of rejection of the transplanted kidney[73] may be observed in primary infections as well as in reactivations.[42] No satisfactory explanation has yet been given of the mechanism(s) involved in the association between viral infection and rejection episodes. In certain cases the rejection phenomenon itself could possibly stimulate expression of a latent virus.

In view of all these uncertainties, it is difficult to adopt a consistent therapeutic approach and particularly to decide whether immunosuppressive therapy ought to be stopped, decreased or even increased. However, in very severe and life-threatening infection, every group agrees with the disruption of immunosuppressive therapy. Various therapeutic attempts have been made—interferon[128] or immunoenhancing agents such as transfer factor or levamasol,[32] vaccination[22, 45] or various antiviral agents[22]—but these efforts have been without effect.

Fungal Infections and Infections Due to Rare Organisms

It is probable that steroids, and perhaps antilymphocyte globulins, rather than azathioprine, are responsible for the very high incidence of mycotic infection and also for various infections due to micro-organisms rarely encountered in human pathology in other circumstances.

The mycoses nearly always appear when infection is treated by antibiotics in a patient who is already receiving azathioprine and steroids. Bone marrow depression is another predisposing factor. For unknown reasons, the incidence in infected males is two to three times that expected from the total male to female ratio.[43, 51, 102]

Infections with *Candida albicans* are the most frequent and generally the least severe of mycoses; however, two out of four patients observed by Gallis et al[43] died. It is often possible to reduce the risk of this type of infection by oral prophylactic antifungal treatment while a patient is receiving high doses of steroids, particularly if he is also receiving antibiotics.

All fungal infections may be observed after transplantation.[43] The usual clinical course of *cryptococcosis* is that of subacute meningitis sometimes associated with pulmonary infiltrates. Cerebrospinal fluid cultures and tests for cryptococcal antigen performed on the cerebrospinal fluid may be positive. Even when a rapid diagnosis is made, allowing treatment by amphotericin B and/or 5-fluorocytosine, the prognosis is very severe.[9, 36, 43]

Diagnosis of *nocardiosis*[43] is demonstrated by the finding of *Nocardia asteroidis* by gram stain in sputum or by thoracotomy with lung biopsy. Patients have fever and pulmonary infiltrates progressing to cavitation, sometimes associated with pleural effusion. Some patients have symptoms which can be attributed to the central nervous system. In general the response to antibiotics is good.[8, 43]

In pulmonary *aspergillosis* (Fig. 8.7), aspergillus can be difficult to culture from sputum and may require biopsy or alveolar washout. While precipitins are commonly positive in patients with aspergillomas or bronchopulmonary aspergilloses, controversy exists about their presence in invasive disease.[85]

Coccidiomycoses have been observed after transplantation in patients originating from the southern United States, Mexico and certain parts of Central and South America.[107]

Other organisms, phycomycosis, chromomycosis and subcutaneous infection with *Phialophora gougeroti*, have been observed but appear to be rare.[43]

Among the organisms responsible for severe infections, *Pneumocystis carinii* can be the cause of pneumonia with acute respiratory insuffi-

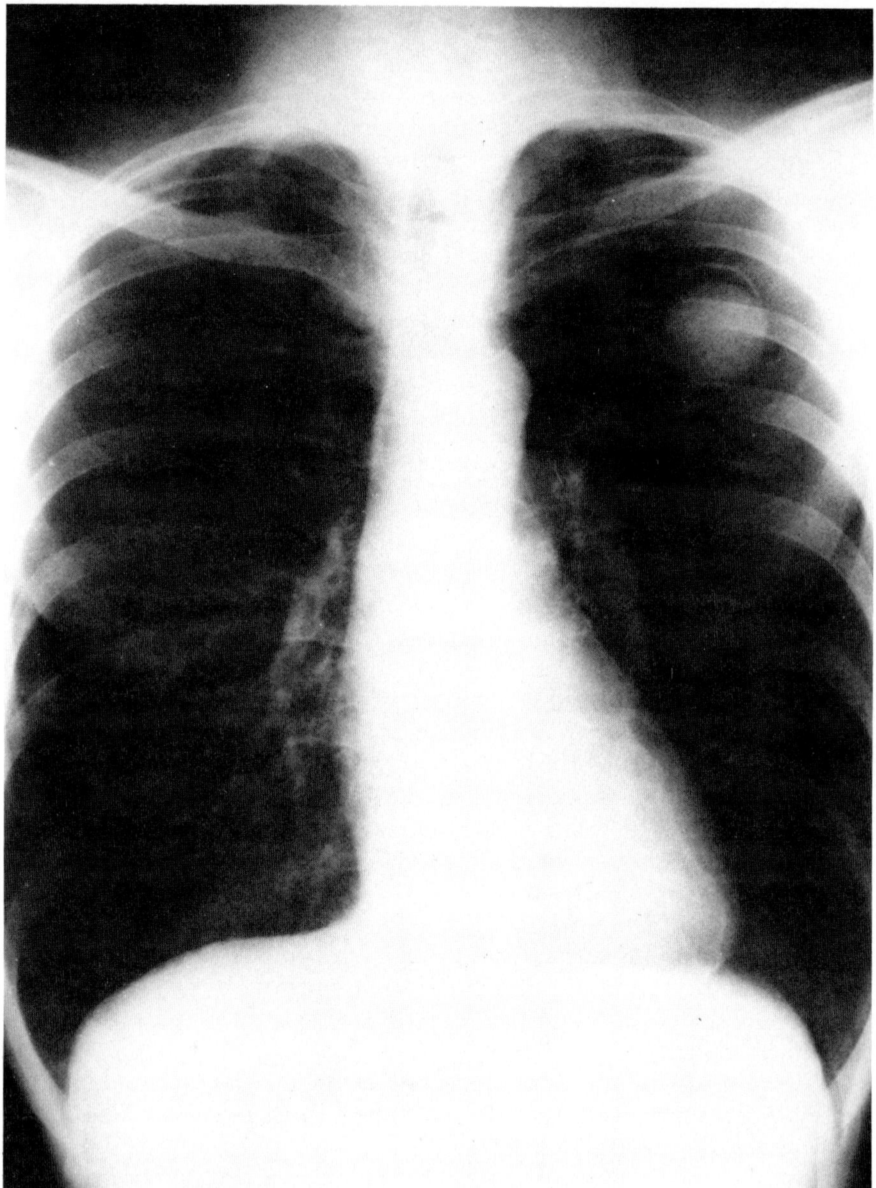

Fig. 8.7. Chest x-ray in a patient with a transplant demonstrating the presence of an aspergilloma in the left lung.

ciency, marked by hypoxia with a remarkable fall in PO_2 and oxygen saturation. Diagnosis is very difficult because attempts to isolate microorganisms from the sputum always produce negative results. Only lung biopsy after thoracotomy or alveolar washout and bronchial brushing can demonstrate the organism. Treatment by pentamidine and by sulfadiazine has been successful in some cases but pentamidine is a difficult drug to handle and should not be used unless diagnosis is certain. The sulfamethoxasol trimethoprime (Bactrim) seems today to be the most efficient drug when used at very high dosage.[68]

PULMONARY COMPLICATIONS

Pulmonary Infections

The lungs are the most frequent site of infection in transplant recipients, and the severity of these infections results in death in about a third of cases. The most severe episodes occur during the first 6 months after transplantation and are directly related to the corticosteroid dosage. All the organisms (see above) detected in immunodeprived individuals can be responsible for lung infection, but their isolation is extremely difficult, which may explain the severity of the prognosis.

The poor prognosis is also due to infectious pulmonary edema that results in acute respiratory insufficiency with severe hypoxemia and hypocapnia; death may occur before results of bacteriologic examinations are available. It is thus important to determine very rapidly the therapy to use and to initiate investigations to determine the agent involved.

The following is the Necker policy when pneumonia is suspected:

1. Immunosuppressive therapy and corticosteroids are disrupted.
2. PO_2, PCO_2 and pH are determined.
3. Routine bacteriologic examinations are performed in the blood and urine, and a primary infectious site is systematically sought.
4. Lung transtracheal puncture, alveolar washout and bronchial brushing under fibroscopic examination are performed as soon as possible.
5. Samples are taken for viral and fungal serodiagnoses.
6. Patients are then routinely subjected to dehydration to maintain hypovolemia, by furosemide if the patient has normal renal function or by hemodialysis or hemofiltration. Very often, dehydration is immediately followed by improvement in chest x-ray and PCO_2.
7. Simultaneously, the patient is subjected to continuous positive airway pressure that will improve his general status and induce a rise in PO_2
8. If the state of the patient permits, it is preferable to await the results of bacteriologic investigations before beginning antibiotherapy. If not, or

if bacteriologic techniques are negative, we are obliged to use a broad spectrum antibiotic, since the organisms most often found in allograft recipients are *Staphylococcus* species, *Streptococcus* species, *K. pneumoniae* and *Escherichia coli*[37] (Table 8.1).

Even lung biopsy may not provide definitive diagnosis. These cases are probably the result of a viral infection which has not been detected. The hypothesis has also been advanced of an autoimmune disease due to the development of antibodies which attack the pulmonary basement membranes as well as the kidney antigens. However, this condition, known as "transplant lungs",[103] has not as yet been elucidated, and it would be unreasonable to increase corticosteroid dosage until it has been clarified.

Tuberculosis

Tuberculosis in a renal transplant recipient is very rare but can occur at any time after transplantation. Publications on this subject stem particularly from French centers, and its frequency is reported to range from less than 1[90] to 6%,[18] although the frequency in the general population in France is 0.7%. In our own series we have observed 15 cases of pulmonary tuberculosis, of which 2 were miliary. The problem of tuberculosis in a transplant recipient does not differ from that in other patients: routine antituberculosis chemotherapeutic agents are effective and it is not necessary to stop immunosuppressive therapy. The only real problem, since it is usual to give isoniazid routinely for protection in transplant recipients who have a previous history of tuberculosis, is to decide whether antibiotic therapy can be stopped at the end of the usual treatment period or should be continued indefinitely. We generally interrupt the treatment; certain authors[90] have noted recurrence in these patients, whereas we have observed recurrence in only one.

Pulmonary Embolism

Most kidney transplantation centers have noted a relative frequency of arterial and venous thrombosis and pulmonary embolism.[25, 46, 86] These complications may occur quite late. In our series 17 embolisms appeared in 16 patients between 10 days and more than 6 years after transplantation. The cause is unknown and there is no obvious coagulation disorder,[122] abnormality of lipid metabolism or evidence of fat embolism.[58]

HEPATIC COMPLICATIONS

Since the first series of renal transplantations, the frequency of liver alterations has been noted in renal allograft recipients by the majority of authors.[34, 49, 81, 97] The various lesions observed are usually considered a consequence of the transplantation procedure. We will successively discuss hepatitis, peliosis and idiopathic portal hypertension.

Hepatitis

Hepatitis is the most frequent type of liver disease in transplant recipients. Clinical manifestations and/or biologic evidence was found in 29% of our patients. Usually it is mixed hepatocellular and cholestatic hepatitis, but the true hepatocellular or cholestatic forms also occur, although rarely. In general, the immunosuppressive drugs are held responsible for the liver lesions, but the deleterious effect of azathioprine or 6-mercaptopurine, either by direct toxic action on the liver[49, 52, 115] or by alteration of the immune response (rendering, for example, patients more susceptible to viruses)[6, 114] remains to be demonstrated.

In fact, it must not be forgotten that before transplantation patients are often treated for a number of years by hemodialysis and that the high incidence of HBsAg in hemodialysis units is well known. It therefore appeared possible that the liver lesions were present before transplantation.

In a prospective study of 64 patients,[28] we routinely performed liver biopsy on the day of transplantation and 1 and 3 years later. Chronic hepatitis was already present in 40% of the patients on the day of transplantation, and an increase of only 12 and 15% in the frequency of this condition was observed 1 and 3 years later. Moreover, at each point of the follow-up, the correlation between the incidence of chronic hepatitis and virus B infection was highly significant.

We therefore conclude that chronic hepatitis cannot be considered a direct consequence of renal transplantation but rather of events prior to transplantation probably related to hemodialysis treatment.

On the other hand, it is quite possible that transplantation can modify the course of pre-existing chronic hepatitis by alteration of immune responses. The normally unusual change from chronic persistent hepatitis, generally considered benign in nontransplant patients,[11] to chronic active hepatitis and to cirrhosis[28, 123] appears to be particularly frequent in renal transplant recipients. It may probably also be observed in hemodialysis patients, perhaps because both in these patients and in allograft recipients an immunodeficiency results respectively from renal failure or from immunodepressive therapy.

In conclusion, in the absence of a control series of liver biopsies in HBsAg positive chronic hemodialyzed patients, it is not possible to determine whether transplantation modifies the course of previous liver lesions. For us, chronic hepatitis in a hemodialyzed patient is not a contraindication to renal transplantation. Moreover, in our experience[30] survival of the transplanted kidney may be significantly better in recipients who carry the hepatitis B antigen than in those who do not.

Lastly, it is interesting to note that the present treatment for chronic hepatitis in nontransplanted patients is the administration of corticosteroids and azathioprine,[113] whereas in graft recipients these drugs not only do not prevent a severe outcome but are considered to be directly responsible for it. It is thus difficult to decide how to handle immunosuppressive therapy when hepatitis occurs. Is it necessary to stop the treatment and run the risk of triggering a rejection episode when there is still little evidence that these drugs are harmful? Or should one continue them, and even at an increased dosage since the immunosuppressive activity of azathioprine is reduced in patients with hepatic dysfunction?[7] In addition, in reaching a decision one must take into account the observation made by our group that disruption of azathioprine during the course of hepatitis was well tolerated in 80% of recipients, even for a period of several years.[26]

Peliosis Hepatis

Peliosis hepatis was first described by Wagner in 1861.[125] It is a very uncommon liver lesion characterized by blood filled cavities bordered by hepatocytic plates. While only 155 cases had been published up to 1978, we observed 12 cases of peliosis hepatis in a series of 500 renal allograft recipients treated at the Necker and Broussais Hospitals between 1965 and 1975.[29] According to the size and the extent of the liver lesions, we distinguished a minor and a major form of peliosis hepatis. The former is clinically latent while the latter is associated with hepatomegaly and portal hypertension. In two of our patients cirrhosis was found on subsequent pathologic examination. This finding is consistent with the view that peliosis hepatis per se can induce the development of cirrhosis.

The incidence of peliosis hepatis in our series is 2.4%. In view of its incidence, the disease is certainly correlated with transplantation. Since peliosis has been reported in patients receiving certain drugs and particularly anabolic, androgenic or estrogenic steroids,[10, 12, 88] and since venoocclusive disease of the liver and sinusoidal dilatation, both hepatic lesions closely related to peliosis, have been reported in patients treated with azathioprine or 6-mercaptopurine,[21, 76] immunosuppressive drugs, azathioprine or corticosteroids, probably play an important role in its pathogenesis.

Idiopathic Portal Hypertension[89]

We have observed two cases in which recurrent hematemesis in renal transplant recipients necessitated a portocaval shunt. The condition of these patients was characterized by increased portal venous pressure in the absence of both histologic lesions of the liver and obstruction of the portal vein. However, in both patients perisinusoidal fibrosis which was not detected by light microscopy was demonstrated by electron microscopy. In these two patients receiving azathioprine, perisinusoidal fibrosis might be the consequence of prolonged administration of this drug, and it is suggested that portal obstruction of hepatic sinusoids by perisinusoidal fibrosis could be the mechanism for increased portal venous pressure.

BONE COMPLICATIONS

Hyperparathyroidism and Disorders of Calcium and Phosphorus Metabolism

In many patients, the biochemical disorders and radiologic changes of hyperparathyroidism regress after transplantation so that parathyroidectomy is rarely needed. This favorable outcome is not consistently observed, however, and its rate and extent are variable.

Whereas early works[57] indicated that parathormone (PTH) in allograft recipients returned to normal within a few months provided graft function was normal, several more recent publications reported persistence of hyperparathyroidism in allograft recipients with normal renal function up to 8 years after surgery.[27, 62, 130]

In our own series, almost half the patients had persistence of hyperparathyroidism, but the abnormalities in these patients were mild and only 13 patients underwent parathyroidectomy.

The mechanism of this persistent abnormality is uncertain, and the reason why parathyroid enlargement and hypersecretion pursue their course in some patients is unknown. A mild alteration of renal function could be involved in some cases; the prolonged parathyroid hyperplasia could provoke or be associated with a poor susceptibility of parathyroid cells to hypercalcemia.[20]

Autonomous or tertiary hyperparathyroidism is perhaps partially responsible for the hypophosphoremia very frequently observed in allograft recipients when renal function is normal. But some studies[20, 35, 77, 82] indicate that hypophosphoremia is above all due to persistent alteration of digestible phosphorous absorption,[35] or more probably to urine leakage of phosphate.[82] The pathophysiology of elevated phosphaturia in transplant patients is unknown. We have shown that in allograft recipients with hypophosphoremia there is an increased production of $1{,}25(OH)_2$ vit D_3 that could explain the hypercalciuria sometimes observed in these patients.

Aseptic Osteonecrosis

First reported by Starzl[119] in 1964, aseptic osteonecrosis in allograft recipients has been observed by most transplantation groups, with an incidence varying from 4 to 41%. In a retrospective study including all patients transplanted at Necker Hospital between June 1959 and October 1978, we observed that among those who received steroid treatment for a minimum of 1 year, 68 patients (49 males and 19 females), i.e., 21%, developed one or more aseptic osteonecrotic lesions, whereas in our overall transplant population for the same period, this incidence was only 14%.

When aseptic osteonecrosis was suspected on the basis of a history of joint pain, diagnosis was based on radiographic and scintigraphic data. The earliest roentgenographic change was the development of a subchondral radiolucent crescent; bone scintigraphy showed hyperfixing focus.

Of the 68 patients cited above, in 38 osteonecrosis had begun within 12 months after transplantation. Two or more affected sites were observed in 88% of the patients, with involvement of the femoral condyles, tibial plateau, shoulder, tali or olecranon; but 39 of the 68 patients (57.8%) demonstrated radiographic evidence of hip joint avascular necrosis, which is the most frequent alteration (Fig. 8.8).

The outcome of osteonecrosis varies. In two-thirds of the patients the progression is frank collapse of the bone, an increase of sclerosis and arthrosis, sometimes with incomplete dislocation of the joint; in one-third of the patients the progression is to osteocondensation without dislocation.

Although the pathogenesis of these bone lesions is still poorly understood, corticosteroid therapy certainly plays a major role. Since the first publication in 1957 relating osteonecrosis to steroid therapy,[99] aseptic necrosis has been described in patients receiving steroids for a diverse group of other disorders treated by corticosteroids that had not been associated with aseptic necrosis prior to the use of corticosteroid therapy.[55] Some centers[87, 132] have found a correlation between the total dose of prednisone administered and the incidence of aseptic necrosis in renal transplant recipients. We did not find this correlation in our own series (see Table 8.2), but in living donor recipients who never received steroids after transplantation (HLA-identical siblings without rejection crises), there was no episode of osteonecrosis.

The way in which steroids produce aseptic necrosis has not been determined.[55] One hypothesis for which there is considerable evidence in both experimental animals and man[40, 41] is that corticosteroids induce hyperlipidemia, fatty infiltration of the liver, systemic fat embolization and occlusion of subchondrial arterioles, leading to ischemic necrosis of

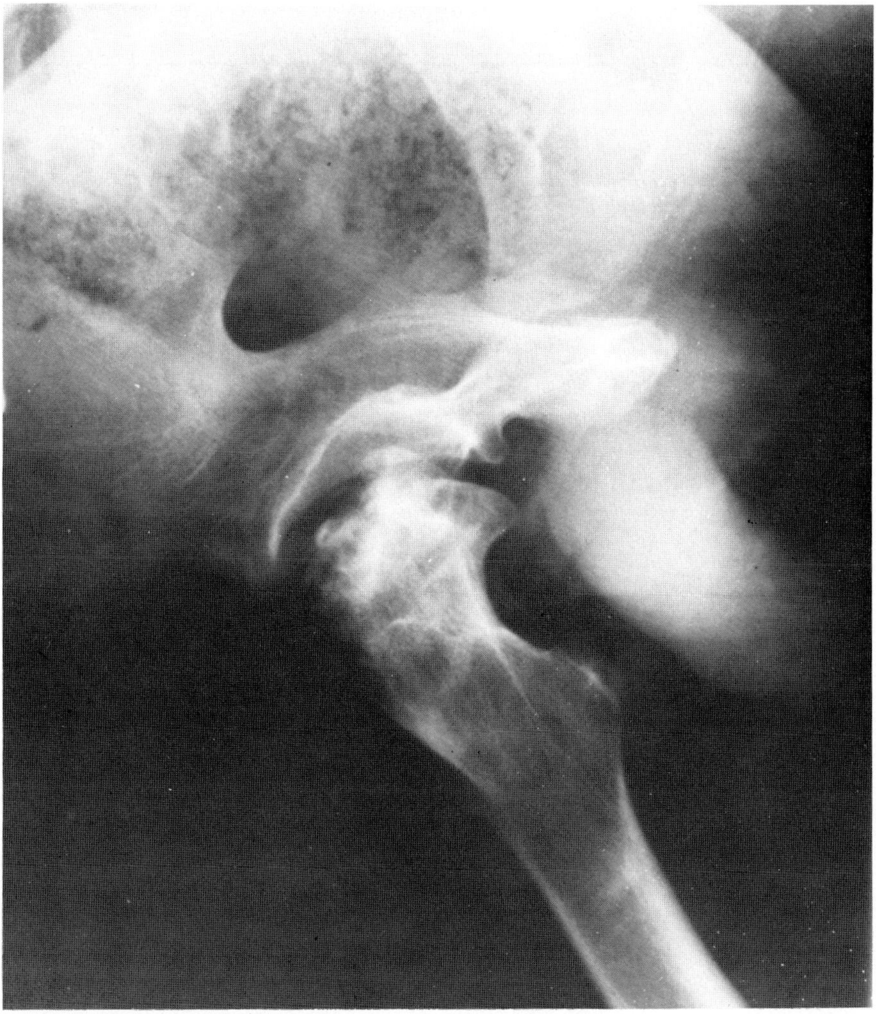

Fig. 8.8. Severe lesions of the right hip as a consequence of aseptic osteonecrosis observed 1 year after transplantation.

bone. However, serum lipids and liver function tests in many series,[112] as well as in our own, are not significantly different in transplanted patients with aseptic necrosis than in those without. Another hypothesis is that bone resorption induced by steroids associated with renal osteodystrophy and inhibition of osteoblastic bone formation due to persistent hyperparathyroidism could lead to trabecular collapse and thus produce bone necrosis.[15, 112]

Both surgical and nonsurgical treatment can be used. The object of

TABLE 8.2
Aseptic necrosis following renal transplantation

Role of Steroids		
Group of Patients	Mean Dosage of Prednisone (g/kg/day)	
68 with aseptic necrosis of bone	0.80	
50 (matched for age, sex, etc.)		N.S.
without aseptic necrosis of bone	0.68	

medical treatment is to limit weightbearing of the joint by the use of a wheelchair and/or of two crutches. At Necker Hospital this treatment is used for 4 to 6 months whenever a patient shows radiologic evidence of osteonecrosis and/or joint hyperfixation in scintigraphy. In our experience this treatment was efficient and sufficed for 40% of these patients.

Of 39 patients with hip lesions, 11 had alterations of one hip and 28 alterations of two; 22 underwent surgical treatment (osteotomy, cupula, Moore prothesis or total hip replacement) with good overall results.[70]

Nevertheless, because of its frequency and severity, aseptic osteonecrosis is often a cause of poor rehabilitation of the transplant recipient. It will certainly not disappear until the day that allografts can be undertaken without corticosteroid therapy.

Other Complications of Steroids Affecting the Skeleton and Joints

High or prolonged steroid dosage can cause severe bone disorders. We have seen vertebral collapse, rib fractures and fracture of the pelvis in patients with no evidence of hyperparathyroidism. In these cases, osteoporosis seems to be entirely explained by the prolonged use of prednisone in high doses.

The growth of children after transplantation is not always satisfactory, and even if the age of bone maturation corresponds to less than 12 years, the proportion of children with normal growth varies considerably from one series to another, from 13 to over 60%.[23] One of the most important factors responsible is the administration of corticosteroids. Thus. many centers use intermittent corticosteroid administration for children, but more experience with this protocol is necessary before final conclusions may be reached.

ARTERIAL HYPERTENSION

The antihypertensive effect of renal transplantation has now been well established. However, in patients who were previously hypertensive its correction can be delayed when they are receiving high doses of prednisone.[50, 119] The persistence or recurrence of hypertension in the transplant recipient, which is more frequently observed in grafts from cadaver donors than in those from living donors, reaches 60% of cases in one small series of 85 patients transplanted in 1970 and 1971 and published by our group in 1977.[64] This may be explained by the discovery of renal arterial stenosis or the advent of chronic rejection or recurrence of glomerulonephritis in the recipient, or it may be due to the original diseased kidney when it is left in place. When hypertension recurs, it is important to determine its exact mechanism so that the best therapeutic choice can be made. In an effort to elucidate the question, we have collected data on intrarenal hemodynamics, renal histopathology and renin secretion rate in 11 normotensive and 51 hypertensive homotransplanted patients.[47, 64] Renin secretion rate and residual output from original in situ kidneys were compared. It is difficult to determine the exact hypertensive mechanism when the original kidney is left in place since many transplant recipients do not develop high blood pressure despite the presence of their own diseased kidney.[65, 131]

Our results were as follows:

1. In the 11 normotensive transplanted patients, renal hemodynamic data were comparable with those obtained in potential kidney donors.

2. In six hypertensive patients having chronic rejection, the mean renal blood flow and the percentage of flow in the first component of the washout curve were reduced. Renin release from the transplant, however, was normal.

3. Eleven hypertensive patients had transplant artery stenosis. In eight of these patients, renin release from the graft as well as peripheral plasma renin activity (PRA) were within normal range. On the contrary, in two of the patients with very tight artery stenosis, renin release from the transplant was elevated. In one patient renin release could not be measured.

4. Thirty-four hypertensive patients had neither renal artery stenosis nor chronic rejection. Twenty-four patients in this group had elevated arteriovenous PRA difference in their own kidney, and peripheral PRA was significantly higher than in normotensive patients; left nephrectomy relieved hypertension in 17 of them and was not effective in two others, while five have so far not undergone nephrectomy.

Conversely, in 10 patients the arteriovenous PRA difference of the patient's own kidney fell within normal range; however, in 7 of them, hypertension was relieved by removal of the in situ kidney.

From this study we concluded that, despite the lack of consistent results, the role of the original diseased kidney in the genesis of hypertension in transplant recipients can be suspected when its renin secretion is much higher than that of the transplant; in these cases, removal of the original kidney will generally be followed by normalization of blood pressure. In contrast, renin secretion by the transplant is rarely increased even if arterial stenosis or chronic rejection are at the origin of renal hypertension. Lastly, nephrectomy of the original kidney may relieve hypertension even in cases where renin release from this kidney is not elevated.

HEMATOLOGIC COMPLICATIONS

Despite the interference of immunosuppressive drugs, kidney transplantation normally leads, within 6 weeks to 3 months, to a complete disappearance of the anemia which was due to uremia.[33] Erythropoietic activity in the serum, which was absent in chronic uremia, also becomes normal after transplantation,[4] as does ^{59}Fe incorporation into red blood cells.[75]

However, certain transplant recipients do not recover normal hematocrit or secondarily develop anemia,[39, 104] even when renal function is normal. Usually this anemia is macrocytic, sometimes megaloblastic, despite normal plasma vitamin B_{12} and folate levels, and it is thought that these patients have a particular bone marrow sensitivity to azathioprine. Moreover, anemia can be increased by the hemolysis often observed in transplant recipients, which is probably due to mild vascular lesions of the graft.[39]

Leukopenia and thrombocytopenia are frequent, due to abnormal bone marrow sensitivity to azathioprine or to an overdosage of this drug, and then frequently associated with or followed by eosinophilia. They require reduction or disruption of Imuran. Thrombocytopenia may be seen in patients treated by antilymphocyte serum. In some cases the existence of a large spleen may suggest peripheral destruction of granulocytes and lead to consideration of splenectomy if splenic sequestration can be proven.

Polycythemia has been described by several authors.[56, 92, 133] In our experience, it can be observed in two different circumstances.

It can occur about 4 months after transplantation and then spontaneously regress after several months.[120] Its mechanism is unknown.

It can sometimes occur in association with hypertension, high plasma renin activity and decreased renal function. It is then thought to be due to the vascular lesions of rejection causing hypoxia of the graft.[61, 129]

Short-lived leukocytosis and thrombocytosis can occur during the course of treating rejection episodes with high doses of steroids.

MALIGNANT TUMORS

It is clearly established that transplant patients are more prone than the general population to develop cancer. The incidence of de novo tumors following transplantation varies according to different authors. In several large series its incidence was found to be between 2[78] and 7%.[109] In our own series it is 3.4%. These figures probably underestimate the problem because they do not make allowance for the fact that a large number of recipients survive only a short time after transplantation and that the length of follow-up for many patients has been short. In an Australian series, where the incidence is very high because of the number of skin or lip cancers due to the oncogenic effects of sunlight, the incidence of cancer in survivors increased progressively with time. The proportion of patients surviving beyond 1, 5, 8 and 10 years who developed cancer were 20, 34, 39 and 57%.[110]

The various types of de novo malignancies occurring in transplant recipients have been particularly studied by Penn[94–96] on data from many series in the Denver Tumor Registry. He estimates that the incidence of cancer for the same age range is approximately 100 times greater than that in the general population.

The most remarkable figure is the high incidence of lymphomas, which occur in 33% of patients with cancer. This is in marked contrast with an incidence of 3 to 4% in the general population. The predominant type of lymphoma is reticulum cell sarcoma, (62%) which is 350 times more common in renal transplant recipients than in the general population.[96] In our own series 6% of patients treated between 1959 and 1964 by total body irradiation died from acute leukemia. Conversely, the types of cancer commonly seen in the general population are infrequent in organ transplant recipients (carcinoma of the prostate, colon and rectum, female breasts, etc.). The most frequently encountered carcinoma involves the skin and lower lip and probably explains the difference between the Australian statistics,[101] where skin cancer is very frequent, and that of the Denver Tumor Registry which includes, among others, European statistics, where this incidence is only 2%.[17]

The skin neoplasm differs from those encountered in the general population because in transplant patients squamous cell carcinomas are far more frequent than basal cell carcinomas.[95, 126]

Premalignant skin lesions, usually in the form of hyperkeratosis, are common in transplant patients, occurring most frequently in areas exposed to sunlight. It is often difficult to distinguish clinically among the various skin lesions, and all suspicious areas should be biopsied. Another source of confusion is warts. In one of our patients, Lutzner[74] found two different human papillomaviruses, HPV_3 being associated with the potentially oncogenic HPV_5.

There is also an unexpectedly high incidence of Kaposi's sarcoma in organ transplant recipients,[95] although in our experience it is difficult to distinguish between them and pseudo-Kaposi lesions.

In the European study,[17] the prognosis appears very severe since 50%

of patients died within 6 months after the discovery of the cancer. In this series, however, skin cancer comprises only 11% of the total. On the contrary, for Penn[95] or for Australian authors,[110] 3% of deaths in transplant recipients are caused by neoplasms. According to the latter authors,[110] patients with cancer may even have a better survival rate during the first 8 years after transplantation than that of patients without cancer.

The role of immunosuppressive agents in the development of malignant tumors in transplant patients is very likely. For example, in 64 recipients of organs from donors who had malignancies, there was a 36% incidence of neoplasia.[94] In these patients, it appears that immunosuppressive therapy permitted the survival, growth and spread of tumor cells inadvertently transplanted with the graft. But it is not the only factor involved, and immunologic responses engendered by the allograft might also play a role.[108]

There is considerable controversy concerning the management of immunosuppressive therapy—whether or not it is necessary to discontinue or reduce immunosuppressive therapy when it is associated with conventional treatment by surgery, and/or radiotherapy and/or chemotherapy. Our own policy is to disrupt immunosuppressive therapy in every case. It is based on reported cases in which tumors regressed completely when immunosuppression was stopped[93, 94] and on our observation that in 80% of cases, disruption of azathioprine was well tolerated and not followed by rejection.[26] Despite this policy, 8 of our 15 patients with cancer have died.

OTHER COMPLICATIONS

Gastrointestinal Complications

In 1969, in a study of nonrenal complications occurring in 97 patients who had received 103 allografts, we reported 13 severe gastrointestinal complications due to steroids, peptic ulcer, perforation and/or gastrointestinal hemorrhage with or without detectable gastric or duodenal ulcer.[25] These complications were responsible for patient deaths in three cases, which represent more than 6% of the mortalities in our series. Since 1969 we have seen only 35 gastric complications in 32 patients, with no deaths.

This improvement is due to three factors: first, in all allograft recipients receiving high doses of steroids, prophylactic therapy with atropine-like drugs and alkaline powders or gels is routinely given; second, gastrointestinal endoscopy is routinely performed when patients have even mild abdominal pain, frequently revealing gastric or duodenal ulcers that were not detected by x-ray examination; third, the introduction of cimetidine, a potent H_2 histamine receptor antagonist, allows good control of gastric hyperacidity and has been successfully used to prevent gastrointestinal ulceration and bleeding in kidney transplant recipients.[59] However, rejection episodes have been reported after the use of cimetidine in transplant recipients,[101] and some authors caution against the use of this drug until more is known about immunologic disorders caused by histamine H_2 receptor antagonists.[101, 134]

In one of our patients 11 years after transplantation, we observed Menetrier disease, for which we completely disrupted immunosuppressive therapy and performed total gastrectomy. The patient underwent chronic rejection and returned to hemodialysis.

Steroid Diabetes

Steroid diabetes is a frequent complication of chronic steroid administration. When the patient receives a high dosage of steroids just after transplantation, sugar is quite consistently found in the urine. This may reflect exacerbation of a prediabetic state or the discovery of a previously latent and unrecognized diabetes. When it is a true steroid diabetes, it is frequently mild and generally may be controlled by diet alone.

Psychiatric Disorders

When patients finally do receive the graft they have long desired, they cannot help worrying about how they will tolerate the transplant, the threat of rejection and the always possible serious complications. Given these conditions, psychiatric complications can occur, especially since the corticosteroids which patients receive after transplantation can trigger latent psychiatric disorders.

Manifestations are usual and are generally mild. In a study of 232 patients who received transplants at Necker Hospital, we noted 21 cases of psychiatric complications.[24] In 14 of these cases the patients were under 25 years of age.

Thrombosis and Thromboembolic Phenomena (cf. p. 248)

Pancreatitis

Severe and fatal pancreatitis has been reported after kidney transplantation.[58, 121] These cases have been considered to be complications of steroid therapy,[13] cytomegalovirus infection[121] or viral hepatitis.[54]

Among two cases of pancreatitis we have observed, one was discovered at autopsy in a patient with hyperparathyroidism and another was the terminal episode in a case of viral hepatitis, but here too autopsy disclosed four hyperplastic parathyroids.

Ophthalmic Complications

Some ophthalmic complications are directly iatrogenic, provoked by corticosteroids, whereas azathioprine is never responsible for eye alterations, and others are due to infections induced by immunosuppression.

Eye Complications Due to Corticosteroids

Low doses of corticosteroids, even during a long period, never provoke *cataract*, but the high doses given during rejection episodes produce subcortical crystalline opacities; these cataracts affect only the posterior pole of the lens. They are not very dense and do not progress; consequently they cause little impairment of visual acuity and do not require surgery.

Long-term steroid therapy may also be responsible for eye hypertonia, but this type of glaucoma is mild and not frequent.

Infectious Complications

Viral infections are frequent and are due to immunosuppression. All transplantation centers observe many cases of cornea herpes simplex or herpes zoster ophthalmicus. They generally do not require disruption of corticotherapy. Uveitis has also been observed, very infrequently but in a highly severe form, due to cytomegalic inclusions disease.

Lastly, we have observed one case of eye and palpebral lesions associated with a Lyell syndrome, due to intolerance of ATG.

Skin Lesions

Most transplant recipients have skin complications, usually related to immunosuppressive therapy. These complications are of different types. We have seen above the high rate of skin and lip tumors, principally in Australia and New Zealand (cf. p. 257). Other skin complications are due to virus, herpes simplex, herpes zoster or wart, to bacterium, sometimes the starting point of septicemia or to fungi, moniliasis, tinea versicolor or trichophytoses. Because of the steroids, the skin is thin and atrophic, with purpura and livedo. Finally, in patients receiving ALS, intolerance reactions can be observed, and one of our patients had a Lyell syndrome.

Most of these complications are induced or aggravated by corticosteroids, which appear to be the most troublesome drugs administered to the transplant recipient.

Because of the severity of these complications, which are actually the major cause of mortality after transplantation, we felt, as early as 1969,[25] that rather than continuing to treat multiple recurrent rejection episodes it is often better to remove the graft and return the patient to hemodialysis before the serious complications of immunosuppressive therapy occur.

REFERENCES

1. ACS/NIH. Organ Transplant Registry. The 11th Report of the Human Renal Transplant Registry. JAMA, *226:*1197, 1973.
2. ACS/NIH. Organ Transplant Registry. The 13th Report of the Human Renal Transplant Registry. Transplant. Proc., *9:*9, 1977.
3. Affre, J., Moreau, J. F., Kreis, H., Crosnier, J., and Michel, J. R. Lithiase urinaire après transplantation rénale. 9 observations. Nouv. Presse Méd., *7:*3223, 1978.
4. Albrecht, P. H., and Greene, J. A., Jr. Serum erythropoietin after renal homotransplantation. Ann. Intern. Med., *69:*908, 1966.
5. Anderson, R. J., Schafer, L. A., Olm, D. B., and Eichkoff, T. C. Infectious risk factors in the immunosuppressed host. Am. J. Med., *54:*453, 1973.
6. Aronoff, A., Gault, M. H., Huang, S. N., Lal, S., Wu, K. T., Moinuddon, M. D., Spence, L., and MacLean, L. D. Hepatitis with Australia antigenemia following renal transplantation. Can. Med. Assoc. J., *108:*43, 1973.
7. Bach, J. F., and Dardenne, M. Serum immunosuppressive activity of azathioprine in normal subjects and patients with liver disease. Proc. R. Soc. Med., *65:*260, 1972.
8. Bach, M. C., Monaco, A. P., and Finland, M. Pulmonary nocardiosis: Therapy with minocycline and with erythromycin plus ampicillin. JAMA, *224:*1378, 1973.
9. Bardana, E. J., Kaufman, L., and Benner, E. J. Amphotericin B and cryptococcal infection. Arch. Intern. Med., *122:*517, 1968.
10. Barrows, G. H., Christopherson, W. M., and Drill, V. A. Liver lesions and oral contraceptive steroids. J. Toxicol. Environ. Health, *3:*219, 1977.
11. Becker, M. D., Scheuer, P. J., Baptista, A., and Sherlock, S. Prognosis of chronic persistent hepatitis. Lancet, *1:*53, 1970.
12. Bhagwat, A. G., and Deodhar, S. D. Experimental hepatic injury. Arch. Pathol., *85:* 346, 1968.
13. Bourne, M. S., and Dawson, H. Acute pancreatitis complicating prednisolone therapy. Lancet, *2:*1209, 1958.
14. Braun, W. E., Banowsky, L. H., Straffon, R. A., Nakamoto, S., Kiser, W. S., Popowneak, K., Hewitt, C. B., Stewart, B. H., Zelch, J. V., Magalhaes, R. L., Lachance, J. C., and Manning, R. F. Lymphoceles associated with renal transplantation. Report of 15 cases and review of the literature. Am. J. Med., *57:*714, 1974.
15. Briggs, W. A., Hampers, C. L., Merrill, J. P., Hager, E. B., Wilson, R. E., Birtch, A. G., and Murray, J. E. Aseptic necrosis in the femur after renal transplantation. Am. Surg., *175:*282, 1972.
16. Caralps, A., Lloweras, S., Masramow, J., Brulles, A., and Gil-Vernet, J. M. Urinary calculi after renal transplantation. Lancet, *I:*544, 1977.
17. Chatelain, C., Frantz, Ph., Luciani, J., Jacobs, C., Petit, J., and Gautier, J. P. Tumeurs et hémopathies malignes chez les insuffisants rénaux traités par transplantation rénale (Etude coopérative de 36 cas). In *Séminaires d'Uro-Néphrologie*, edited by R. Küss and M. Legrain, p. 184. Masson, Paris, 1979.

18. Chebat, J., Gluckman, J. C., Legrain, M., and Küss, R. Les complications pulmonaires infectieuses observées après transplantation rénale. Ann. Med. Interne, *124:*99, 1973.
19. Cheeseman, S. H., Stewart, J. A., Winkle, S., Cosimi, A. B., Tolkoff-Rubin, N. F., Russell, P. S., Baker, G. P., Herrin, J., and Rubin, R. H. Cytomegalovirus excretion 2–14 years after renal transplantation. Transplant. Proc., *11:*71, 1979.
20. Christensen, M. S., and Nielsen, H. E. Parathyroid function after renal transplantation: interrelationships between renal function, serum calcium and serum parathyroid hormone in normocalcemic long-term survivors. Clin. Nephrol., *8:*472, 1977.
21. Clark, P. A., Hsia, Y. E., and Huntsman, R. G. Toxic complications of treatment with 6-mercaptopurine. Two cases with hepatic necrosis and intestinal ulceration. Br. Med. J., *1:*393, 1960.
22. Condie, R. M., Hall, B. L., Howard, R. J., Fryd, D., Simmons, R. K., and Najarian, J. S. Treatment of life-threatening infections in renal transplant recipients with high-dose intravenous human IgG. Transplant. Proc., *11:*66, 1979.
23. Crosnier, J., and Broyer, M. Treatment of chronic renal failure in children. In *Nephrology*, edited by J. Hamburger, J. Crosnier and J. P. Grünfeld, p. 1361. John Wiley & Sons, New York, 1979.
24. Crosnier, J., and Descamps, B. Conditions de vie et possibilités de réadapter des patients porteurs d'un transplant rénal. Réadaptation, *217:*24, 1975.
25. Crosnier, J., Leski, M., Kreis, H., and Descamps, B. Non renal complications of kidney allotransplantations. In *Proceedings of the Fourth International Congress on Nephrology*, vol. 3, p. 270. Karger, Stockholm, 1969.
26. Dandavino, R., Trunet, P., Descamps, B., and Kreis, H. Prolonged withdrawal of azathioprine in kidney transplantation. Transplant. Proc., *10:*655, 1978.
27. David, D. S., Sakai, S., Brennan, B. L., Riggio, R. A., Cheigh, J., Stenzel, K. H., Rubin, A. L., and Sherwood, L. M. Hypercalcemia after renal transplantation long-term follow-up data. N. Engl. J. Med., *289:*398, 1973.
28. Degos, F., Degott, C., Bedrossian, J., Camilieri, J. P., Barbanel, C., Duboust, A., Rueff, B., Benhamou, J. P., and Kreis, H. Is renal transplantation involved in post transplantation liver disease? A prospective study. Transplantation, *29:*100, 1980.
29. Degott, C., Rueff, B., Kreis, H., Duboust, A., Potet, F., and Benhamou, J. P. Peliosis hepatis in recipients of renal transplants. Gut, *19:*748, 1978.
30. Descamps, B., N'Guyen, A. T., and Kreis, H. New insights into immunologic selection of human cadaver renal allograft recipients based on immune response capacity criteria. Transplant. Proc., *10:*497, 1978.
31. Descamps, P., Bedrossian, J., Nocky, D., Duboust, A., Idatte, J. M., Lagrange, P., Acar, J., Leroux-Robert, C., Sraer, J. D., Kourilisky, O., Meyrier, A., Dupuy, C. A., Huraux, J. M., Nicolas, J. C., and Bricourt, F. Renal transplantation and viral infections. Clinical and virological correlations. Biomedicine, *28:*113, 1978.
32. Drew, W. L., Blume, M. R., Miner, R., Silverberg, I., and Rosenbaum, E. H. Herpes zoster; transfer factor therapy. Ann. Intern. Med., *79:*747, 1973.
33. Dunea, G., Nakamoto, S., Staffon, R. A., Figueroa, J. E., Versaci, A., Shibergaki, M., and Kolff, W. J. Renal transplantation in 24 patients. Br. Med. J., *1:*7, 1965.
34. Evans, D. B., Millard, P. P., and Hebertson, B. M. Hepatic dysfunction associated with renal transplantation. Lancet, *2:*929, 1968.
35. Farrington, K., Vargheze, Z., Newman, S. P., Ahmed, K. Y., Fernando, O. N., and Moorhead, J. F. Dissociation of absorption of calcium and phosphate after successful cadaveric renal transplantation. Br. Med. J., *1:*712, 1979.
36. Fass, R. J., and Perkins, R. L. 5-Fluorocytosine in the treatment of cryptococcal and candida mycoses. Ann. Intern. Med., *74:*535, 1971.
37. Fauchère, J. L., Berche, P., Kreis, H., Dandavino, R., Descamps, J. M., and Crosnier, J. Accidents infectieux bactériens après transplantation rénale. Résultats et intérêt

d'une surveillance bactériologique systématique. Nouv. Presse Med., *8:*1991, 1979.

38. Fauchère, J. L., Berche, P., Véron, M., Kreis, H., and Crosnier, J. Infection expérimentale de Klebsiella Pneumoniae chez la souris immunodéprimée par le cyclophosphamide et traitée par la gentamicine. Ann. Microbiol. (Inst. Pasteur), *129D:*433, 1978.
39. Fisher, A. M. Problèmes hématologiques rencontrés dans les suites des transplantations rénales. Thèse Médecine, Paris, 1979.
40. Fisher, D. E., and Bickel, W. H. Corticosteroid induced avascular necrosis—a clinical study of seventy seven patients. J. Bone Joint. Surg. (Am.), *53A:*859, 1971.
41. Fisher, D. E., Bickel, W. H., Holley, K. E., and Ellefson, R. D. Corticosteroid induced necrosis. II. Experimental study. Clin. Orthop., *84:*200, 1972.
42. Frala, M., Payne, J. E., and Berne, T. V. Epidemiology of cytomegalovirus infection after transplantation and immunosuppression. J. Infect. Dis., *132:*421, 1975.
43. Gallis, H. A., Berman, R. A., Cate, T. R., Hamilton, J. D., Gunnells, J. C., and Stickel, D. L. Fungal infection following renal transplantation. Arch. Intern. Med., *135:*1163, 1975.
44. Gil-Vernet, J. M. Le remplacement du rein:Technique chirurgicale. 63e Session Association Française d'Urologie, p. 221. Masson, Paris, 1969.
45. Glazer, J. P., Friedman, H. M., Grossman, R. A., Barker, C. F., Starr, S. E., Plotkin, S. A. Cytomegalovirus vaccination and renal transplantation. Lancet, *1:*90, 1978.
46. Goodman, N., Daves, M. L., and Rifkind, D. Pulmonary roentgen findings following renal transplantations. Radiology, *89:*621, 1967.
47. Grünfeld, J. P., Kleinknecht, D., Moreau, J. F., Kamoun, P., Sabto, J., Garcia Torres, R., Osorio, M., Kreis, H. Permanent hypertension after renal homotransplantation in man. Clin. Sci. Mol. Med., *48:*391, 1975.
48. Haber, M. H., and Putong, P. B. Ureteral vascular rejection in human renal transplants. JAMA, *192:*417, 1965.
49. Hamburger, J., Crosnier, J., and Dormont, J. Experience with 45 renal homotransplantations in man. Lancet, *1:*985, 1965.
50. Hamburger, J., Crosnier, J., Dormont, J., Réveillaud, R. J., Hors, J. H., and Alsina, J. Homotransplantation rénale humaine. Résultats personnels chez 52 malades. II. Histoire Naturelle du greffon dans les cas de tolérance prolongée. Presse Med., *73:*2873, 1965.
51. Hart, P. D., Russell, E., and Remington, J. S. The compromised host and infection: II. Deep fungal infection. J. Infect. Dis., *120:*169, 1969.
52. Haxhe, J. J., Alexander, G. P., and Kestens, P. J. The effect of Imuran and Azaserine on liver function tests in the dog. Arch. Intern. Pharmacodyn. Ther., *168:*366, 1967.
53. Hill, R. B., Jr., Dahrling, B. E., Starzl, T. E., and Rifkind, D. Death after transplantation. An analysis of sixty cases. Am. J. Med., *42:*327, 1967.
54. Hume, D. M. Kidney transplantation. In *Human Transplantation*, edited by F. T. Rapaport and J. Dausset, p. 110. Grune and Stratton, New York, 1968.
55. Ibels, L. S., Alfrey, A. C., Huffer, W. E., and Weil, R. Aseptic necrosis of bone following renal transplantation: Experience in 194 transplant recipients and review of the literature. Medicine, *57:*25, 1978.
56. Jepson, J. H., de Leeuw, N. K. M., Gault, M. H., Dossetor, J. B., and Manasc, B. Characteristics of erythropoiesis following human renal homotransplantation. Transplant. Proc., *3:*353, 1971.
57. Johnson, J. W., Hattner, R. S., Hampers, C. L., Bernstein, D. S., Merrill, J. P., and Sherwood, L. M. Secondary hyperparathyroidism in chronic renal failure. Am. J. Med., *215:*478, 1971.
58. Jones, F. P., Engleman, F. P., and Najarian, J. S. Systemic fat embolism after renal homotransplantation and treatment with corticosteroids. N. Engl. J. Med., *273:*1453, 1965.

59. Jones, R. H., Rudge, C. J., Bewick, M., Parsons, V., and Weston, M. J. Cimetidine: prophylaxis against upper gastrointestinal haemorrhage after renal transplantation. Br. Med. J., *1:*398, 1978.
60. Kincaid-Smith, P., Hare, W. S. C., Morris, P. J., and Marshall, V. C. Renal artery stenosis due to the vascular lesions of rejection in cadaveric allografts. Proc. Eur. Dial. Transplant. Assoc., *6:*235, 1969.
61. Kisher, C. T., and Kleinman L. I. Primary benign erythrocytosis and abnormal renal perfusion. Lancet, *1:*1162, 1971.
62. Kleenkoper, M., Ibels, L. S., Ingham, J. P., McCarthy, S. W., Mahary, J. F., Stewart, J. H., and Posen, S. Hyperparathyroidism after renal transplantation. Br. Med. J., *3:* 680, 1975.
63. Kreis, H. Procedure for performing renal transplantation. In *Nephrology*, edited by J. Hamburger, J. Crosnier and J. P. Grünfeld, p. 1311. John Wiley & Sons, New York, 1979.
64. Kreis, H., Lefèvre, J. J., Grünfeld, J. P., Moreau, J. F., and Sabto, J. Explorations au cours de l'hypertension artérielle permanente après transplantation rénale. In *Transplantation et Immunologie Clinique*, edited by J. L. Touraine, J. Traeger, and R. Triau. Simep, Villeurbanne, 1977.
65. Küss, H., Legrain, M., Mathey, G., Nedey, R., and Camey, M. Homotransplantation rénale chez l'homme hors de tout lien de parenté. Survie jusqu'au dix-septième mois. Rev. Fr. Etud. Clin. Biol., *7:*1048, 1962.
66. Lacombe, M. Arterial stenosis complicating renal allotransplantation in man. A study of 38 cases. Ann. Surg., *181:*283, 1975.
67. Lagrange, Ph., Acar, J. F., Idatte, J. M., Bedrossian, J., and Brisset, J. M. Infections au cours des transplantations rénales. Pathol. Biol., *21:*981, 1973.
68. Lau, W. K., and Young, L. S. Trimethoprine-sulfamethyxazole treatment of pneumocystis carinii pneumonia in adults. N. Engl. J. Med. *295:*716, 1976.
69. Leapman, S. B., Vidne, B. A., Butt, K. M. H., Waterhouse, K., and Kountz, S. L. Nephrolithiasis and nephrocalcinosis after renal transplantation: A case report and review of the literature. J. Urol., *115:*129, 1976.
70. Lecestre, P., Dabos, N., Benoit, J., and Ramadier, J. O. L'ostéonécrose aseptique chez le transplanté rénal à propos de 27 cas opérés. Rev. Chir. Orthop., *63:*373, 1977.
71. Light, J. A., and Burke, D. S. Association of cytomegalovirus (CMV) infectious with increased recipient mortality following transplantation. Transplant. Proc., *11:*79, 1979.
72. Linnemann, C. C. Jr., Dunn, C. R., First, M. R., Alvira, M., and Schiff, G. M. Late onset of fatal cytomegalovirus infection after renal transplantation. Arch. Intern. Med., *138:*1247, 1978.
73. Lopez, C., Simmons, R. L., Mauer, M., Park, B., Najarian, J. S., and Good, R. A. Role of virus infections in immunosuppressed renal transplant patients. Transplant. Proc., *5:*803, 1973.
74. Lutzner, M. A., Croissant, O., Ducasse, M. F., Kreis, H., Crosnier, J., and Orth, G. Two different human papillomaviruses HPV-3 and HPV-5 found in the same warty lesion occurring in a renal allograft recipient (to be published).
75. Mc Main, P. B., Hoffman, G. C., Nakamoto, S., and Kolff, W. J. Erythropoiesis and renal homotransplantation. Can. Med. Assoc. J., *93:*241, 1965.
76. Marubbio, A. T., and Danielson, B. Hepatic veno occlusive disease in a renal transplant patient receiving azathioprine. Gastroenterology, *69:*739, 1975.
77. Massry, S. G., Coburn, J. W., Lee, D. B. N., Jowsey, J., and Kleeman, C. R. Skeletal resistance to parathyroid hormone in renal failure studies in 105 human subjects. Ann. Intern. Med., *78:*357, 1973.
78. Matas, A. J., Simmons, R. L., Kjellstrand, C. M., Buselmeier, T. J., and Najarian, J. S. Increased incidence of malignancy during chronic renal failure. Lancet, *1:*883, 1975.

79. Matas, A. J., Simmons, R. L., and Najarian, J. S. Chronic antigenic stimulation, herpes virus and cancer in transplant recipients. Lancet, *1:*1277, 1975.
80. Montgomerie, J. Z., Kalmanson, G. M., and Guze, L. B. Renal failure and infection. Medicine, *37:*1, 1968.
81. Moore, T. C., and Hume, D. M. The period and nature of hazard in clinical renal transplantation. I. The hazard to patient survival. Ann. Surg., *1:*170, 1969.
82. Moorhead, J. F., Ahmed, K. Y., Varghese, Z., Wills, M. R., Baillod, R. A., and Tatler, G. L. V. Hypophosphataemic osteomalacia after cadaveric renal transplantation. Lancet, *1:*694, 1974.
83. Moreau, J. F., Leski, M., Beurton, D., Cukier, J., Michel, J. R., and Kreis, H. Lymphocèles obstructives après transplantation. Ann. Radiol., *16:*471, 1973.
84. Murphy, J. F., McDonald, F. D., Dawson, M., Reite, A., Turcotte, J., and Fekety, F. R., Jr. Factors affecting the frequency of infection in renal transplant recipients. Arch. Intern. Med., *136:*670, 1976.
85. Murray H. W., Moore, J. O., and Luff, R. D. Disseminated aspergillosis in a renal transplant patient. Diagnostic difficulties re-emphasized. Johns Hopkins Med. J., *137:* 235, 1975.
86. Murray, J. F., Barnes, B. A., and Atkinson, J. Fifth report of the human kidney transplant registry. Transplantation, *5:*752, 1967.
87. Murray, W. R. Hip problems associated with organ transplants. Clin. Orthop., *90:*57, 1973.
88. Nadell, J., and Kosek, J. Peliosis hepatis. Twelve cases associated with oral androgen therapy. Arch. Pathol. Lab. Med., *101:*405, 1977.
89. Nataf, C., Feldmann, G., Lebrec, D., Degott, C., Descamps, J. M., Rueff, B., and Benhamou, J. P. Idiopathic portal hypertension (perisinusoidal fibrosis) after renal transplantation. Gut, *20:*531, 1979.
90. Neff, T. A., and Hudgel, D. W. Miliary tuberculosis in a renal transplant recipient. Am. Rev. Respir. Dis., *108:*677, 1973.
91. Nesbit, R., Blake, D. D., Ekstrand, K., and James, P. M. Lymphocele following renal transplantation. Values of ultrasonography in diagnosis and follow up studies. South. Med. J., *69:*303, 1976.
92. Nies, B. A., Cohn, R., and Schrier, S. Erythremia after renal transplantation. N. Engl. J. Med., *273:*785, 1965.
93. Penn, I. Chemical immunosuppression and human cancer. Cancer *34:*1474, 1974.
94. Penn, I. Malignancies associated with immunosuppression or cytotoxic therapy. Surgery, *83:*492, 1978.
95. Penn, I. Malignant tumors in organ transplant recipients. *Séminaires d'Uro-Néphrologie*, edited by R. Küss and M. Legrain, p. 173. Masson, Paris, 1979.
96. Penn, I. Tumor incidence in human allograft recipients. Transplant. Proc., *11:*1047, 1979.
97. Penn, I., Hammond, W., Bell, P., McGuire, R., Hutt, M., and Starzl, T. E. Hepatic disorders in renal homograft recipients. Curr. Top. Surg. Res., *1:*67, 1969.
98. Pfeffermann, R., Vidne, B., Leapman, S., Butt, K., and Kountz, S. L. Urologic complications in renal primary and retransplantation. Experience with 202 consecutive transplants. Am. J. Surg., *131:*242, 1976.
99. Pietrogrande, V., and Mastromarino, R. Osteopatia da prolongato trattamento cortisonico. Orthop. Travmatol., *25:*791, 1957.
100. Porter, K. A., Thomson, W. B., Owen, K., Kenyon, J. R., Mowbray, J. F., and Peart, W. S. Obliterative vascular changes in four human kidney homotransplants. Br. Med. J., *II:*639, 1963.
101. Primack, W. A. Cimetidine and renal allograft rejection. Lancet, *1:*824, 1978.
102. Rifkind, D. Marchioro, T. L., Schneck, S. A., and Hill, R. B. Systemic fungal infections

complicating renal transplantation and immunosuppressive therapy. Am. J. Med., *43:* 28, 1967.
103. Rifkind, D., Starzl, T. E., Marchioro, T. L., Waddell, W. R., Rowlands, D. T., Hill, R. B. Transplantation pneumonia. JAMA *189:*114, 1964.
104. Roman, J., Wheby, M. S., Atuk, N. O., and Westervelt, F. Anemias with renal transplantation. JAMA, *221:*1283, 1972.
105. Salvatierra, O., Kountz, S. L., and Belzer, F. O. Prevention of ureteral fistula after renal transplantation. J. Urol., *112:*445, 1974.
106. Schiff, M., Jr., McGuire, E. J., Weiss, R. M., and Lytton, B. Management of urinary fistulas after renal transplantation. J. Urol., *115:*251, 1976.
107. Schroter, G. P. J., Bakshandeh, K., Husberg, B. S., and Weil, R. Coccidiomycosis and renal transplantation. Transplantation, *23:*485, 1977.
108. Schwartz, R. S., Beldotti, L. Malignant lymphomas following allogenic disease: transition from an immunological to a neoplastic disorder. Science, *149:*1511, 1965.
109. Sheil, A. G. R. Cancer in renal allograft recipients in Australia and New Zealand. Transplant. Proc., *9:*1133, 1977.
110. Sheil, A. G. R., Mahoney, J. F., Horvath, J. S., Johnson, J. R., Tiller, D. J., May, J., and Stewart, J. H. Cancer and survival after cadaveric donor renal transplantation. Transplant. Proc., *11:*1052, 1979.
111. Smellie, W. A. B., Vinik, M., and Hume, D. M. Angiographic investigation of hypertension complicating human renal transplantation. Surg. Gynecol. Obstet., *128:*963, 1969.
112. Solomon, L. Drug induced arthropathy and necrosis of the femoral head. J. Bone Joint Surg., *55B:*246, 1973.
113. Soloway, R. D., Summerskill, W. H. J., and Baggentoss, H. A. Clinical, biochemical and histological remission of severe chronic active liver disease. A controlled study of treatments and early prognosis. Gastroenterology, *63:*820, 1972.
114. Sopko, T., and Anuras, S. Liver disease in renal transplant recipients. Am. J. Med., *64:* 139, 1978.
115. Sparberg, M., Simon, N., and Delgreco, F. Intrahepatic cholestasis due to azathioprine. Gastroenterology, *57:*439, 1969.
116. Spencer, E. S. Clinical aspects of cytomegalovirus infection in kidney graft infections. Scand. J. Infect. Dis., *6:*315, 1974.
117. Starzl, T. E. *Experience in Renal Transplantation*. Saunders, Philadelphia, 1969.
118. Starzl, T. E., Groth, C. G., Putnam, C. W., Penn, I., Halgrimson, C. G., Flatmark, A., Gecelter, L., Brettschneider, C., and Stonington, O. G. Urological complications in 216 human recipients of renal transplants. Ann. Surg., *172:*1, 1970.
119. Starzl, T. E., Marchioro, T. L., Porter, K. A., Moore, C. A., Rifkind, D., and Waddell, W. C. Renal homotransplantation. Late function and complications. Ann. Intern. Med., *61:*470, 61.
120. Swales, J. D., and Evans, D. B. Erythraemia in renal transplantation. Br. Med. J., *2:* 80, 1969.
121. Tilney, N. L., Collins, J. J. Jr., and Wilson, R. E. Hemorrhagic pancreatitis: A fatal complication of renal transplantation. N. Engl. J. Med., *275:*1051, 1966.
122. Van Kaulk, K. K., Von Kaulla, E., Wasantapuck, S., Marchioro, T. L., and Starzl, T. E. Blood coagulation in uremic patients before and after hemodialysis and transplantation of the kidney. Arch. Surg., *92:*184, 1966.
123. Van Waes, L., Segers, J., Van Egmond, J., Van Nimmen, L., Barbier, F., Wieme, R., and Demeulenaere, L. Chronic liver disease and hepatitis B antigen: a prospective study. Br. Med. J., *3:*444, 1974.
124. Vidne, B. A., Leapman, S. B., Butt, K. M., and Kountz, S. L. Vascular complications in human renal transplantation. Surgery, *79:*77, 1976.

125. Wagner, E. Fall von blutecystem der leber. Arch. Heilkunde, *2:*369 1861.
126. Walder, B. K., Robertson, M. R., and Jeremy, D. Skin cancer and immunosuppression. Lancet, *2:*1282, 1971.
127. Walsh, A. Some practical problems in kidney transplantation. Transplant. Proc., *1:* 170, 1969.
128. Weimar, W., Lameiger, L. D. F., Edy, V. G., and Schellekens, H. Prophylactic use of interferon in renal allograft recipients. Transplant. Proc., *11:*69, 1979.
129. Westerman, M. P., Jenkins, J. L., Dehker, A., Kreutner, A., and Fisher, B. Significance of erythrocytosis and increased erythropoietin secretion after renal transplantation. Lancet, *2:*755, 1967.
130. Wilson, R. E., and Roth, S. I. Persistent hypercalcemia six years after a renal homograft. N. Engl. J. Med., *294:*793, 1974.
131. Woodruff, M. F. A., Robson, J. S., Ross, J. A., Nolau, B., and Lambie, A. J. Transplantation of a kidney from an identical twin. Lancet, *I:*1245, 1961.
132. Woods, J. E., de Weerd, J. H., Johnson, W. J., Anderson, C. F., and Shorter, R. G. Experience in human renal allotransplantation. Surg. Gynecol. Obstet., *134:*394, 1972.
133. Wu, K. K., Gibson, T. P., Freeman, R. M., Bonney, W. W., Fried, W., and Degowin, R. L. Erythrocytosis after renal transplantation. Its occurence in two recipients of kidneys from the same cadaveric donor. Arch. Intern. Med., *132:*898, 1973.
134. Zammick, M., and Toledo Pereyra, L. H. Cimetidine for kidney transplantation: experimental observation. Surgery, *86:*611, 1979.

CHAPTER NINE

Results of Renal Transplantation

Jean Crosnier, Patrice Rioux and Anh Thu N'Guyen

International multicenter results—Local results (Necker Hospital)—Renal transplantation in children—Conclusions.

Despite all the problems involved in renal transplantation and all the complications which can occur in a renal allograft recipient, transplantation remains the treatment of choice whenever possible for the majority of patients with terminal renal failure.

We will first discuss results reported in the last (13th) report of the Human Renal Transplant Registry[2] which includes 25,108 renal transplants performed in 301 centers throughout the world, and more specifically those in the more recent report of the European Dialysis and Transplant Association (EDTA) covering the years ending December 31, 1978.[4]

But overall results from many different centers can only very imperfectly reflect the real possibilities of renal transplantation. We will, therefore, also discuss the results obtained in 471 transplants performed in 437 patients at Necker Hospital between June 1959 and June 1977.

INTERNATIONAL MULTICENTER RESULTS

The Ninth Report of the EDTA includes 20,773 transplants performed in 19,534 patients up to December 31, 1978. Of these, 17,462 were from cadaver donors and 3107 from living donors.

The annual death rate of patients with functioning first grafts from cadavers is 4.5%. It is higher in the older age groups: 13.33% in patients over 55 years of age against 2.14% in patients between 15 and 34 years of age. The annual death rate is also much higher in the first 3 months (27.6%) than after 2 years (3.1%). The major causes of death are infections, which are responsible for 40% of all deaths when there is a functioning transplant.

Cumulative patient and graft survival for 5782 first grafts from cadaver donors performed between 1976 and 1978 are shown in Figure 9.1. Patient

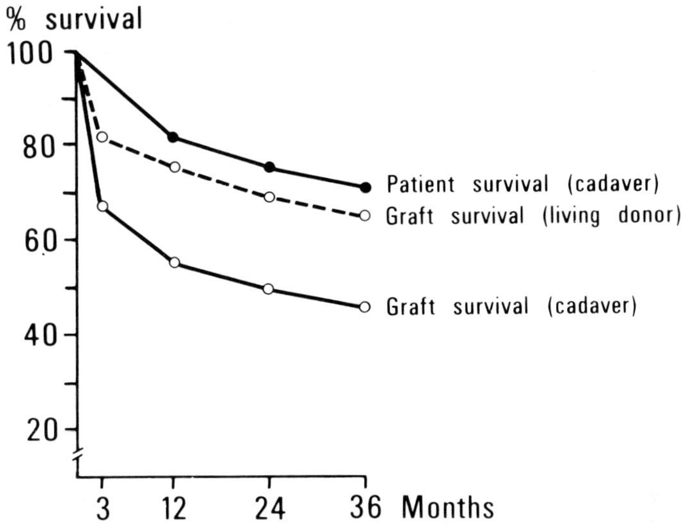

Fig. 9.1. European patient and graft survival in 5782 first cadaver transplants performed between 1976 and 1978 compared with graft survival of transplants with living donors (based on statistics contained in ref. 4).

survival is 81.1% at 1 year and 70.6% at 3 years; graft survival is 55.6% at 1 year and 45.7% at 3 years. These results are at least 5% better at 1 year and 10% better at 3 years than those of patients transplanted between 1973 and 1975.

This improvement is at variance with the data reported in the 13th Human Renal Transplant Registry, indicating that the rate of graft success decreased between 1969 and 1974. On the contrary, it agrees with the results observed at the Johns Hopkins Hospital.[27]

This report does not show any significant change in graft survival between first and second cadaver grafts. On the other hand, third grafts continue to fail at a very high rate, and only 35% and 29% continue to function after 1 and 3 years.

The graft survival of transplants from living donors is better than that from cadavers: 75% at 1 year and 65% at 3 years (Fig. 9.1).

Human Leukocyte A (HLA) Histocompatibility

Until 1973, the analysis of pooled worldwide results did not demonstrate any significant benefit derived from matching for HLA antigens on the outcome of renal transplantation. In 1974 the 12th Human Transplant Registry[1] first reported a significant difference in the survival of grafts removed from cadaver donors having three or four antigens identical to those of the recipient, as compared to those having fewer in common. It is easy to understand that the analysis of results from a large number of centers is difficult to interpret in view of the multiple variables involved.

We have seen (p. 46) that all preliminary data strongly suggest that matching for HLA-DR (D-related) may influence graft survival, but it is still too early to draw any definite conclusions.

Kidney Graft Survival and Pretransplant Blood Transfusions

A recent study managed by Terasaki's group[19] including 1636 patients transplanted in 61 centers in the United States and Canada, corroborates the relationship of graft survival and the number of blood units transfused (Table 9.1).

Rehabilitation

A comparison of rehabilitation made in 1978 between 2958 survivors of transplantation from cadaver donors and 11,372 hospital hemodialysis patients[4] shows that 63% of the former work fulltime (and 15% part-time), against 37% (and 22% part-time) of the hospital hemodialysis patients.

The report also investigated the hospitalization of patients with functioning cadaver transplants. In the first year almost 90% were hospitalized less than 3 months, and after 5 years almost 80% were never hospitalized.

Rehabilitation of these patients was superior to that of hospital hemodialysis patients at each point, and it thus appears that transplantation has an important economic advantage over hospital hemodialysis.

LOCAL RESULTS (NECKER HOSPITAL)

Between June 1959 and June 1977, 471 transplants were performed at Necker Hospital in 437 patients.* Of the total number, 32 had two transplants and 2 had three. Male patients made up 284 of the total and 153 recipients were females. In 307 cases the graft came from a cadaver and in 164 cases from a living donor.

Overall Results

Overall results of these 471 transplantations appear in Figure 9.2. Survival at 1, 2, 5, 10 and 20 years are respectively 77, 73, 68, 59 and 55% for the patient and 61, 56, 46, 37 and 33% for the graft. Actually, these data have no real value except as history, for they include many varying

* We limited our patient population to those transplanted no later than June 1977 so as to have a follow-up period of at least 2 years for evaluating outcome.

TABLE 9.1
Effect of pretransplant blood transfusions on graft outcome in first cadaver transplantation[19]

No. of Units Transfused	No. of Patients Studied	Graft Survival Rates (% ± SE)	
		1 Year	2 Years
0	615	45 ± 2	35 ± 2
1	101	50 ± 5	48 ± 5
2–5	426	56 ± 3	51 ± 3
6–10	233	59 ± 3	53 ± 4
11–20	137	64 ± 4	56 ± 5
>20	124	69 ± 4	67 ± 4
		$P < 0.0001$	$P < 0.0001$

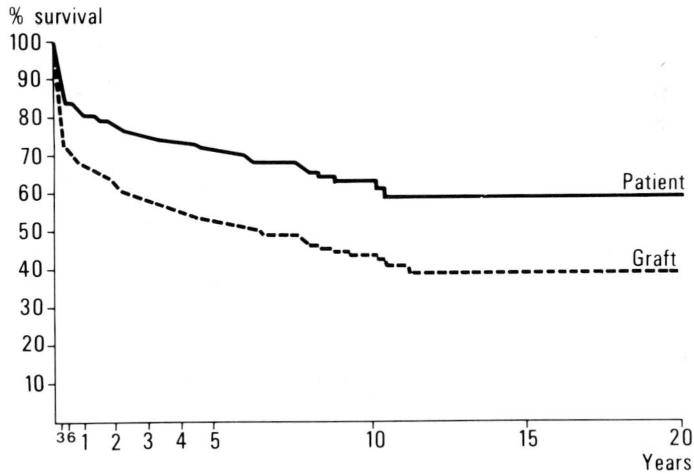

Fig. 9.2. Overall actuarial patient and graft survival at Necker Hospital since June 1959.

factors: living donor or cadaver kidney, age of the recipient, recent or long-standing transplantation, compatibility between donor and recipient, first or repeated transplantation, etc.

Date of the Transplantation

Figure 9.3 and Table 9.2 show that patient and graft survival differ significantly ($P < 0.001$) according to whether transplantation was performed before 1969 (139 patients), i.e., during our first 10 years' experience in transplantation, or after 1969 (325 patients).

The death rate of patients remains a major preoccupation of transplantation teams, although it has been considerably reduced during recent years. In our series, recipient mortality reached 35% during the

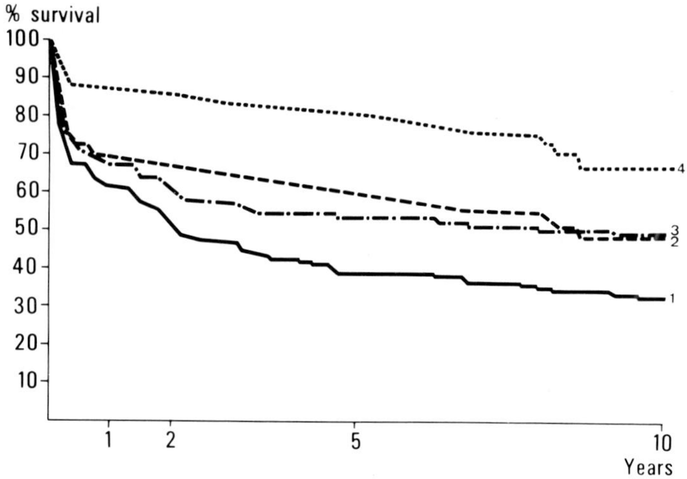

Fig. 9.3. Kidney and patient survival are significantly different according to whether transplantation was performed before or after 1969 (Necker Hospital).
1, overall kidney survival before 1969
2, overall kidney survival after 1969
3, overall patient survival before 1969
4, overall patient survival after 1969

TABLE 9.2
Patient and graft survival in transplantation before or after 1969

	1 Year		2 Years		5 Years		10 Years	
	Before 1969	After 1969	Before 1969	After 1969	Before 1969	After 1969	Before 1969	After 1969
Patient Survival (%)	65	85	59	84	51	79	47	65
Graft Survival (%)	60	66	50	63	38	56	31	45
								$P < 0.001$

years preceding 1969 and was still 15% for the years after 1969. Since 1976, however, it has varied between 5 and 10%.

Living Donor or Cadaver Kidney

Figures 9.4 and 9.5 show patient and graft survival in the cases of living donor or cadaver kidney before or after 1969 (to have a sufficient number of patients in each group we stopped the actuarial curve at 7 years).

Several remarks may be made:

1. The difference between the results of transplantation performed before and after 1969 is observed both for transplantation from living donors and for transplantation from cadavers.

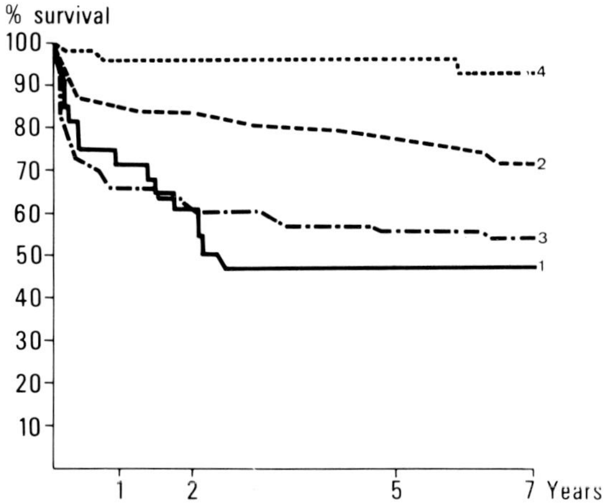

Fig. 9.4. Patient survival at Necker Hospital after transplantation performed before and after 1969.

1, cadaver kidney transplantation before 1969 } $P < 0.01$
2, cadaver kidney transplantation after 1969

3, living donor kidney transplantation before 1969 } $P < 0.0001$
4, living donor kidney transplantation after 1969

2. Whereas during the first period there was no difference between results obtained with cadaver kidneys and living donor kidneys, during the period after 1969 the results of living donor transplants, with graft survival reaching 83% at 7 years, are much better than with cadaver donors. This is due to two reasons: mortality before 2 years was very high before 1969 in both living donor and cadaver kidney recipients (Fig. 9.4); and, whereas before 1969 living donors were sometimes HLA-identical with recipients but very often were only haploidentical or even HLA-different, conversely, since 1969, all living donors were HLA-identical siblings. The good results observed with HLA-identical siblings explain why at Necker Hospital kidneys are removed from living donors only when this donor is an HLA-identical sibling. In all other cases we prefer to have recourse to cadaver kidneys.

This fact explains why the majority of transplantations at Necker Hospital since 1969 have been performed with cadaver kidneys; thus, all the correlations we will discuss hereafter in this chapter concern only cadaver kidney transplantation since 1969.

Sex of Recipient

Necker Hospital data (Fig. 9.6) confirm studies[21] showing that the sex of the recipient does not seem to affect significantly allograft survival. However, we have previously shown[10] that when the survival of compat-

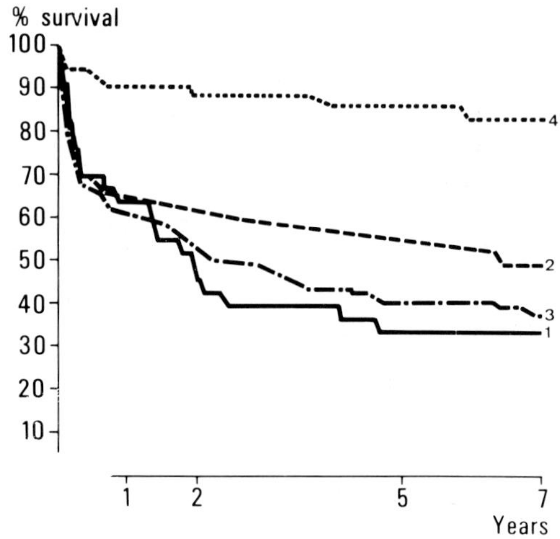

Fig. 9.5. Graft survival at Necker Hospital according to whether transplantation was performed before or after 1969.

1, cadaver kidney transplantation before 1969 } $P < 0.01$
2, cadaver kidney transplantation after 1969 }

3, living donor kidney transplantation before 1969 } $P < 0.0001$
4, living donor kidney transplantation after 1969 }

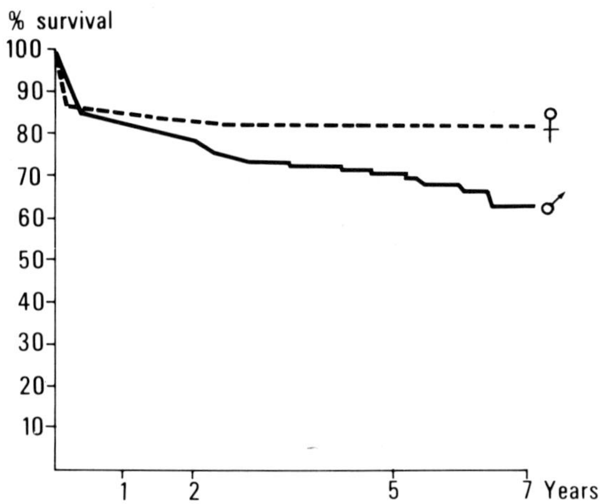

Fig. 9.6. Patient survival at Necker Hospital in 197 males and 107 females (N.S.).

ible and noncompatible transplants are studied separately, female recipients of noncompatible kidneys have significantly poorer graft survival compared to overall results; on the other hand, female recipients of compatible kidneys have the best results. Among males, compatibility does not appear to play a role in graft survival. These results are contrary to those reported by Opelz and Terasaki[18] in a multicenter study.

Repeated Transplantation

We did not note a significant difference in the graft survival of 31 repeated transplantations and 275 first grafts (Fig. 9.7). There are few reports from single centers having large enough series to be significant. The largest is the Göteborg group,[12] who find no difference between results of 74 repeated transplants and those of first transplants. Results reported in the 12th Transplant Registry[1] on 772 second transplants are also similar. Morris[16] underlines the fact that the fate of a second graft is dependent on the source of both the first and the second grafts, the cause of graft loss and the length of survival of the first graft.

Age of the Recipient

We compared patient survival and graft survival in a group of 245 patients, dividing them into those between 10 and 40 years of age and those between 40 and 50. Figure 9.8 shows a significant difference in patient survival between the two groups, but not in kidney survival. These data could suggest that deaths due to complications are more frequent in the older patients, but that if these patients survive, they better tolerate the kidney. On the other hand, no difference is observed among recipients in each decade range within the 10 to 40-year-old group.

HLA Histocompatibility

In our experience, histocompatibility has no influence on patient sur-

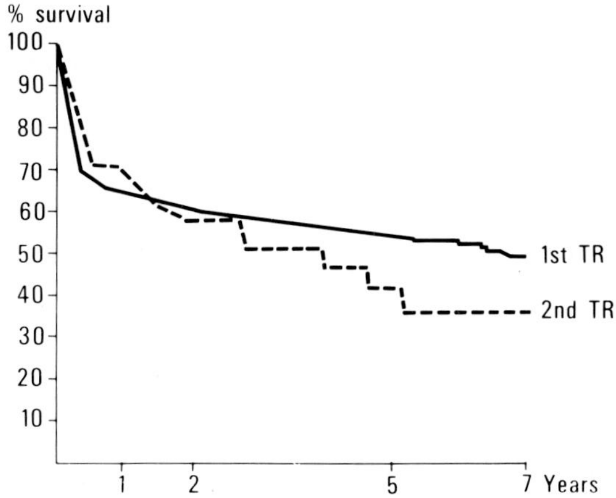

Fig. 9.7. Graft survival at Necker Hospital in 275 first cadaver grafts and 31 repeated transplantations (N.S.).

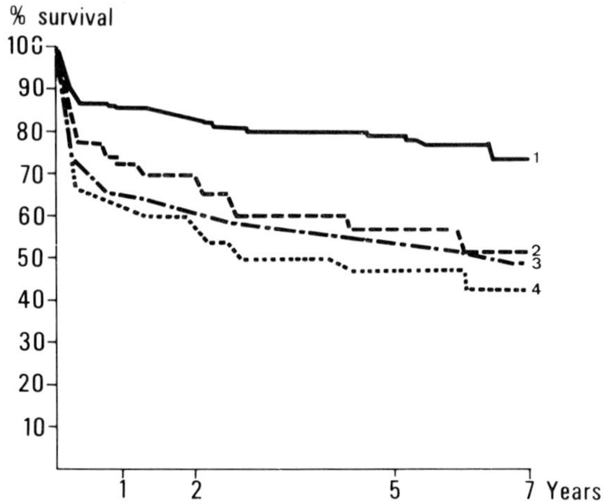

Fig. 9.8. Influence of the age of the recipient on patient and graft survival.
1, patient survival in patients under 40 years of age
2, patient survival in patients over 40 years of age } $P < 0.002$

3, kidney survival in patients under 40 years of age
4, kidney survival in patients over 40 years of age } N.S.

vival. Even for graft survival, it is well known how difficult it is to assess the influence of histocompatibility. Analysis of data from a large number of centers is difficult to interpret in view of the multiple variables involved. But even when considering the results from individual centers, it is surprising to note the disparity of observations among various homogeneous groups, some of them[10, 23] showing a significantly better survival of compatible grafts, while in others it was impossible to demonstrate any real advantage of HLA matching.[3, 14, 25] This difference in results clearly suggests the large number of other factors which play a role in the outcome of cadaver kidney transplantation; in these circumstances any attempt to correlate graft outcome with a single factor runs the risk of bias by the unknown influence of the other factors. Our results, shown on Figure 9.9, concern 161 patients with zero or one mismatch and 104 patients with two, three or four mismatches. Kidney survival in the two groups is significantly different, and the difference increases with time, probably because during the first months the nonimmunological complications play a more important role than does histocompatibility in the survival of the graft.

We have seen (p. 43) that several groups[8, 17, 26] have shown an imbalance of strength among the various loci in the HLA region and that identity for antigens at the HLA-B locus plays a more important role than that at the HLA-A locus in terms of graft survival. It is thought that the reason for this imbalance is that the genes of the B locus are actually more closely associated to those of the D locus than those of the A locus.

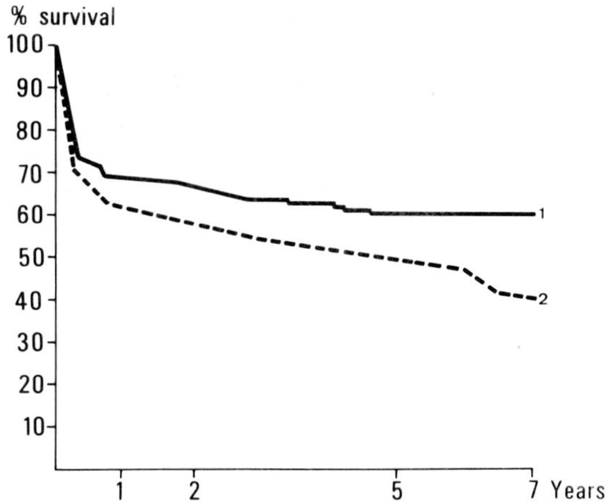

Fig. 9.9. Graft survival at Necker Hospital according to HLA matching.
1, 161 patients with 0 or 1 mismatch
2, 104 patients with 2, 3 or 4 mismatches $\} P < 0.05$

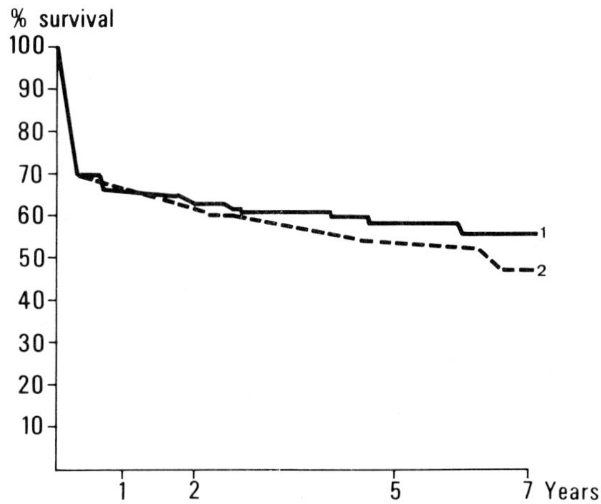

Fig. 9.10. Graft survival:
1, in locus B matched recipients
2, in recipients having 2 antigens in common with their donor either at the A locus or one at each locus

However, such a more important role of the B locus is not apparent in the results observed at Necker Hospital. Figure 9.10 shows that, the total number of mismatches being the same, there is no difference between the graft survival of 101 patients with identical HLA-B locus antigens and that of 164 patients with different antigens at this locus. This lack of influence of the B locus was also observed whether A locus antigens were compatible or different. Other groups[24] have also failed to find a greater strength of B locus antigens.

A prospective study of the influence of the D locus on graft survival is underway in our group, but results are not yet interpretable (cf. p. 46).

Influence of Preimmunization

In 1976, in a retrospective study on 191 patients, we demonstrated that preformed anti-HLA cytotoxic antibodies in recipient serum are pejorative to allograft survival only in presensitized incompatible recipients, whereas, on the contrary, the best results are seen in subjects with circulating antibodies but who are HLA-compatible (Figure 9.11*A*).[10]

Since 1978 we have undertaken a prospective study on the role of transfusions and compatibility in transfused recipients. Our patients received an established protocol of transfusions (cf. p. 151) and were divided according to graft results into three groups: responder and compatible (13 patients); nonresponder and compatible (22 patients); and nonresponder and incompatible (24 patients). Based on our 1976 results discussed in the preceding paragraph, since that period all our responders have received only compatible kidneys.

Figure 11*B* shows that kidney survival is not significantly different among the three groups: 83.5% for responders and 75.36 and 71.53%, respectively, in the groups of nonresponders.

Social and Professional Rehabilitation

In almost two-thirds of cases, transplantation leads to successful social and professional rehabilitation and, in this regard, is more successful than treatment by center hemodialysis. Transplantation not only allows patients to survive but usually also permits them to live a full and totally normal life.

We particularly studied daily time devoted to medical care in 440 patients treated by center hemodialysis and 221 treated by transplantation between 1970 and 1979. This study shows that, except during the 1st year, this time is unimportant and almost negligible in the transplant recipient, whereas it is 42 days per year for the dialysis patient (Table 9.3).[5]

These data probably explain why 78% of allograft recipients are again working fulltime at the end of 2 years and 68% were doing so at the end of 1 year.[5, 7] The interval varies greatly according to the social and professional level of the patient. Among skilled workers, 90% have returned to fulltime work after only 1 year, against 54% of executives and professional people.[7, 13] Professional reorientation was necessary in only

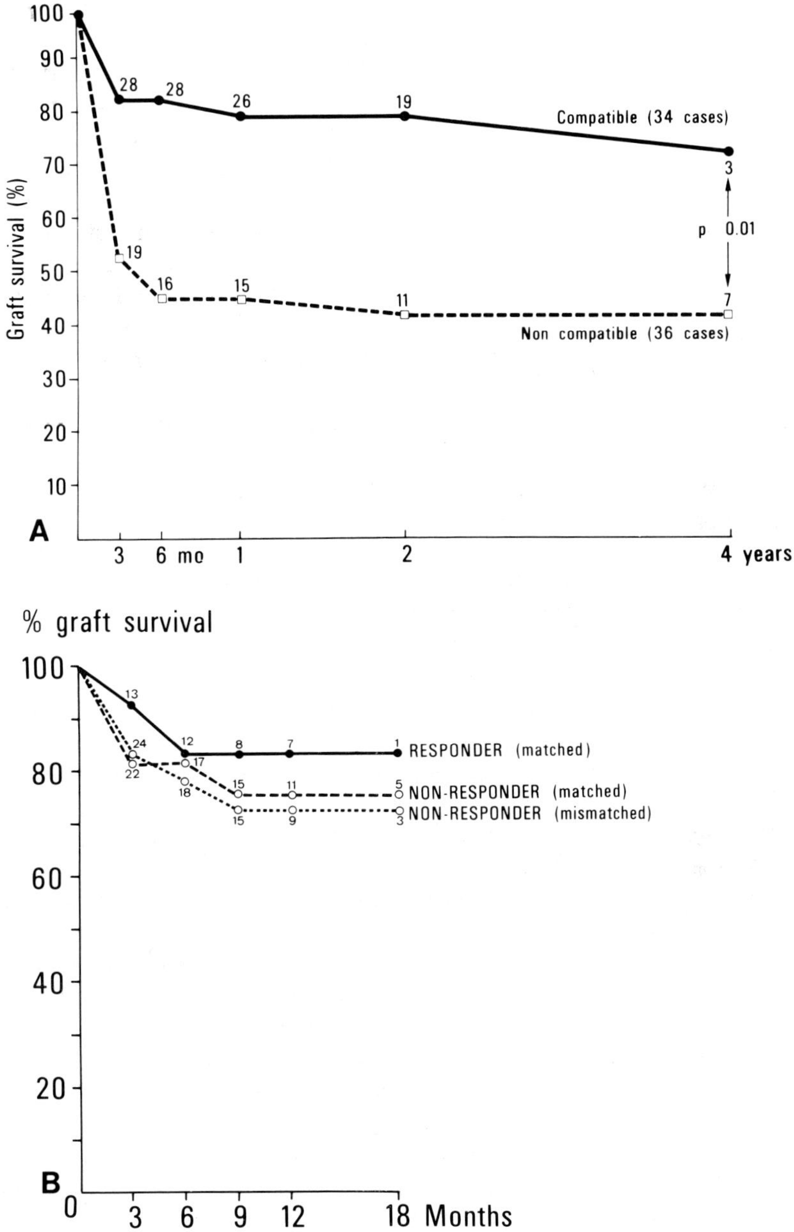

Fig. 9.11. Kidney survival according to anti-HLA preimmunization of recipient. *A*, better results in HLA compatible recipients with circulating antibodies[10] ($P < 0.01$); *B*, nonsignificant difference in kidney survival of responder and compatible recipients, nonresponder and compatible recipients, nonresponder and incompatible recipients.

TABLE 9.3
Mean number of hospital days for patients treated by hemodialysis or by transplantation

	Year After Initiation of Treatment or Surgery					
	1	2	3	4	5	6
440 Patients treated by hemodialysis						
Hospitalization	35.8	13.9	13.5	7.6	9.6	8.3
Dialysis	32	32	32	32	32	32
Total	67.8	45.9	45.5	39.6	41.6	40.3
221 Patients treated by transplantation						
Hospitalization	86	7.3	4.9	2.9	3.1	0
Outpatient consultation and investigations	22.1	10	3.6	3.6	1.8	2.8
Total	108.1	17.3	8.5	6.5	4.9	2.8

16% of cases. Finally, the length of nonworking time after transplantation is in direct relation to that time before transplantation.[7, 13]

RENAL TRANSPLANTATION IN CHILDREN

Actuarial curves show that graft survival is better in recipients who are less than 15 years old when compared with the overall population of graft recipients.[20]

In the group at Enfants Malades Hospital in Paris,[6] success in cadaver renal transplantation (as of 2 years after surgery) has been obtained in more than 70% of cases, with failure almost always being limited to the first 2 or 3 months.

Certain complications appear to be more specifically observed in children. For example, arterial hypertension seems to be more frequent after renal transplantation in children than in adults.[15]

The most important problem is perhaps that of growth. Following a transplant, the growth of children is not always satisfactory[11] and depends on several factors. It is poor if renal insufficiency due to chronic rejection or any other cause persists. Uncontrolled hypertension may also hinder growth. The administration of corticosteroids very often limits growth possibilities, and it is possible that in this case hope rests with the use of intermittant corticosteroid administration.[22] Finally, growth is, of course, possible only if bone maturation is not too advanced. If it is that of a child over 12 or 13 years of age, puberty occurs more or less rapidly and induces an insufficient growth peak.

CONCLUSIONS

Although each chapter of this book has emphasized the unknown in the mechanisms of rejection, the debate as to donor selection and the influence of histocompatibility, the present impossibility of an actual immunologic monitoring of the recipient and the many problems in the management of renal transplantation, every year during the past 20 years has brought some progress. Today renal transplantation is the only treatment allowing the uremic patient to live a normal life, and the proportion of these patients increases every year.

REFERENCES

1. ACS/NIH Organ Transplant Registry. The 12th Report of the Human Renal Transplant Registry. JAMA, *233:*787, 1975.
2. ACS/NIH Organ Transplant Registry. The 13th Report of the Human Renal Transplant Registry. Transplant. Proc., *9:*9, 1977.
3. Belzer, F. O., Perkins, H. A., and Fortman, J. L. Is HLA typing of clinical significance in cadaver renal transplantation? Lancet, *1:*774, 1974.
4. Brunner, F. P., Brynger, H., Chantler, C., Douckerwolcke, R. A., Hathway, R. A., Jacobs, C., Selwood, M. H., and Wing, A. J. Combined report on regular dialysis and transplantation in Europe IX 1978. Proc. Eur. Dial. Transplant Assoc., *16:*4, 1979.
5. Crosnier, J. Indications respectives de la transplantation rénale et de l'hémodialyse périodique. Bull. Acad. Natl. Med., *163:*553, 1979.
6. Crosnier, J., and Broyer, M. Treatment of chronic renal failure in children. In *Nephrology*, edited by J. Hamburger, J. Crosnier and J. P. Grünfeld, p. 1361. John Wiley & Sons, New York, 1979.
7. Crosnier, J., and Descamps, B. Conditions de vie et possibilités de réadaptation des patients porteurs d'un transplant rénal. Réadaptation, *217:*24, 1975.
8. Dausset, J., Festenstein, H., Hors, J., Busson, M., Olivier, R. T. D., Paris, A. M. I., and Sachs, J. A. Serologically defined HLA antigens and long term survival of cadaver kidney transplants. A study of 918 cases. N. Engl. J. Med., *290:*979, 1974.
9. Descamps, B., and Kreis, H. Recipient presensitization: a critical survey. In *Advances in Nephrology*, edited by J. Hamburger, J. Crosnier and M. H. Maxwell, vol. 6, p. 443. Year Book Medical Publishers, Chicago, 1976.
10. Descamps, B., N'Guyen, A. T., and Kreis, H. New insights into immunologic selection of human cadaver renal allograft recipients based on immune response capacities. Transplant. Proc., *10:*497, 1978.
11. Grushkin, C. M., and Fine, R. M. Growth in children following renal transplantation. Am. J. Dis. Child., *125:*514, 1973.
12. Gustafsson, A. Regrafting in human kidney transplantation. Scand. J. Urol. Nephrol. (Suppl.) 22, 1974.
13. Kreis, H. Procedure for performing renal transplantation. In *Nephrology*, edited by J. Hamburger, J. Crosnier and J. P. Grünfeld, p.1311. John Wiley & Sons, New York, 1979.
14. Luciani, J., Frantz, P., Sanici, K., Thibault, P., Min, C. L., Degoulet, P., Chatelain, C., and Küss, R. Transplantation d'un rein de cadavre. La logistique du prélevement et le traitement immédiat du receveur. In *Séances d'UroNéphrologie*, edited by R. Küss and M. Legrain, p. 77. Masson, Paris, 1980.
15. Malekzadeh, M. H., Brennan, P., Payne, V. C., and Fine, R. M. Hypertension after renal transplantation in children. J. Pediatr., *86:*370, 1975.

16. Morris, P. J. Results of renal transplantation. In *Kidney Transplantation. Principles and Practice*, edited by P. J. Morris, p.377. Grune and Stratton, New York, 1979.
17. Oliver, R. T. D., Sachs, J. A., Festenstein, H., Pegrum, G. D., and Moorhead, J. F. The influence of HLA matching antigenic strength, and immune responsiveness on the outcome of 349 cadaver renal grafts. Lancet, *2:*1381, 1972.
18. Opelz, G., and Terasaki, P. J. Influence of sex on histocompatibility matching in renal transplantation. Lancet, *2:*419, 1972.
19. Opelz, G., Terasaki, P. J., Graves, B., Sasaki, M., Langston, M., Cohn, M., and Mickey, M. R. Correlation between number of pretransplant blood transfusions and kidney graft survival. Transplant. Proc., *11:*145, 1979.
20. Parsons, F. M., Brunner, F. P., Burck, H. C., Graser, W., Gurland, H. J., Harlen, H., Scharer, K., and Spies, G. W. Combined report, including pediatrics, on regular dialysis and transplantation in Europe. Proc. Eur. Dial. Transplant Assoc., *11:*3, 1974.
21. Parsons, F. M., Brunner, F. P., Burck, H. C., Graser, W., Gurland, H. J., Harlen, H., Scharer, W., and Spies, G. W. Statistical review. Proc. Eur. Dial. Transplant Assoc., *12:* 3, 1975.
22. Potter, D. E., Holliday, M. A., Wilson, C. J., Salvatierra, O., and Belzer, F. O. Alternate day steroids in children after renal transplantation. Transplant. Proc., *7:*79, 1975.
23. Sandberg, L. The ABC antigens of the HLA system in primary cadaveric kidney transplantation. Renal transplantation. Scand. J. Urol. Nephrol. (Suppl.), *38:*13, 1976.
24. Thompson, J. S., Corry, R. J., Lawton, R. L., Bonney, W. W., and Kaloyanides, G. J. Effect of prospective HLA haplotype matching on renal transplantation. Transplant. Proc., *9:*205, 1977.
25. Van Hoof, J. P. The relative importance of HLA matching in kidney transplantation. Thesis, Pasmans, Den Haag, 1976.
26. Van Hoof, J. P., Schippers, H. M. S., Van der Steen, G. J., and Van Rood, J. J. Efficacy of HLA matching in Euro Transplant. Lancet, *2:*1385, 1972.
27. Williams, G. M. Progress in clinical renal transplantation. Transplant. Proc., *11:*4, 1979.

CHAPTER TEN

Heterotransplantation*

Michel Leski

Basic data on kidney xenografts—Attempts at clinical application: Heterotransplantation of monkey kidneys to man.

BASIC DATA ON KIDNEY XENOGRAFTS

The transplantation of kidneys from other species could be an attractive solution to some of the difficult problems of obtaining human kidneys for homotransplantation. Clinical efforts at heterotransplantation have not been very successful and experimental work gives little hope for the near future of long-term success with heterotransplantation.

The earliest efforts at kidney heterotransplantation date from the beginning of the century.

In 1902, Ullman[41] reported the first transplantation of a kidney from a dog to a goat. Many further attempts followed in man and animals.

In man, Jaboulay[13] in 1906 tried on two occasions to graft kidneys from a pig and a goat to uremic women. Unger,[42] in 1910, and Schonstadt, in 1913, tried grafting monkey kidneys. Neuhof[23] transplanted a lamb kidney in 1923 to treat a case of mercurial anuria. All these transplantations, without immunosuppressive treatment, and the earliest without vascular suture, failed immediately.

In animals, renal xenografts were also attempted,[1, 2, 44] with equally bad results. Only Avramovici[1] reported function for several days with cat kidneys grafted into dogs, but when Brull et al[2] tried the same experimental protocol there was immediate acute rejection.

Since 1957,[4, 8] further researches in renal heterotransplantation have been undertaken in many laboratories, and there is now better understanding of xenograft rejection mechanisms.

Role of Species and Order of the Donor Animal

Way et al[43] and Perper and Najarian,[27, 28] on the basis of their own

---

* This chapter, which originally appeared in the first edition of *Renal Transplantation, Theory and Practice*, has been retained in the present edition mainly for historical reasons.

work and of that of many other laboratories, have shown that the rapidity of failure of heterotransplantation is directly related to the distance separating the two species in zoologic classification. In particular, all heterotransplants between animals of different order are inevitably rejected hyperacutely, whereas heterografts within the same zoologic order (Primates, Artiodactyla, Carnivora, etc.) behave more like homotransplants.

The principal difference between interordinal heterotransplantations, which fail very rapidly, and intraordinal heterotransplantations, which fail more slowly, is that circulating antibodies play a predominant part in the former, whereas they are less important in the latter and so there is time for cell-mediated immunity to take effect.[16, 32] The clinical and histologic features of the hyperacute rejection of interordinal heterotransplantation are similar to those found in man when homotransplantation is performed in the presence of circulating cytotoxic antibodies. Renal blood flow ceases in a few minutes and the kidney becomes purple and infarcted. Histologic examination reveals diffuse hemorrhagic infarction, fibrinoid necrosis of the arterioles and thrombosis in the vessels and glomeruli. There is no round cell infiltration in the interstitial tissues. The demonstration of immunoglobulin deposits on the walls of the arteries may be difficult and requires very special techniques.[10]

In contrast, rejection of intraordinal transplants is slower; urine may be secreted for several days. Histologic examination shows few vascular lesions but a massive interstitial infiltration with mononuclear cells.[28]

Furthermore, some animals have higher levels of circulating cytotoxic antibodies than others and they are the worst graft recipients. For example, dogs reject pig kidneys much faster than pigs reject dog kidneys.[43] Egdahl et al reported a similar finding in 1957 with skin heterografts between rats and rabbits.

Role of Circulating Antibodies and of Complement

Circulating *cytotoxic antibodies*, active in the presence of complement, are the agents responsible for hyperacute rejection. These antibodies are present before transplantation. They can be shown to be cytotoxic to all nucleated cells of the donor animal.[27] In more closely related species, the formation of these antibodies may be induced or increased by preliminary sensitization.[29] These antibodies cannot be absorbed on erythrocytes. They are thermostable.[16] They are mainly IgG, but also include IgM.[22]

Many methods have been used in an attempt to diminish the level of circulating cytotoxic antibodies and it has been found that heterotransplant survival is prolonged in direct proportion to the extent of the reduction in the level of circulating antibodies. The principal techniques used have been hemodilution in dogs,[19] selective plasmapheresis[18, 20] perfusion of the recipient with homogenates of donor kidneys[10, 27] and *ex vivo* perfusion of the donor liver by the recipient.[20, 26] This last method seems the most effective.

Other circulating antibodies (hemolysins, hemagglutinins and precipitins of plasma proteins) can be found in the blood of animals before grafting. They play a less important role than cytotoxic antibodies, as shown by the fact that their absorption does not modify the evolution of the graft.[27, 29] Nevertheless, the level of heterospecific hemolysins has been shown to fall after heterotransplantation.[10, 22]

Complement plays an important part in hyperacute rejection of heterografts because circulating cytotoxic antibodies are active only in the presence of complement. Gewurz et al[10] have demonstrated a significant drop in total complement levels and in the levels of the different fractions (C_1, C_4, C_2) in renal vein blood. These facts have been widely confirmed.[10, 15, 16, 18, 20, 22, 28] The constriction of the renal artery which occurs almost immediately after the circulation is restored is due to liberation of anaphylatoxin, a degradation product of C_5.[16] There is a marked prolongation of heterotransplant survival if complement is inactivated by cobra venom (C_3 inhibitor), by carrageenin (C_1 inhibitor) or by injection of aggregated human globulins.[10, 20]

Changes in Coagulation Factors and Blood Cells

Histologic examination of heterografted kidneys gives clear evidence of *coagulation phenomena*: vascular thromboses, platelet aggregates, and intra- and extravascular fibrin deposits. Furthermore, many authors[10, 17, 20, 27] have shown that platelet and fibrinogen levels are lowered by more than 50% in the renal vein of the heterograft.

However, the intervention of coagulation factors is probably only secondary to the antigen-antibody-complement reaction and intensive anticoagulant therapy is totally ineffective in preventing rejection. This has been shown with Malaysian viper venom,[20] or with Arvin,[36] injection of antiplatelet serum,[36] perfusion with a platelet-free fluid[15] and heparin.[10, 36]

Comparison of *blood counts* in arterial and venous blood[10, 17, 20] shows that the platelet and leukocyte counts drop by more than 50% during passage of the blood through the heterograft. In contrast, the red cell count is unchanged.

Although there is no cell infiltration in hyperacute rejection, with the single exception, described above, of the slower rejection of intraordinal heterotransplants, Land et al[15] have shown that the presence of leukocytes accelerates the process even in hyperacute rejection. These results have been confirmed by Linn and associates.[16] Perper[27] has demonstrated the presence of cytotoxic antibodies on the spleen cells of heterografted animals.

Effect of Drugs on Renal Xenografts

It has already been pointed out that heparin does not improve graft survival significantly.[10, 36] Steroid therapy has proved equally ineffective.[8, 10, 17, 26] Azathioprine and 6-mercaptopurine, possibly effective in skin heterografts,[3] have produced no appreciable effect in renal xenografts, even in experimental intraordinal heterotransplantation.[10, 17, 26, 27] Nevertheless, these therapeutic measures have succeeded in producing at least temporary regression of rejection of monkey kidneys heterografted into man.[34, 35, 37, 38]

Antilymphocyte globulin is effective in skin heterografts in rodents but does not delay rejection of a baboon kidney in a macaque,[7] although it prolongs survival of goat heart grafts in calves.[6] Many other drugs (antihistamines, antiserotonins, etc.) have been tried without success.[17, 21]

Attempts to Induce Tolerance to Renal Heterotransplants

In 1957, Egdahl et al[8] induced specific tolerance to rabbit skin grafts in the rat by injecting the fetus with spleen cells from the future donor. In 1965, Marceau and associates[17] fed dog γ-globulins to newborn pigs and obtained partial tolerance to subsequent kidney transplantation. Owen[24, 25] treated rabbits for 5 weeks by injecting small doses (0.5 μg/kg/day) of guinea pig liver antigen. These rabbits subsequently tolerated guinea pig kidneys for periods from 5 to 25 days, although the control animals rejected the kidney on the 1st day. The same technique also prolongs the survival of pig kidneys in dogs, chimpanzee skin grafts in macaques and rabbits and pig skin grafts in dogs. Messmer et al[19] obtained less, but very significant, prolongation of survival of pig kidney grafts in dogs, by 6 weeks of preliminary treatment at a higher dosage (3 mg/kg/week).

ATTEMPTS AT CLINICAL APPLICATION: HETEROTRANSPLANTATION OF MONKEY KIDNEYS TO MAN

Between 1963 and 1965 several monkey kidneys were transplanted into man by American and French groups experienced in kidney homotransplantation. All the patients died, after an interval which varied from days to 9 months, and the method has been abandoned.

Clinical Evolution of Monkey Kidney Heterotransplants

On 16 February 1963, Hitchcock et al[11] transplanted a baboon (*Papio doguera*) kidney into a patient whose cadaver graft had failed 3 days earlier. The baboon kidney was implanted into the upper thigh. Immunosuppressive therapy consisted of azathioprine (4 mg/kg/day) and 6-diazo-5-oxo-L-norleucine at a dose of 0.05 mg/kg/day. Three liters of urine were put out in the first 24 hours but excretory function was poor, with a creatinine clearance below 10 ml/min. Urine output fell, and on the 4th day there was evidence of thrombosis of the renal artery. The patient died rapidly from diffuse hemorrhages.

In October 1963, Reemtsma et al[33] transplanted both kidneys from a rhesus monkey into the right iliac fossa by the en bloc technique. This technique was later adopted in nearly all clinical heterotransplantations. The immunosuppressive treatment comprised azathioprine, azaserine, actinomycin and steroids. There was a rapid onset of diuresis with an output of 35 liters in the first 24 hours. But renal function diminished and ceased on the 8th day. The patient died on the 12th day from septicemia.

During the following months, Reemtsma's group[31] performed 12 transplantations with chimpanzee kidneys. Only the first six have been reported in detail.[35] In these six, the immunosuppressive treatment included high doses of azathioprine, actinomycin C, prednisone and local radiation. The kidneys functioned immediately in all but one case, where there was erythrocyte incompatibility (A donor and O recipient), this patient received a second graft 2 days later from a compatible chimpanzee. There was considerable diuresis in the first 24 hours, but not more than 8 liters. Excretory function of the transplanted kidneys was good, except during rejection crises. Creatinine clearance was frequently more than 60 ml/min. In the five cases with good function, there were one or more rejection crises which responded to steroid therapy and local radiation in the same manner as homotransplant crises. These six patients died at periods ranging from 18 days to 10 months after transplantation and in all cases infection was a major cause of death. "In the first six chimpanzee-to-man grafts, rejection appeared to be a less serious problem than infection."[31]

In the six subsequent cases, there was early and irreversible rejection.

Starzl's group[37–39] at the University of Colorado performed, in December 1963 and January 1964, six transplantations with kidneys from baboons (*Papio doguera*). Immunosuppressive therapy including azathioprine, actinomycin C, prednisone and local radiation was given in the highest dosage that could be tolerated. The surgical technique used was the en bloc technique of Reemtsma. All six cases had satisfactory function on the 1st day with diuresis reaching a maximum of 9 liters in 24 hours. Creatinine clearance reached 90 ml/min in one case but the mean was 30 to 40 ml/min (apart from rejection crises) and then diminished progressively. Rejection crises occurred early in five of the six cases. These crises seemed to respond favorably to combined treatment with local radiation, actinomycin C and steroids in high doses, but relapsed rapidly as soon as any attempt was made to reduce the dose of steroids and immunosuppressive drugs. The duration of graft function varied from 19 to 60 days. The patients all died between the 20th and the 99th day. In five of the six cases, death was ascribed to infection.

Three other transplantations with chimpanzee kidneys were reported by Fries[9] and Traeger et al.[40] In one case it seemed that the en bloc transplantation technique was responsible for immediate failure. The implantation of a large transplant into a space too small to contain it led to embarrassment of venous return and vascular thrombosis. The two remaining grafts survived 7 days and 49 days. Urinary output in the first 24 hours was 30 liters in the first case and 11 liters in the second. As with other reported cases of heterotransplantation, there was progressive deterioration of renal function after a rejection crisis and fatal infective complications in one case.

Hume[12] reported a case of transplantation of chimpanzee kidneys which survived for only 3 days, but the remarkable feature of this case was the extreme polyuria (54 liters in 24 hours) and the difficulty in compensating for the huge potassium loss (600 mEq/day).

Immunologic Studies on Kidney Heterotransplantation from Monkey to Man

De Witt[5] studied nine patients grafted with chimpanzee kidneys.

In every case, he found circulating cytotoxic antibodies against the blood lymphocytes, lymphocytes extracted from the lymph nodes and the hepatocytes of the chimpanzees. These antibodies are thermostable, active in the presence of complement, absorbable on erythrocytes and nucleated cells of chimpanzees but not absorbable on human tissues. The appearance of these antibodies and variations in the serum levels are strictly correlated with the appearance and progess of rejection crises.

On the other hand, the serum level of heterohemagglutinins, present before transplantation, does not vary with renal function. There is evidence of a biphasic anamnestic response, unrelated to the rejection crises. These antibodies are thermolabile, active in the absence of complement, and absorbable by chimpanzee red cells but not absorbable by the nucleated cells.

In the two patients who received grafts from chimpanzees incompatible in the erythrocyte group, anti-A isoantibodies were isolated. Variation in levels of these antibodies was suggestive of a monophasic anamnestic response. These antibodies were thermostable, active in the absence of complement. They could be absorbed on the red cells and nucleated cells of chimpanzees and of group A men.

Very similar results have been reported in patients receiving baboon kidneys.[14, 37]

It would thus appear that cytotoxic antibodies play a dominant role in the rejection of heterotransplants.

Anatomopathologic Study of Heterotransplants

Porter[30] has made an anatomic and histologic study of baboon kidneys and several chimpazee kidneys.

In the baboon kidneys that functioned for a maximum of 60 days, the lesions were very similar in all cases. All the kidneys were very swollen, with more or less confluent hemorrhages on the surface. In five cases out of six, there was no thrombosis in the main renal vessel. Histologic examination revealed 1) dense and diffuse interstitial infiltration with round cells, of which more than half had pyroninophilic cytoplasm; 2) diffuse interstitial edema; 3) localized hemorrhagic infarcts and disseminated hemorrhagic infiltration of the interstitial tissue; 4) major vascular lesions: subintimal fibrinoid necrosis of the interlobular arteries and afferent arterioles, subintimal edema, deposits of fibrin and platelets on the intima of the arterioles, rupture of the internal elastic lamina of the arteries, thromboses of arterioles and arteries; and 5) tubular necrosis, regenerating in places. There was no significant lesion in the glomeruli.

According to Porter, these lesions differ from those seen in homotransplantations by the intensity of cell infiltration and the severity of the vascular lesions.

Surprisingly, histologic examination of the first chimpanzee heterotransplant revealed no sign of rejection: neither cell infiltration nor vascular lesion. Similar observations were made in another chimpanzee heterotransplant that had functioned for 9 months and in which the only vascular lesions were endothelial proliferation of the interlobular arteries.

In contrast, in six other rapidly rejected chimpanzee heterotransplants,[31] the same lesions were found as in the baboon kidneys: massive swelling, hemorrhagic infarction, cell infiltration and vascular lesions.

REFERENCES

1. Avramvici, A. Les transplantations de rein. Lyon Chir., *21:*734, 1924.
2. Brull, L., Louis-Bar, D., and Marson, F. G. W. Auto- and homotransplanted kidneys grafted on the same dog: A functional comparison. Arch. Int. Physiol., *64:*269, 1956.
3. Calne, R. Y. Observations on renal homotransplantation. Br. J. Surg., *48:*384, 1960.
4. Calne, R. Y. *Renal Transplantation.* Arnold, London, 1963.
5. De Witt, C. W. Serologic response of humans to chimpanzee tissue. Fed. Proc., *24:*573, 1965.
6. Donawick, W. J., Shaffer, C. F., Dodd, D. C., Buchanan, J. W., and Fregin, G. F. Cardiac and skin heterograft rejection: Suppression with antilymphocyte serum. Third Inter-

national Congress of Transplantation Society, The Hague, 1970. Transplant. Proc., *3:* 551, 1971.

7. Dubernard, J. M., Bonneau, M., Bomel, J., Montagard, J., Blitz, M., Latour, M., Blanc-Brunat, N., Fries, D., Brochard, J. C., Banssilon, V., Banssilon, G., and Capodicasa, G. Renal and skin xenografts from baboons to macaques. Effect of antilymphocyte globulins. Third International Congress of Transplantation Society, The Hague, 1970. Transplant. Proc., *3:*545, 1971.
8. Egdahl, R. H., Good, R. A., and Varco, R. L. Studies in homograft and heterograft survival. Surgery, *42:*228, 1957.
9. Fries, D. Personal communication, 1970.
10. Gewurz, H., Clark, D. S., Finstad, J., Kelly, W. D., Varco, R. L., Good, R. A., and Gabrielsen, A. E. Role of the complement system in graft rejection in experimental animals and man. Ann. NY Acad. Sci. *129:*673, 1966.
11. Hitchcock, C. R., Kiser, J. C., Telander, R. L., and Seljeskog, E. L. Baboon renal grafts. JAMA, *189:*934, 1964.
12. Hume, D. M. Discussion. American Surgical Association Meeting, Hot Springs, Virginia, 1964. Ann. Surg., *160:*409, 1964.
13. Jaboulay, M. Greffe de reins au pli du coude par sutures artérielles et veineuses. Lyon Méd., *107:*575, 1906.
14. Kirkpatrick, C. H., and Wilson, W. E. C. Immunologic studies of baboon to man renal heterotransplantation. In *Experience in Renal Transplantation*, edited by T. E. Starzl, p. 284. Saunders, Philadelphia, 1964.
15. Land, W., Schillin, A., Aldenhoff, J., Lamerz, R., Pielsticker, K., Mendler, N., and Brendel. W. *In vitro* studies on the mechanism of hyperacute xenograft rejection. Third International Congress of Transplantation Society, The Hague, 1970. Transplant. Proc., *3:*888, 1971.
16. Linn, B. S., Jensen, J. A., Pardo, V., Davies, D., and Franklin, L. Relationship between structural and functional changes in rejecting renal xenograft. Third International Congress of Transplantation Society, The Hague, 1970. Transplant. Proc., *3:*527, 1971.
17. Marceau, J. P., Hallenbeck, G. A., Zollman, P. E., Butler, H. C., and Shorter, R. G. A comparison of autoplastic allogenic and xenogenic perfusion of isolated kidneys. J. Surg. Res. *5:*492, 1965.
18. Merkel, F. K., Bier, M., Beavers, C. D., Merriman, W. G., Wilson, C., and Starzl, T. E. Modification of xenograft response by selective plasmapheresis. Third International Congress of Transplantation Society, The Hague, 1970. Transplant. Proc., *3:*534, 1971.
19. Messmer, K., Hammer, C., Land, W., Fiedler, L., Klövekorn, W. P., Holper, K., Lob, G., Merzel, D., and Brendel, W. Modification of hyperacute xenogeneic kidney rejection. Third International Congress of Transplantation Society, The Hague, 1970. Transplant. Proc., *3:*542, 1971.
20. Moberg, A. W., Shons, A. R., Gewurz, H., Mozes, M., and Najarian, J. S. Prolongation of renal xenografts by the simultaneous sequestration of preformed antibody, inhibition of complement, coagulation and antibody synthesis. Third International Congress of Transplantation Society, The Hague, 1970. Transplant. Proc., *3:*538, 1971.
21. Mowbray, J. F., and Kenyon, J. R. An experimental study on the action of 5-hydroxytryptamine antagonists on the recently transplanted autograft, homograft and heterograft. Bull. Soc. Int. Chir., *20:*604, 1961.
22. Mozes, M. F., Gewurz, H., Gunnarson, A., Moberg, A. W., Westberg, N. G., Jetzer, T., and Najarian, J. S. Xenograft rejection by dog and man: Isolated kidney perfusion with blood and plasma. Third International Congress of Transplantation Society, The Hague, 1970. Transplant. Proc., *3:*531, 1971.
23. Neuhof. H. *The Transplantation of Tissues,* p. 260. Appleton, New York, 1923.

24. Owen, E. R. Prolonged survival in heterografted kidneys with transplantation antigen pretreatment. Nature *219:*970, 1968.
25. Owen, E. R. Xenograft protection by low-dose, antigen-induced tolerance. Third International Congress of Transplantation Society, The Hague, 1970. Transplant. Proc., *3:* 562, 1971.
26. Perper, R. J., May, J., Way, L. W., and Najarian, J. S. Experimental renal heterotransplantation in closely related species. Fed. Proc., *24:*573, 1965.
27. Perper, R. J., and Najarian, J. S. Experimental renal heterotransplantation. I. In widely divergent species. Transplantation, *4:*377, 1966.
28. Perper, R. J., and Najarian, J. S. Experimental renal heterotransplantation. II. Closely related species. Transplantation, *4:*700, 1966.
29. Perper, R. J., and Najarian, J. S. Experimental renal heterotransplantation. III. Passive transfer of transplantation immunity. Transplantation, *5:*514, 1967.
30. Porter, K. A. Pathological changes in transplanted kidneys. Renal heterotransplants. In *Experience in Renal Transplantation,* edited by T. E. Starzl, p. 345. Saunders, Philadelphia, 1964.
31. Reemtsma, K. Heterotransplantation. In *Human Transplantation,* edited by F. T. Rapaport and J. Dausset, p. 357. Grune and Stratton, New York, 1968.
32. Reemtsma, K. Heterotransplantation: Theoretical considerations. Third International Congress of Transplantation Society, The Hague, 1970. Transplant. Proc., *3:*49, 1971.
33. Reemtsma, K., McCracken, B. H., Schlegel, J. U., and Pearl, M. A. Heterotransplantation of the kidney: Two clinical experiences. Science, *143:*700, 164.
34. Reemtsma, K., McCracken, B. H., Schlegel, J. U., Pearl, M. A., De Witt, C. W., and Creech, O. Reversal of early graft rejection after renal heterotransplantation in man. JAMA, *187:*691, 1964.
35. Reemtsma, K., McCracken, B. H., Schlegel, J. U., Pearl, M. A., Pearce, C. D., De Witt, C. W., Smith, P. E., Hewitt, R. L., Flinner, R. L., and Creech, O., Jr. Renal heterotransplantation in man. Ann. Surg., *160:*384, 1964.
36. Slapak, M., Greenbaum, M., Bardarvil, W., Saravis, C., Joison, J., and McDermott, W. V., Jr. Effect of heparin, arvin, liver perfusion and heterologous antiplatelet serum on rejection of pig kidney by dog. Third International Congress of Transplantation Society, The Hague, 1970. Transplant. Proc., *3:*558, 1971.
37. Starzl, T. E. Renal heterotransplantation. In *Experience in Renal Transplantation,* edited by T. E. Starzl, p. 262. Saunders, Philadelphia, 1964.
38. Starzl, T. E. Discussion. American Surgical Association Meeting, Hot Springs, Virginia, 1964. Ann. Surg., *160:*409, 1964.
39. Starzl, T. E., Marchioro, T. L., Peters, G. N., Kirkpatrick, C. H., Wilson, W. E. C., Porter, K. A., Rifkind, D., Ogden, D. A., Hitchcock, C. R., and Waddell, W. R. Renal heterotransplantation from baboon to man: Experience with 6 cases. Transplantation *2:*752, 1964.
40. Traeger, J., Fries, D., Perrin, J., Saubier, E., Vicaria, E., Cuche, M., and Laurent, G. Hétérotransplantation chez l'homme, premiers résultats. Proceedings of the European Dialysis Transplant Association, 1965, vol. II, p. 214. Excerpta Medica, Amsterdam, 1966.
41. Ullman, E. Experimentelle nierentransplantation. Wien. Klin. Wschr., *15:*281, 1902.
42. Unger, E. Nierentransplantationen. Berlin. Klin. Wschr., *47:*573, 1910.
43. Way, L. W., May, J., and Perper, R. J. Experimental renal heterotransplantation in various species. Fed. Proc. *24:*572, 1965.
44. Williamson, C. S. Further studies on the transplantation of the kidney. J. Urol., *16:*231, 1926.

CHAPTER ELEVEN

Psychological, Moral and Legal Problems

Jean Crosnier

Recipients: psychological problems before and after transplantation—Living donors: moral and legal problems—Transplants of organs from cadavers: legislation in France, the United States and other countries.

Like all new therapeutic methods, but to a far greater degree, organ transplantation raises many problems: moral, psychological, social, cultural and legal. The emotional atmosphere surrounding the discussion of these problems may be ascribed to various factors. First, organ exchange challenges many traditional concepts, for the individual and for society. In particular, heart transplantation, or more exactly heart removal from cadavers, has stimulated ardent discussion, and very often absolute opposition, that could for some be extended to renal transplantation. Second, despite remarkable progress in the last 20 years, the results of transplantation are still somewhat unpredictable, complications are frequent, failure is not rare and mortality has not reached zero. Third, patients with terminal renal failure can be treated either by renal transplantation or by chronic hemodialysis. Although mortality at 3 years is nearly the same with the two methods,[3] the risk in transplantation is much greater during the first 6 months.

Each individual case poses difficult problems, and these problems present physicians with a load of responsibility rarely encountered in other fields of medicine. Disturbed by the weight of this responsibility, physicians have turned for aid to moral philosophers and lawyers. These experts do not often find entirely satisfactory solutions. But gradually, from individuals and through group deliberations throughout the world, agreement on certain basic attitudes has emerged.

The problems can be considered under three headings: the recipient, the living donor and the removal and transplantation of cadaver organs.

PSYCHOLOGICAL PROBLEMS OF THE RECIPIENT

Before Transplantation

As with any surgical procedure, it is necessary to have the recipient's consent. It is conceivable that a patient might refuse to consider all forms of treatment of terminal renal failure, both dialysis and transplantation. If theoretically this decision must be respected, the validity of such a refusal by a seriously ill patient is always open to question, and physicians have often persuaded patients to accept these types of treatment.

In fact, the true problem is to help each patient choose between dialysis and transplantation. And for the patient such a choice is possible only if he has been thoroughly informed as to the results, the complications, the risks and the constraints of each of these two techniques, both short-range and long-range.

If the patient desires transplantation, in the great majority of cases in our group it is a question of cadaver kidney transplantation. We propose transplantation from living donors only when the patient has a family member who is an HLA(human leukocyte A)-identical and volunteer sibling (cf. p. 58); but in this case we have had some patients refuse to accept a sibling kidney in favor of a cadaver graft so as not to expose a relative to any risk.

The true problem for patients desiring a transplantation, at least in France, is that they often have to wait for several years. During this time they are treated by hemodialysis, and often discouragement and even anxiety occur. We have seen (p. 151) that it is frequently necessary to convince these patients that this long delay is due to the necessity of finding a compatible cadaver kidney donor, on which depends the successful outcome of the transplantation.

After Transplantation

We have seen (p. 259) that psychological and even psychiatric problems are relatively common in the recipient after transplantation.[1, 4] They are usually mild, however, and the depressive state is rarely so severe as to interfere with treatment and rehabilitation of these patients.

Psychotic problems are usually due to anxiety over rejection and return to hemodialysis treatment, but they are often aggravated by a latent preexisting psychotic disorder disclosed by steroid therapy. Theoretically, the more serious problems could be foreseen to some extent by preoperative psychological examination, but the poor physical condition of these patients can invalidate such tests.

LIVING DONORS

Considerable attention has been paid to the moral problems involved in transplantation from living donors[6, 8, 14]; legal problems, at least in France, have now been resolved (cf. below).

Moral Problems

According to traditional medical ethics, a mutilating operation is acceptable only when performed for the benefit of the person undergoing the surgery and when the risk of operating is less than the risk of not operating. However, in the case of a graft from a living donor, the operation benefits only the recipient and even entails certain risks for the donor. On the other hand, it is generally held that an individual has not only the right but an actual obligation to help another in danger, even at the risk of his own life. And if one may risk his life for a fellow man, it is difficult not to accept the idea that he may sacrifice one of his kidneys for the same purpose. Theologians such as Tesson[13] and Cunningham (cited by Tesson[13]) have concluded that there is no moral objection to donating a kidney in the hope of saving a relative's life.

The role of the physician in this situation is to ascertain whether the project is reasonable, i.e., that the risk to which the potential donor is exposing himself is extremely low and that the possibility of the graft being successful is good. The physician also must make sure that the donor has been fully informed and is entirely free in his decision.

Risks Run by the Donor

The immediate risk of unilateral nephrectomy in a healthy subject has been put at 0.05%.[7] The long-term risk, taking into account the possibilities of injury to a solitary kidney that may compromise survival, has been estimated at about 0.07%.[9] The overall risk, between 0.1 and 0.2%, is therefore slight but not negligible, and cases of fatal complications in living donors have already been reported.

The figures quoted above are only averages. The individual risk must be weighed in each case. All possible operative and postoperative difficulties must be taken into account: age over 50, obesity, venous diseases in the lower limbs, anatomical anomalies which may increase the operative risk, the risks of preliminary investigations, especially renal arteriography, etc.

Whether or not to perform transplantation from a living donor must also take into account the alternative offered by hemodialysis, since transplantation is no longer the only means of saving a patient. The patient can continue living an almost normal life on dialysis while awaiting a suitable cadaver donor, whereas transplantation from a living donor would only provide a more rapid return to a more normal life. Under these circumstances, only a very strong possibility of success, near 100%, would for us justify the use of a living donor today.

Probability of a Successful Graft

The current results of kidney transplantation have been discussed in an earlier chapter.

1. Transplantation performed with a kidney removed from an HLA-identical sibling constitutes the ideal situation, with a possibility of success near 100%. For us, it is the only case where transplantation from a living donor should be accepted and even recommended.
2. In all other cases, treatment by hemodialysis while awaiting a compatible cadaver kidney appears to us to be the only reasonable decision. However, in certain very special cases such as severe and life-threatening complications in hemodialysis or the problem of growth retardation in children, an HLA semi-identical donor, parent or sibling, may be accepted if the mixed lymphocyte culture shows a degree of cell transformation which indicates the absence of frank stimulation.

Freedom of Decision by the Donor

The donor should be a well balanced individual, fully aware of the risk he runs and the uncertain outcome of the graft. He must be able to make his decision in complete freedom. It is essential to be certain that he is a genuine volunteer and is receiving no external pressure, especially from his family. The best way to be sure is to give the possible donor adequate time for reflection and to inform him that he need not hesitate to change his mind at any time, and that in this case the transplantation team will give some technical reason for not performing the graft so that no one will know of his decision. In such circumstances, well balanced adults can refuse to donate a kidney, especially since they know that the secret of their decision will be scrupulously kept. Like other groups, we have encountered many such cases.

It is also essential to be sure of the mental stability of the potential donor, and particular inquiry should be made into any history of psychological disorders. A psychiatrist can be very helpful in this matter,[1] but with a little experience it is not difficult for the physician to form an accurate opinion.[5] Mentally defective persons, prisoners and children must not be accepted as donors. It is, however, difficult to establish an age limit because psychological maturity is at least as important as physical age in determining the ability to make a decision; moreover, in especially favorable circumstances such as that of identical twins, there may be less hesitation about accepting a donation before maturity.

In our view, unrelated donors should not be accepted. It is our experience that only mentally abnormal individuals offer a kidney to a transplantation center for grafting to a total stranger. It would be possible, on the other hand, to consider a transplant between husband and wife or between close friends; but the very slight chance of finding perfect histocompatibility between two such individuals greatly limits such transplantation.

Psychological Effect of Transplantation on the Donor

How do the donors themselves react to the fact that they have given a kidney? Our experience tallies with that of Eisendrath et al,[5] who found that they rarely experience regret, even when the graft fails; in most cases, despite the anxieties of the operative period, their action is for them a source of immense satisfaction and pride. They do sometimes complain that all the attention is devoted to the recipient, whereas they have little of the limelight. This is a minor difficulty which is easily resolved. Sometimes anxious or hypochondriac individuals complain of various troubles at the site of their nephrectomy and may make demands for various types of disability benefits.

Legal Problems

Until the end of 1976, there was no law authorizing the donation of organs by living volunteers in France, and it was theoretically possible to consider such acts as "self-inflicted injury" and to legally punish the volunteer donor and the accessory surgeon. On December 22, 1976, a law was enacted in France[10] authorizing the removal of organs from a donor who has reached the age of legal consent, providing the decision is completely voluntary (cf. below).

Legal authority for the removal of organs from living donors also exists in most other countries. This legislation is usually principally concerned with the removal of cadaver organs, but generally a brief mention of living donors is made, merely stipulating that the donor must give his consent and that organ removal cannot be the object of any monetary counterpart.

CADAVER KIDNEYS

Removal of a kidney from a cadaver donor should entail no ethical problems. In 1970, the International Society of Transplantation[11] published the following guidelines: "It is merely desirable to make use of all organs and tissues after death that could save life and lead to curing individuals in danger" but "...if the patient had stated during his lifetime his aversion to such a donation, this will be entirely respected."

Legal Problems

Each country has its own rules or laws concerning removal of cadaver organs, and in practice most laws require that organ removal coincide with the will of the individual as expressed before his death. In France, the law of December 22, 1976,[10] authorizes the removal of organs from cadavers of persons who have not expressed refusal of such a procedure during their lifetimes.

Law 76-1181 of December 22, 1976
Concerning Removal of Organs

The National Assembly and Senate have adopted, and the President of the Republic issues the following law:

Article 1. An organ to be used for transplantation for therapeutic purposes in a human subject may be removed from a living person who is of age and in full possession of his mental faculties, and who has freely and expressly consented to its being removed.

If the prospective donor is a minor an organ may be removed only if he or she is a brother or sister of the recipient. In this case consent to organ removal must be given by his or her legal representative, and the procedure must in addition be authorized by a committee composed of at least three experts. Two of the experts must be doctors, of whom one must have practiced for 20 years. The committee will first examine all foreseeable consequences, physical and psychological, of the procedure. If the minor's wishes can be consulted, refusal on his part to donate an organ must in all cases be respected.

Article 2. An organ to be used for therapeutic or scientific purposes may be removed from the cadaver of a person who has not during his lifetime made known his refusal of such a procedure. If, however, the cadaver is that of a minor or a mentally defective person, organ removal for transplantation must be authorized by his legal representative.

Article 3. Organ removal as referred to in the preceding articles cannot be the object of any monetary counterpart. This does not exclude reimbursement of any contingent expenses incurred (by the hospital concerned).

Article 4. A decree of the Council of State will specify: 1) How a donor referred to in article 1 or his legal representative will be informed of the possible consequences of his decision, and how he will express his consent. 2) How the refusal or the authorization referred to in article 2 will be expressed. 3) The conditions that hospitals must satisfy to be authorized to carry out organ removal as referred to in article 2 and to figure on an approved list to be drawn up by the Minister of Health. 4) The procedures and methods to be used for diagnosing death.

Article 5. The provisions of this present law should in no way obstruct the application of provisions of Law 49-890 of July 8, 1949, which concerns corneal grafts or those of the sole chapter in Book VI of the Public Health Code concerning the therapeutic use of human blood, plasma, and its derivatives. This above law will be enacted as Law of the State.

Paris, December 22, 1976 Valéry Giscard d'Estaing

For the President of the Republic:

Raymond Barre Olivier Guichard
Prime Minister Minister of Justice

Simone Veil
Minister of Health

1. Expression of Refusal. The decree, published March 31, 1978, states that an individual may use any means to express his opposition to organ removal during his lifetime. Moreover, all hospitals must have a register in which each patient admitted may express his refusal or any individual with proof may testify to such an opposition.

2. Diagnosis of Death. The problem of defining death has been debated extensively. Cessation of circulation and respiration has long been the basis for this definition; however, some cases, for example, brain injury or some cerebral vascular accidents, do not fulfill the traditional criteria of death, while death actually occurs in the sense that the brain is irretrievably destroyed. In these cases, it seems legitimate to declare the patient dead and to seek consent for organ removal.

Even in these cases it is necessary for physicians to conform to strict rules. In France, these rules were clearly set out as early as 1968 in a Circular from the Minister of Social Affairs (Circular 67 of April 24, 1968):

> a) The occurrence of death may be established by the presence of irreversible changes in the nervous system, based on the following points: clinical history, absence of spontaneous respiration, absence of reflexes, lack of muscular tone, mydriasis and disappearance of all electroencephalographic signals in a normothermic patient who has had no sedative drug. Treatment may not be abandoned nor may an organ be removed until death, defined according to the above criteria, has been established.
> b) The death certificate must be signed by two doctors who are totally unconnected with any transplantation team.

The same rules are expressed in the Decree of March 31, 1978, again specifying that the death certificate cannot be established either by the doctors who will perform the organ removal or by those who will perform the transplant.

Few other countries have established such precise rules. For European countries, however, the Council of Europe on May 11, 1978,[2] passed a resolution aimed at the harmonization of laws connected with "removal, grafts and transplantation of human products." The content of this resolution is very close to that of the French law.

Other countries have already enacted laws similar to that of France. The Spanish Government, for instance, adopted such a law on October 17, 1979.

On the other hand, the Italian law of December 26, 1975, which has been considered progressive in that country, is in fact too limiting and is responsible for the lack of development of organ transplantation in Italy.

In the United States, the situation was particularly confused for some years due to the great differences from state to state, some on the lines of common law, others more precise and modern. After lengthy study, the Uniform Anatomical Gift Act was presented on July 30, 1968.[11] It set out a pattern of a law to be enacted by individual states after debate and approval by the state legislatures. Because of the widespread feeling that such a uniform law was necessary and because of the extensive preliminary discussion, the authors of the project hoped that it would be adopted at an early date, without significant change, by most American states. A detailed commentary on the main points of the Act can be found in the publications of Sadler and Sadler,[11] who were instrumental in establishing the project.

The project was very successful and was passed into Law by the legislatures of most States.[12] Generally, only minor changes were made by individual state legislatures. At the same time, the public was encouraged to donate organs voluntarily, and a uniform model of a card to be carried on the person was circulated. This card has legal validity if signed by the person himself and by two witnesses in his presence. The almost uniform character of the law across the country has considerably facilitated organ exchanges among states in regionalized dialysis and transplantation programs.

This brief review of existing legislation indicates the variety of solutions proposed. Two main trends can be distinguished:

In France and in most European countries, laws allow the removal of cadaver organs without reference to the wishes of the relatives and do not mention voluntary donation. On the other hand, American laws require formal permission from a member of the family before an organ can be removed, and the law envisages public campaigns to encourage the voluntary donation of organs after death.

In conclusion, the ideal is a law in harmony with the character and traditions of each country and fully in accord with medical opinion. This would greatly increase the availability of cadaver organs to provide for the needs of patients who might be saved from death and restored to normal life by kidney transplantation.

REFERENCES

1. Colomb, G., and Hamburger, J. Psychological and moral problems of renal transplantation. Int. Psychiatry Clin., *4:*157, 1967.
2. Conseil de l'Europe. Harmonisation des législations des états membres relatives aux prélèvements, greffes et transplantation de substances d'origine humaine. Rapport des Affaires Juridiques Resolution, *78:*29, Strasbourg, 1978.
3. Crosnier, J. Indications respectives de la transplantation rénale et de l'hémodialyse périodique. Bull. Acad. Natl. Med., *163:*553, 1979.
4. Crosnier, J., and Descamps, B. Condition de vie et possibilités de réadaptation des patients porteurs d'un transplant rénal. Réadaptation, *217:*24, 1975.

5. Eisendrath, R. M., Guttmann, R. D., and Murray, J. E. Psychological considerations in the selection of kidney transplant donors. Surg. Gynecol Obstet., *129:*243, 1969.
6. Elkinton, J. R. Moral problems in the use of borrowed organs, artificial and transplanted. Ann. Intern. Med., *60:*309, 1964.
7. Hamburger, J. Reflexions sur la transplantation du rein chez l'homme. Brux. Med., *41:* 1405, 1961.
8. Hamburger, J., and Crosnier, J. Moral and ethical problems in transplantation. In *Human Transplantation*, edited by F. J. Rapaport and J. Dausset, p. 37. Grune and Stratton, New York, 1968.
9. Hamburger, J., Crosnier, J., and Dormont, J. Problèmes moraux posés par les méthodes de suppléance et de transplantation d'organes Rev. Fr. Etud. Clin. Biol., *9:*587, 1964.
10. Loi n° 76 1181 du 22 Décembre 1976 relative aux prélèvements d'organes. J. Officiel de la République Franc., du 23 décembre 1976.
11. Sadler, A. M., and Sadler, B. L. Transplantation and the law: The need for organized sensitivity. Georgetown Law J., *57:*5, 1968.
12. Sadler, A. M., Sadler, B. L., and Stason, E. B. Transplantation and the law. Progress toward uniformity. N. Engl. J. Med., *282:*717, 1970.
13. Tesson, E. Greffe humaine et morale. Cahier Laennec, *1:*28, 1956.
14. Wolstenholme, G. E. W., and O'Connor, M. *Ethics in Medical Progress with Special Reference to Transplantation*. Churchill, London, 1966.

APPENDIX I

Surgical Techniques

Michel Lacombe

SURGICAL TECHNIQUES IN MAN

Removing Donor Kidney

Donor nephrectomy is a delicate procedure requiring great care. The object is to remove the kidney without damaging it, to preserve the greatest possible length of artery and vein and to avoid interfering with the blood supply of the ureter. Gentle dissection is mandatory in order to avoid vascular or parenchymatous lesions of the graft. Ease of the recipient operation and good function of the transplant in the immediate postoperative period depend essentially on the quality of the donor operation.

Living and cadaver donors present entirely different practical conditions.

Nephrectomy in a Living Donor

The surgical advantages of a living donor are that the anatomic arrangement of the renal vessels is known in advance from preoperative angiography, and the operation can be synchronized with the transplant procedure to reduce the ischemic time to a minimum.

Preoperative Studies. Intravenous pyelography and abdominal aortography are indispensable for the surgeon.

Intravenous Pyelography. Ideally it should be quite normal. A minor abnormality of one kidney, such as malformation of the ureteropelvic junction, will not preclude the use of that kidney, but a serious abnormality or any bilateral changes, even minor, makes the donor unacceptable. Intravenous pyelography will also reveal any ureteral duplication. This is not in itself an obstacle to transplantation but will add technical difficulties during the transplantation procedure.

Aortography. Aortography (by the Seldinger technique with selective opacifications) reveals the arrangement of the renal arteries on each side (duplication, length of the arterial trunk, early branching). This information is essential because of the technical complications if multiple arterial anastomoses are needed. Aortography also gives information about the renal parenchyma (homogeneity of the nephrogram, thickness of the renal cortex, regularity of its limits) whose integrity must be confirmed before the operation.

Choice of Side. The choice of side depends in part on the results of the preceding examinations. The arrangement of the renal arteries is paramount, but the state of the pelvis and ureter is also important.

All things being equal, the left kidney is preferred because of the greater length of renal vein on the left side which makes venous suture easier in the recipient; the left kidney will be turned over when placed in the recipient's right iliac fossa and so the vein will lie behind the artery—the best position for the venous anastomosis. If the donor is a young woman, Hume[10] prefers to take the right kidney because of the greater risk of urologic complications on that side if she should subsequently become pregnant.

Again, other factors being equal, a kidney with a single artery is preferred to one with two arteries.

Where function is not equal on the two sides, or where one kidney presents an abnormality such as renal artery stenosis or malformation of the ureteropelvic junction, which might cause trouble at a later date, the paramount interests of the donor require that the poorer or abnormal kidney be taken, even if this means a more difficult transplantation (Fig. I.1). Where both kidneys present even minor abnormalities, future risks make the donor unacceptable.

Operative Techniques. The donor nephrectomy and the preparation of the transplant bed in the recipient are carried out simultaneously by two surgical teams in adjoining operating rooms. The work of the two teams is synchronized so that the kidney is removed at the moment the recipient team is ready for it. The donor operation is begun first because it takes longer than the preparation of the transplant bed in the recipient. However, if bilateral nephrectomy is to be performed in the recipient, the two operations should begin at about the same time. Some surgeons, such as Gil-Vernet,[8] prefer to do both nephrectomy and transplantation themselves. This provides advance knowledge of the arrangement of the renal vessels and facilitates implantation of the kidney in the recipient. Although ischemia time is lengthened, it does not adversely affect the function of the grafted kidney or the final outcome of the transplantation.

Removal of a Left Kidney. The *incision* must be large for good exposure of the kidney and its pedicle. The level of the incision depends on the corpulence of the donor, on the position of the kidney and on the level at which the renal artery arises. A flank incision with resection of the 12th rib[32, 39] or an incision in the 11th intercostal space is generally adequate. This has been the usual approach in our series.

Thoracoabdominal incisions[32] and resection of the 11th rib[33, 34] give

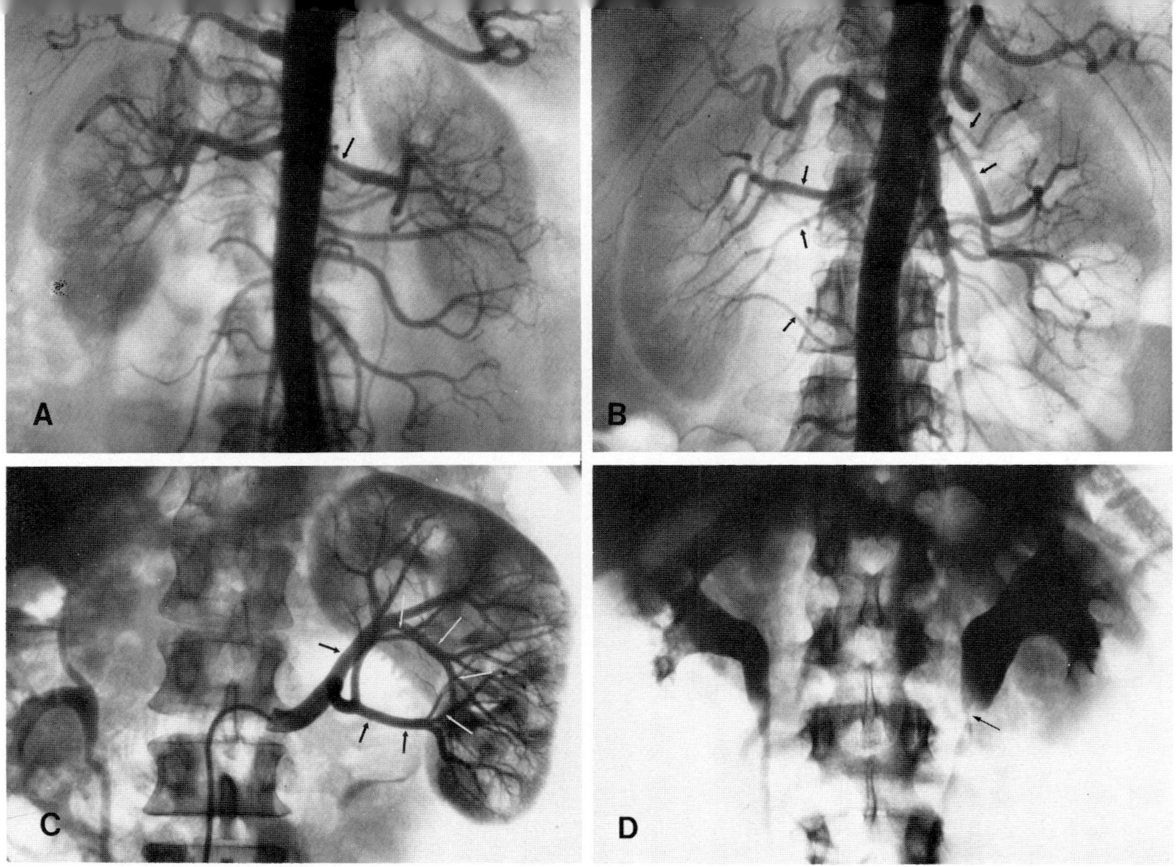

Fig. I.1. Choice of kidney in a living donor. *A*, on the left, atheroma of the renal artery (arrow); on the right, a normal kidney with no arterial anomaly. The left kidney was taken. *B*, on the right, three renal arteries (*arrows*); on the left, two renal arteries (*arrow*) arising from a very short common trunk. The left kidney was taken. *C*, parapelvic cyst in the left kidney (*arrows*), right kidney normal. The left kidney was taken. D, on the left, malformation of the ureteropelvic junction (*arrow*), right kidney normal. The left kidney was taken.

excellent exposure, but they are more traumatic and rarely necessary unless the kidney is very high or very big.

The pleura should be preserved intact, but if it is opened accidentally the pleural cavity must be drained.

The *preliminary stage* of the removal begins with exposure of the kidney after opening the renal fascia. The perirenal fat is separated from the kidney capsule, and the small vessels which traverse the capsule are coagulated. The anterior surface of the kidney should be freed first, then the upper pole, to permit easier downward displacement. The ureter is dissected with great care to preserve the ureteric vessels, especially the very fragile veins. Dissection continues up toward the renal pelvis, freeing the lower pole of the kidney, until the renal vein is exposed. The vein lies anteriorly and is approached from in front, then followed medially as far as the origin of the superior mesenteric artery. The main tributaries, the suprarenal vein above and the gonadal vein below, are tied and divided close to the renal vein; it is not uncommon to find a renal azygolumbar arch on the posterior aspect of the vein. If present, this is also tied and divided. It is rare to find two renal veins; they nearly always unite close to the origin of the superior mesenteric artery. The posterior aspect of the kidney is then freed and the kidney is turned forward to facilitate dissection of the renal artery, which is followed to its origin from the aorta; there is rarely any branch other than a small suprarenal artery which must be tied and cut. The nerves and lymphatics of the kidney are coagulated and divided during this dissection. It is important to avoid traction on the kidney or renal artery to avoid causing spasm and renal ischemia; infiltration of procaine around the artery[1, 10] helps to prevent spasm and facilitates dissection.

At this stage the kidney is attached only by its artery, vein and ureter.

The *actual removal* is performed when the recipient team is ready.

The ureter is tied and divided low down, below the pelvic brim, for subsequent ureterovesical anastomosis. Ten centimeters are sufficient for ureteroureteral anastomosis.

The artery is then clamped at its origin and divided; multiple renal arteries are tied and divided separately. The kidney can now be lifted out further to facilitate clamping of the vein. There is no need to clamp the artery on the renal side because there is little danger of air embolism; trauma to the artery by the clamp is thus avoided.

Finally the vein is clamped with a De Bakey clamp and divided medially as far as possible to provide the maximum length for subsequent anastomosis.

The kidney is now passed to the perfusion team.

The stumps of the renal vessels are secured by simple ligature or by suture. The wound may be closed with suction drainage or without drainage if hemostasis is perfect.

Removal of a Right Kidney. The exposure may be through a flank incision without rib resection; this incision is usually sufficient because of the lower position of the right kidney. The technique is similar to that described for the left side.

We have, however, often used the midline transperitoneal approach, which gives more direct access to the origin of the renal vessels from the aorta and vena cava. The operation is carried out in a slightly different manner.

The *preliminary stage* is dissection of the renal vessels before mobilizing the kidney.

The inferior vena cava is isolated and raised in a sling. The renal vein, the most anterior structure in the pedicle, is freed to its junction with the vena cava. Unlike the left renal vein, the right renal vein is very short and receives no major tributary; the presence of two renal veins is more common than on the left, and may pose special problems.

The artery lies posteriorly. Dissection begins at the origin of the artery medially to the vena cava; the vessel is found in the angle between the left renal vein and the vena cava. Dissection proceeds laterally, the retrocaval segment of the artery being displayed by using the sling to retract the vena cava alternately to the right and left.

The ureter is dissected as on the left side.

Finally, the kidney is freed from its bed but should not be lifted out of the wound for fear of kinking the vessels, especially the artery.

The *actual removal* is similar to that on the left side. However, to give the greatest possible length of vein, a lateral clamp is placed on the inferior vena cava and a patch of vena cava is excised with the renal vein. The vena cava is then closed by suture. Venous anomalies are more common on the right but present no serious difficulty. If double renal veins enter the vena cava close together, the patch of vena cava can include the orifice of both veins; if their junctions with the vena cava are too far apart, they are divided separately; if one of the veins is less than 5 mm caliber it may be tied without any ill effect because of the anastomoses in the intrahilar venous network.

Removal of Cadaver Kidneys

Cadaver kidneys are seldom taken from subjects who die unexpectedly of cardiac arrest without previous respiratory assistance. These circumstances are not propitious for obtaining good quality kidneys; ischemic damage to the kidney is quickly irreversible and does not allow sufficient time to organize the operation. Maintaining the circulation by external cardiac massage or by mechanical ventricular assistance[3, 37] in the interval from death to removal of the kidney is not satisfactory. Perfusing the kidneys in situ through a catheter in the aorta by the femoral route[7] with cold solutions requires complex perfusion devices.

Cadaver kidneys are usually taken from subjects who die from irreversible brain damage. Survival of the donor is artificially prolonged by mechanical ventilation and maintenance of blood volume. The kidneys can thus be removed in the most favorable conditions because renal ischemia is avoided by these resuscitative measures. Preliminary aortography is rarely possible and the surgeon therefore has no warning of possible anatomic abnormalities. Surgical exploration is the first stage of the donor operation and recipient surgery must not begin until it has been verified that the kidneys are suitable for transplantation.

The subject is placed supine with a support under the lowest ribs. Normally both kidneys are removed.

Some surgeons use a transverse incision two to three finger breadths above the umbilicus, joining the tips of the 11th ribs.[4] A vertical midline incision[5] from xiphoid to pubis is simpler, quicker and less hemorrhagic and, with a good rib retractor, gives comparable access.

The best access to the great vessels and both kidneys is by eviscerating the small bowel and the right and transverse colon outside the abdomen. The parietal peritoneum is incised around the cecum and the right colon and along the root of the small bowel mesentery up to the jejunoduodenal angle (Fig. I.2). The small bowel and the right and transverse colon are mobilized and retracted upward and to the left. The duodenum and the pancreas are completely freed from the retroperitoneum to the midline after dividing the ligament of Treitz and ligating and cutting the inferior mesenteric vein. The superior mesenteric artery is then ligated and divided. The intestine can now be removed from the peritoneal cavity; it is protected with moist packs and placed under self-retaining retractors.

The aorta and the inferior vena cava are dissected free below and above the renal pedicles and encircled with rubber vessel loops (Fig I.3). Both vessels are tied and divided 4 to 5 cm below the left renal vein, care being taken that a polar renal artery does not originate from the aorta below the ligature. Anterior traction on the two vessels allows freeing of the posterior walls up to their suprarenal segment. All lumbar vessels are tied and cut. The suprarenal vein, the gonadal vein and the azygolumbar arch are divided close to the left renal vein.

Division and upward retraction of the inferior vena cava provide perfect exposure of the retrocaval segment of the right renal artery, whereas mobilization of the cava and left renal vein allows good access to the left renal artery. The arrangement of the renal arteries may now be determined, but the dissection of the arteries is undertaken at a later stage.

Both kidneys are now freed from their bed but should not be lifted out of the wound for fear of kinking the vessels, especially the arteries. Both ureters are dissected and cut at the level of the pelvic brim.

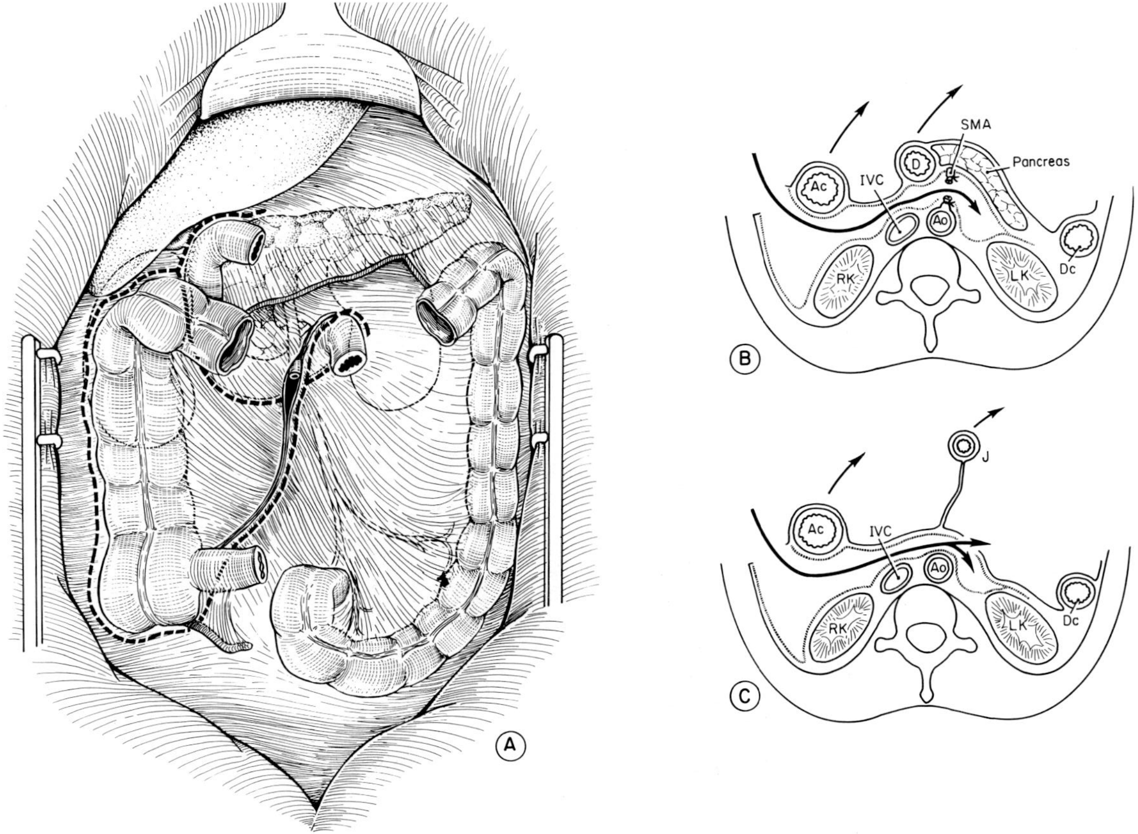

Fig. I.2. Exposure of the kidneys in the cadaver donor. *A*, incisions in the posterior parietal peritoneum. *B*, mobilization to the left of ascending colon, duodenum and pancreas. *C*, mobilization to the left of ascending colon, root of the small bowel mesentery and small bowel. *RK*, right kidney; *LK*, left kidney; *Ao*, aorta; *IVC*, inferior vena cava; *SMA*, superior mesenteric artery; *Ac*, ascending colon; *D*, duodenum; *J*, jejunum; *Dc*, descending colon.

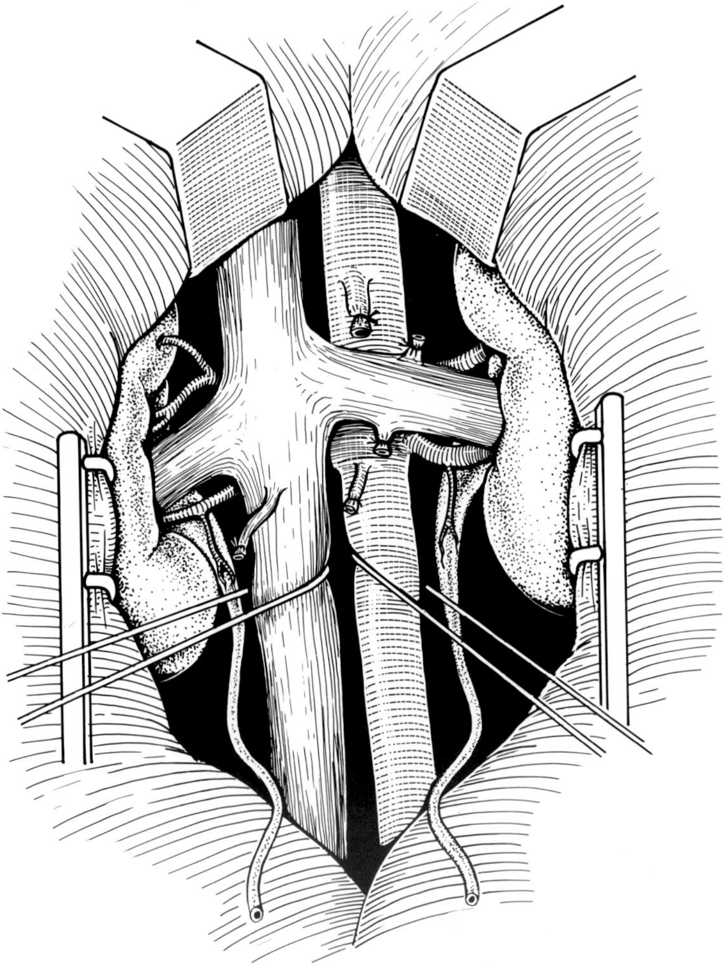

Fig. I.3. Exposure of both kidneys and great vessels in the cadaver donor. The aorta and inferior vena cava have been isolated and tapes placed around them.

At the end of this preliminary stage two situations may be observed:

1. Favorable circumstances: blood pressure of the donor is stable, urinary output is adequate and arrangement of the renal vessels is simple with one artery on each side. Dissection of the kidneys and of their vessels is completed. Each kidney is then removed successively and perfused exactly as in removal from a living donor.

2. Unfavorable circumstances: blood pressure of the donor falls, cardiac arrythmias or circulatory arrest appear, urinary output ceases, arrangement of the vessels is complex with multiple arteries. Protection of the kidney against ischemic damage must be undertaken immediately by in

situ cooling of the kidneys before their removal.[2] Canulas are introduced in the aorta and in the vena cava (Fig. I.4). Both vessels are cross clamped above the renal pedicles and Collins' solution at 4°C is perfused through the aortic canula, the venous blood flowing through the caval canula. In a few minutes both kidneys are cooled. The aorta and the vena cava are divided between two clamps above the renal pedicles. Perfusion is continued while the dissection is completed. Both kidneys with their ureters and an adequate length of abdominal aorta and vena cava are removed

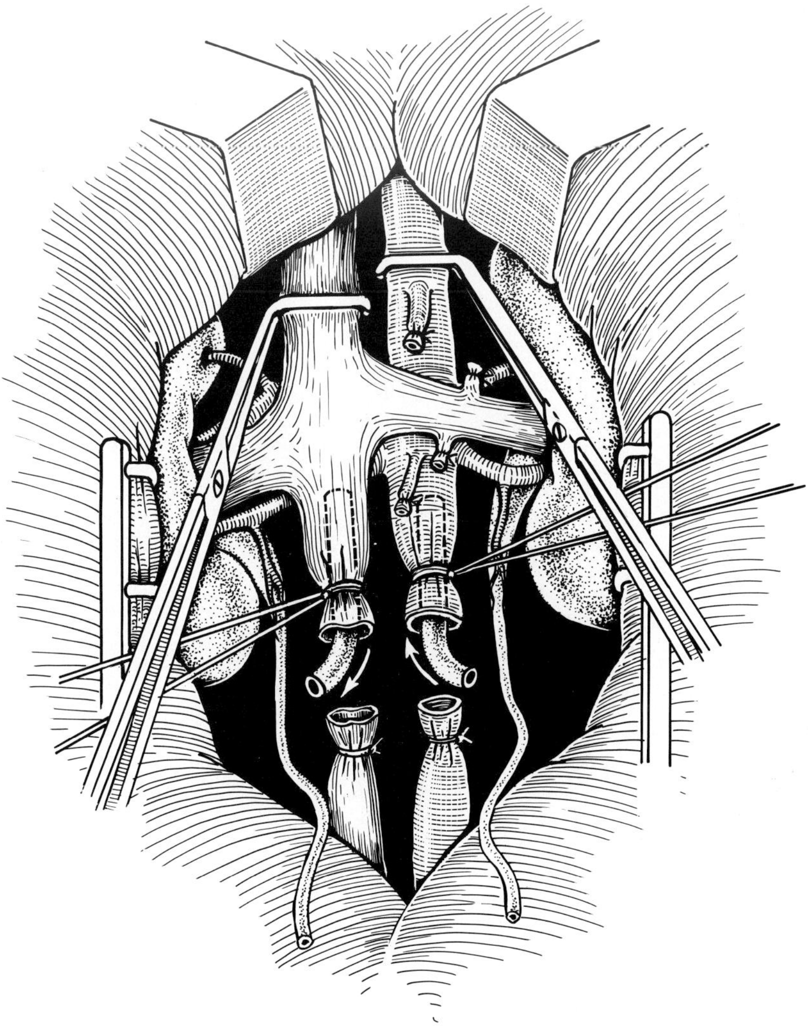

Fig. I.4. Disposition for in situ perfusion of both kidneys in the cadaver donor. See text for details.

en bloc and quickly immersed in iced Collins' solution. The two kidneys are then separated by cutting the aorta and the vena cava vertically along their sagittal axes (Fig. I.5). Large aortic and caval patches including the openings of the renal vessels are thus preserved. In situ cooling must begin to protect against ischemic damage as soon as the donor's condition becomes precarious. This is necessary because transplanting a nonviable organ creates a life-threatening risk for the recipient.[17]

After the kidneys have been removed, the respirator may be switched off and other resuscitative measures stopped.

Anatomic Anomalies

Anatomic anomalies may modify surgical tactics and techniques.

Vascular anomalies are important, both in removing the kidney and in subsequent transplantation. They present few problems if both kidneys are removed en bloc with the adjacent great vessels and prepared ex vivo as described above.

In other cases, if multiple renal arteries arise close together, a patch of aorta including the arterial openings is resected; if the arterial origins are

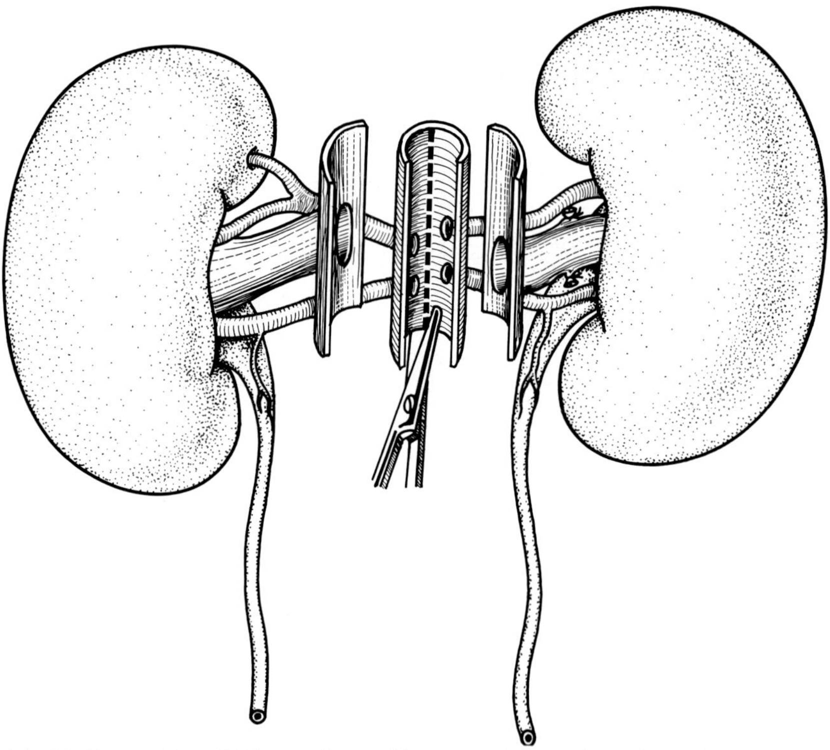

Fig. I.5. Preparation of kidneys after en bloc removal from the cadaver donor.

at a distance from one another, they are taken separately. An independent polar artery supplying a significant volume of kidney will have to be anastomosed; it is thus essential to take the full length of this artery including a patch of aorta to facilitate its reimplantation. Ligature should be considered only for a very small polar artery supplying a minute segment of the kidney. If there are two veins they can be taken separately or together with a patch of vena cava according to their arrangement.

Ureteral anomalies can cause difficulties. If the ureter is completely duplex, the two ureters are taken separately, but when the two ureters join lower down, it may be possible to take the terminal common ureter.

Whatever anomaly is encountered, it must be reported in detail to the transplantation team, whose responsibility it is to make the final decision about proceeding with transplantation.

Other Sources of Kidneys

In rare cases, kidneys which have normal parenchyma but must be removed from otherwise normal patients because of some vascular abnormality, an ectopic position or an incurable ureteral fistula can be used as transplants.

Rare too, are kidneys taken from anencephalic newborns. En bloc removal and transplantation should be made in such cases, as in transplanting pediatric kidneys to adult recipients.[14, 16, 31]

Heterotransplantation from primates[30, 33, 36] has now been abandoned.

Transplantation

The technical problems of renal transplantation are those of any major surgery. But, because of the defective healing and impaired defense mechanisms in patients treated with immunodepressive drugs, the following points are particularly important:

1. Rigorous hemostasis is essential to prevent hematoma, which could become infected or compress the graft. This hemostasis may be difficult because of the bleeding tendency in so many of these patients.

2. Strict asepsis must be observed in every stage of the operation. The large bladder opening necessary for ureterovesical reimplantation is a possible source of contamination and should not be considered unless the bladder is sterile. In the early postoperative period, aseptic precautions must be continued so as to avoid any external contamination, especially from drains, tubes or catheters.

Choice of Site for Implanting Kidney

Transplantation in the normal anatomic position in the left loin, as recommended by Küss,[16] is very attractive in theory. The kidney is placed in its normal position with restoration of a normal urinary tract; the surgery is simplified by using a single incision to remove the recipient kidney and transplant the donor kidney into the same bed and by avoiding any dissection of the iliac vessels. Transplantation in situ has always been done on the left side. After removing the patient's own left kidney, the transplant kidney is placed in the renal bed; the transplant artery is anastomosed end-to-end, either to the stump of the recipient's renal artery if this is big enough or to the splenic artery (a splenectomy has been frequently associated); the donor vein is anastomosed to the stump of the recipient's renal vein; the donor ureter is anastomosed to the recipient ureter (Fig. I.6).

This technique has rarely been used (three cases in Küss' series and one case in our own series), and should be considered only exceptionally.

It has the disadvantage that postoperative supervision of the graft is more difficult. Swelling of the kidney is almost impossible to detect and biopsy is not easily performed. In the event of surgical complications, reoperation is more difficult.

Transplantation in the right iliac fossa[4, 16, 18, 23] is the procedure of choice. It is true that the superficial placement of the kidney might make it vulnerable to trauma, but the operative technique is simple and straightforward and postoperative observation of the graft is easy. There is no difficulty in palpating the kidney and assessing changes in volume, nor is there any technical problem in biopsy. If there is any local complication, further surgery presents no undue difficulty.

According to the level of vascular reimplantation, two positions are possible for the transplant kidney:

1. Pelvic transplantation: the kidney is placed in a low position. The donor renal artery is anastomosed end-to-end to the recipient's internal iliac artery, which is divided close to its termination. The renal vein of the transplant is anastomosed end-to-side to the external or common iliac vein of the recipient. This is the routine transplantation technique that has been used in the majority of cases throughout the world, including our own series. The only problems that may arise are that the recipient's internal iliac artery is not suitable for anastomosis with multiple arteries with an aortic patch or may be too small or severely calcified or atheromatous.

2. Low lumbar transplantation: the kidney is placed in a higher position. The donor artery is anastomosed to the side of the common iliac artery or to the terminal part of the aorta, and the vein is anastomosed to the upper end of the common iliac vein or to the beginning of the inferior vena cava. This technique was originally advocated by Starzl et al[35] for grafting adult kidneys into children. Many surgeons[16, 27] adopted this technique; it is Gil-Vernet's[8] technique of choice in all cases. Indeed, this

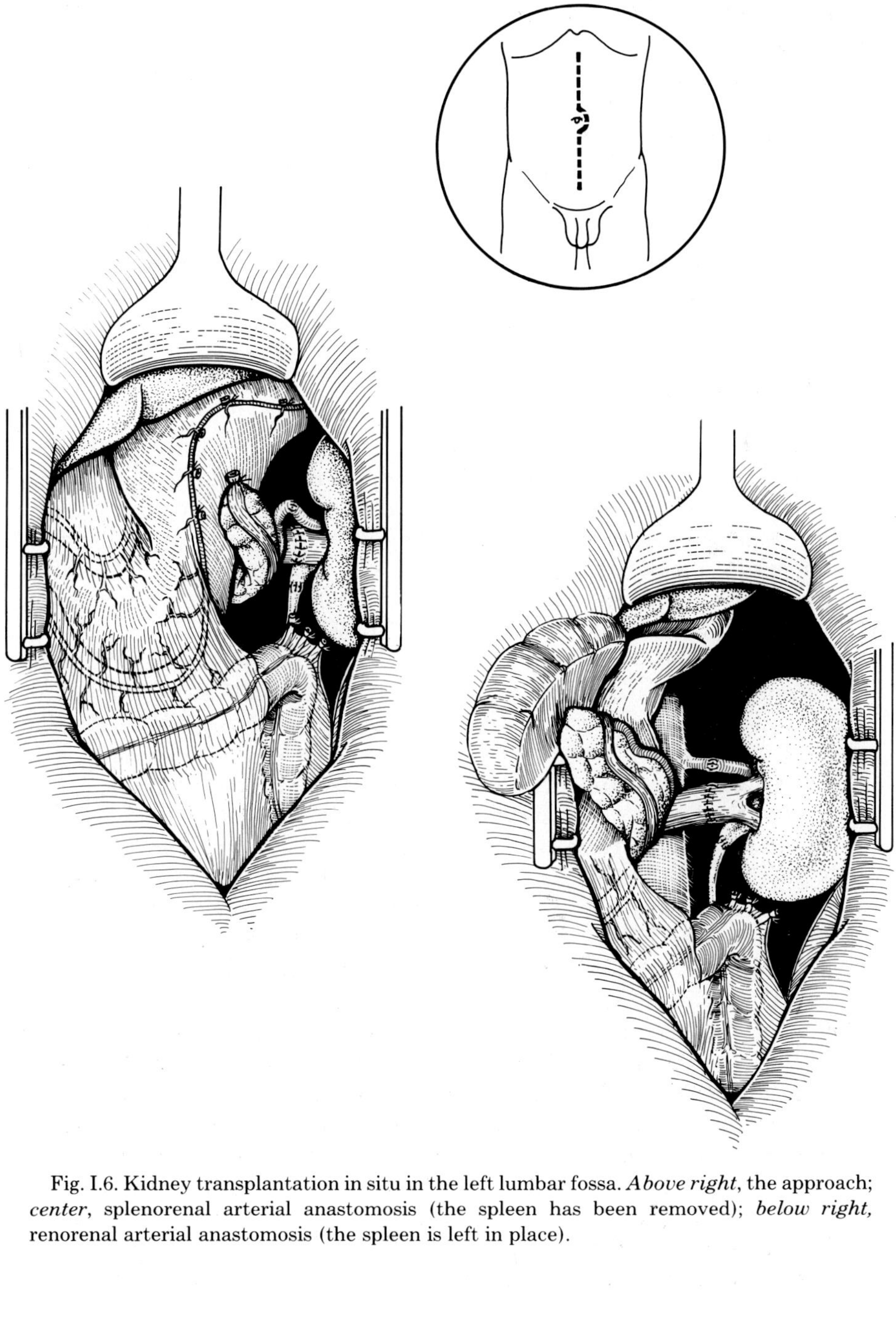

Fig. I.6. Kidney transplantation in situ in the left lumbar fossa. *Above right*, the approach; *center*, splenorenal arterial anastomosis (the spleen has been removed); *below right*, renorenal arterial anastomosis (the spleen is left in place).

is the only possible technique when the recipient's internal iliac artery is unsuitable for anastomosis or when an aortic patch of the donor has to be anastomosed.

In both techniques, the ureter may be joined to the recipient ureter or reimplanted directly into the bladder.

Transplantation in the left iliac fossa is technically identical but may be more difficult because the common iliac vein is situated more deeply in the pelvis, so that the venous anastomosis may be more difficult to perform.

For this reason, we have used the left iliac fossa only for second transplantations after failure of a graft on the right side. Many groups[10, 11] routinely use the left iliac fossa when transplanting a right kidney.

Technique of Transplantation

The technique of the actual transplantation can be divided into three stages: preparation of the kidney bed and the recipient vessels, revascularization of the kidney and restoration of urinary tract continuity.

We shall describe the common routine with implantation in the right iliac fossa on the pelvic vessels.

The preliminary stage includes preparation of the arterial anastomosis, the venous anastomosis and the urinary anastomosis (Fig. I.7).

1. *The incision* is made obliquely in the right iliac fossa. At the lower end it comes near the pubic spine. The incision is continued upward to the costal margin if the donor's right kidney is to be removed at the same session; otherwise the incision stops short of the costal margin. The approach is extraperitoneal and strict hemostasis is essential.

2. *The iliac vessels are displayed* without any difficulty. The ureter is reflected with the peritoneum. As a first stage the arteries are displayed and isolated with slings. The external and the common iliac artery are mobilized, then the internal iliac artery is freed throughout its length, with ligature of a few small posterior branches. If the internal iliac artery is short, its major branches are tied, but if the main trunk of the artery is sufficiently long, the distal ligature may be applied to the trunk itself. The artery is clamped near its origin and divided at the deepest possible level close to the ligature. The arterial stem is retracted medially and the venous axis, which is bound down to the wall of the pelvis, is freed from below upward until sufficient space has been gained for applying vascular clamps and performing venous anastomosis. The veins are surrounded by a dense lymphatic network and the lymph vessels must be tied with nonabsorbable ligatures during the dissection to prevent lymphorrhea or subsequent lymphocele formation.

If the ureter is to be implanted into the bladder, the bladder is exposed

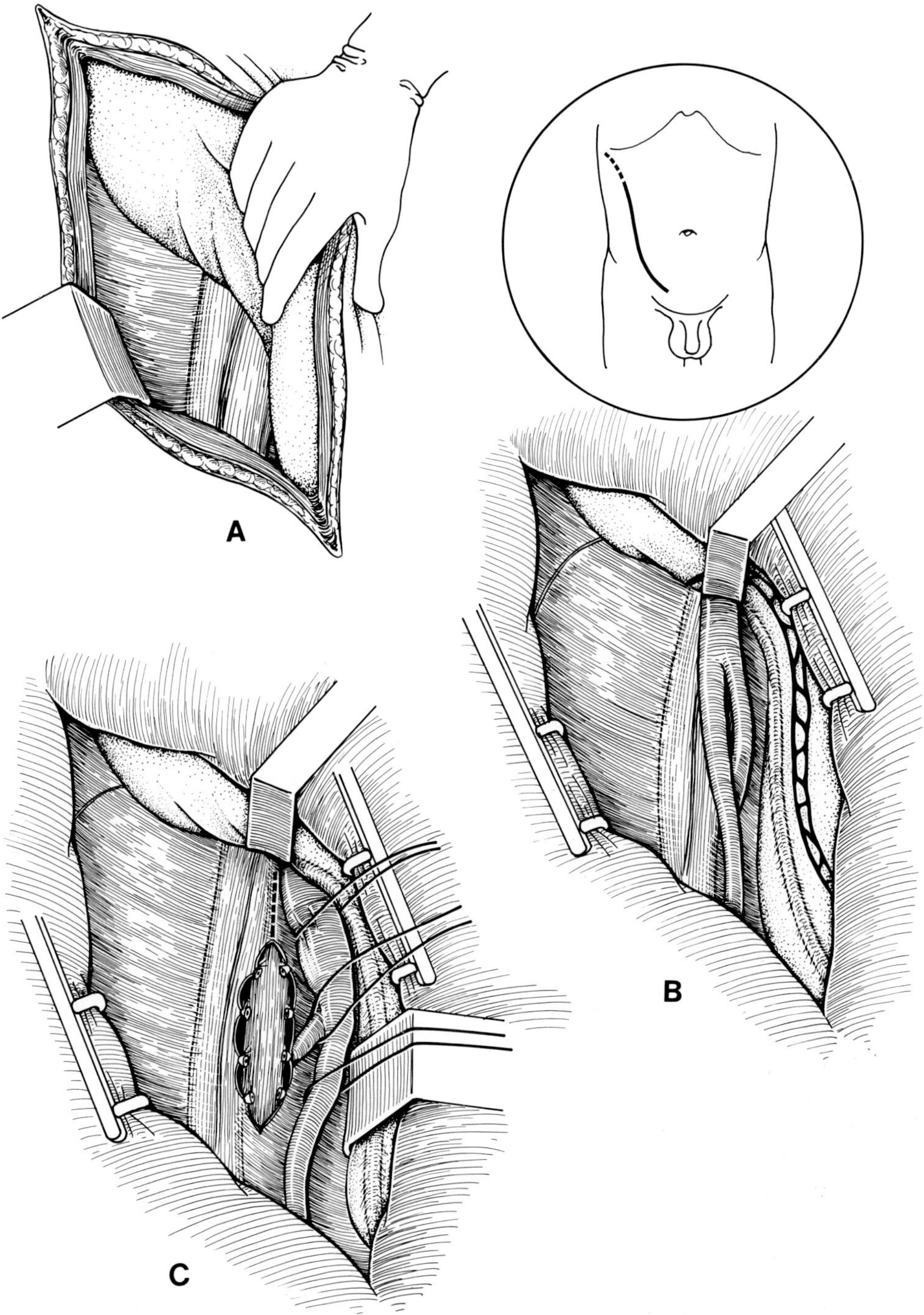

Fig. I.7. Kidney transplantation in the right iliac fossa. Preliminary stage. *Inset*: the incision (the dotted line indicates the extension required if the right kidney is to be removed during the same session). *A*, reflection of the peritoneum. *B*, exposure of the arteries. *C*, dissection of the arteries completed, beginning the vein dissection.

at this stage by downward extension of the pelvic dissection. If ureteroureteral anastomosis is envisaged, the ureter is identified along the peritoneum, but its dissection takes place later.

At this stage everything is ready for the vascular anastomoses. After division of the internal iliac artery, its lumen is washed out with heparinized saline and its adventitia is excised. The venous axis is then clamped, using a Satinsky type clamp to give broad lateral occlusion.

The actual transplantation now begins. The perfused and cooled kidney is brought to the operating table. When the transplant is a cadaver kidney coming from another center, its vessels must be carefully inspected and prepared for the sutures before it is placed in the iliac fossa. Reimplanting a polar artery in the main trunk, if necessary, is thus easier.

The kidney is placed where it lies most naturally. Usually the left kidney is turned over so that its anterior surface faces posteriorly. A right kidney may be placed with normal orientation, but as the renal vein is short and lies anteriorly, the arrangement of vascular anastomoses is more convenient if the kidney is turned head downwards, its anterior face lying posteriorly. We have frequently placed the kidney in this orientation and have never observed complications attributable to it. The hairpin course of the ureter does not affect the function of the transplant.

1. *The venous anastomosis*, being the deepest, is done first (Fig. I.8). Its site is chosen where the renal vein most easily meets the iliac vein. At this site an ellipse of iliac vein, equal in length to the diameter of the renal vein, is removed. A suture is placed at each angle of the anastomosis and tied. The posterior layer of the anastomosis is done from within the venous lumen and the anterior layer from the outside. The suture is a continuous over and over stitch with 5/0 monofilament nylon. The reimplanted renal vein usually passes lateral to the arterial axis. When the venous anastomosis is complete a bulldog clamp is placed on the renal vein and the clamp is removed from the iliac vein in order to restore venous return from the leg.

2. *The arterial anastomosis* comes next (Fig. I.9). The end of the renal artery is gently dilated and cut obliquely to enlarge the anastomosis. Depending on its site of origin and its length, the internal iliac artery is passed either in front or behind the external iliac artery. With the latter arrangement, the iliac axis rotates more easily and the beginning of the internal iliac artery is less liable to kink if this artery is short; on the other hand, if stenosis of the renal artery subsequently develops, reoperation will be extremely difficult. This is the reason we prefer to place the hypogastric artery anterior to the external iliac. When the internal iliac artery is short, angulation at its origin is frequent with that arrangement; in that case, we prefer anastomosis of the renal artery to the common iliac. The end of the recipient artery is often larger than the end of the donor renal artery, but it may be possible to adapt the internal

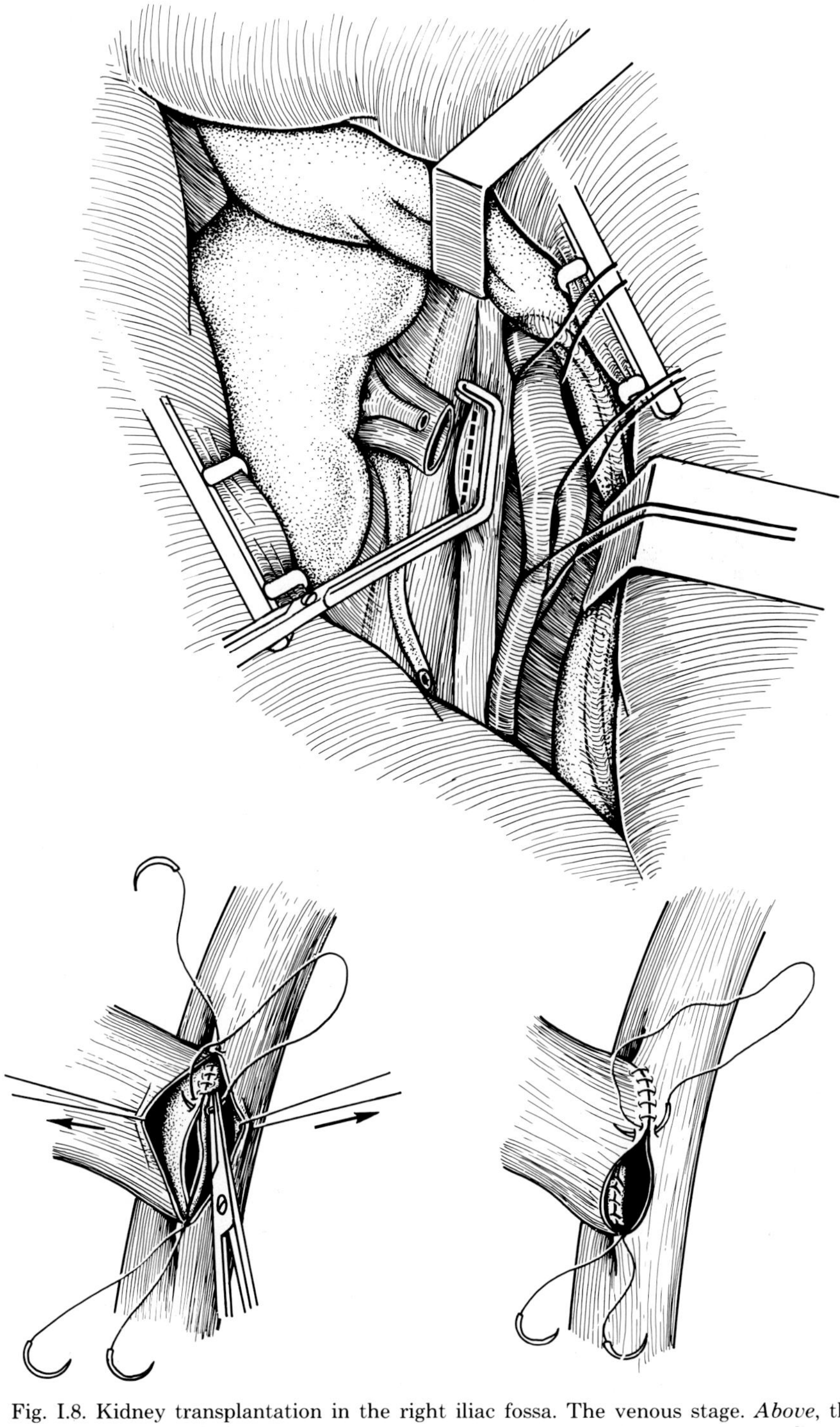

Fig. I.8. Kidney transplantation in the right iliac fossa. The venous stage. *Above*, the kidney in place, outline of the incision in the vein; *below*, details of the venous anastomosis.

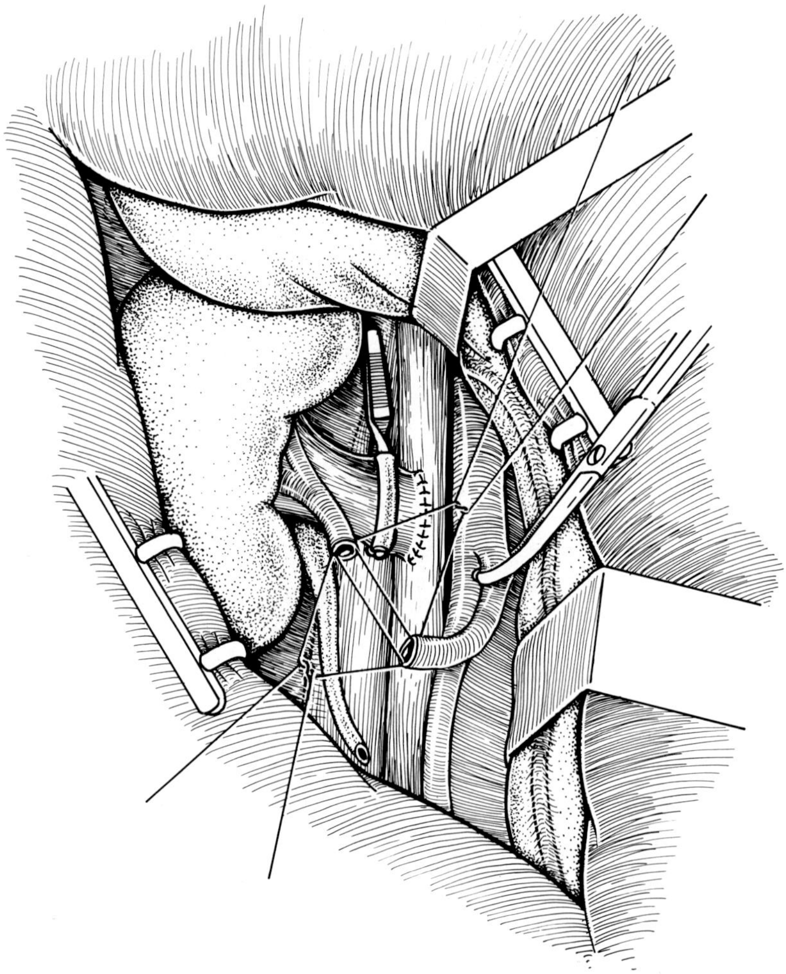

Fig. I.9. Kidney transplantation in the right iliac fossa. End-to-end anastomosis of the renal artery to the internal iliac artery. Preferably, the internal iliac artery may be passed in front of the external iliac axis.

iliac artery directly to the obliquely cut renal artery; otherwise the latter is cut more obliquely so that the vessels will run in a smooth curve, allowing a natural flow. The anastomosis is done with a simple continuous stitch, or a separate continuous stitch may be used for each half. This is preferable to the Blalock stitch, which can cause stenosis. In children, interrupted sutures are preferable. Before completing the anastomosis, the vessels are flushed with heparinized saline to remove any air, avoiding even minimal gas embolism of the kidney.

The clamps can now be removed. The venous clamp is removed first to avoid undue tension in the kidney; the internal iliac clamp is then removed while a clamp is left on the renal artery so that the anastomosis is put under tension and any last traces of air are evacuated. Finally the clamp is removed from the renal artery. The kidney rapidly resumes its normal color and becomes tense. After some seconds the ureter begins to contract and within minutes urine appears.

Circumferential capsulotomy of the kidney, formerly advocated[10, 12] when the kidney was very tense, has been abandoned for fear of bleeding and rupture of the transplanted kidney.

3. *Re-establishment of the urinary tract* completes the procedure. There are many possible methods.

Implantation of the ureter into the bladder or ureteroneocystostomy is preferred by many.

The advantage of this technique is that it can be used in every type of case and indeed it must be used if the recipient ureters are absent (congenital absence or surgical removal) or unsuitable because of hypoplasia or dilatation due to reflux, stenosis or infection.

This technique is, however, relatively complicated and technically difficult. The wide opening in the bladder can be dangerous. There is risk of contaminating the operation site if the bladder is not perfectly sterile, so this technique must not be used if there is any question as to bladder infection. Furthermore, there may be inadequate vascularization at the distal extremity of the donor ureter with a risk of ureteral necrosis and subsequent fistula or stricture. The ureter may also become stenosed in its intramural course. Even if the anastomosis is satisfactory, there may be problems with the healing of the cystotomy wound. We have seen this breakdown on several occasions.

An antireflux technique (Fig. I.10) such as that described by Paquin[26] or by Leadbetter et al[21] and Politano and Leadbetter[28] is recommended. The bladder is opened near the fundus and the lateral wall of the bladder is pierced by a hemostat some 4 or 5 cm above and lateral to the right ureteral orifice. From this point, a submucosal tunnel 3 to 4 cm long is made with a curved clamp in the direction of the normal ureteral orifice. The mucosa is incised at the lower end of the tunnel. The ureter is then pulled through the hole in the bladder wall and along the submucosal tunnel. Any excess length is removed. The end of the ureter is slit along one side to enlarge the new orifice. The cut end of the ureter is then anastomosed to the vesical mucosa with interrupted catgut sutures. The anastomosis is reinforced by fixing the ureter with a few interrupted sutures where it enters the bladder wall. The ureteroneocystostomy is facilitated by using a trocar to bore the submucosal tunnel and passing the ureter through its sheath.[29] Care must be taken to avoid torsion of the ureter. It is also important to be sure that the opening in the bladder

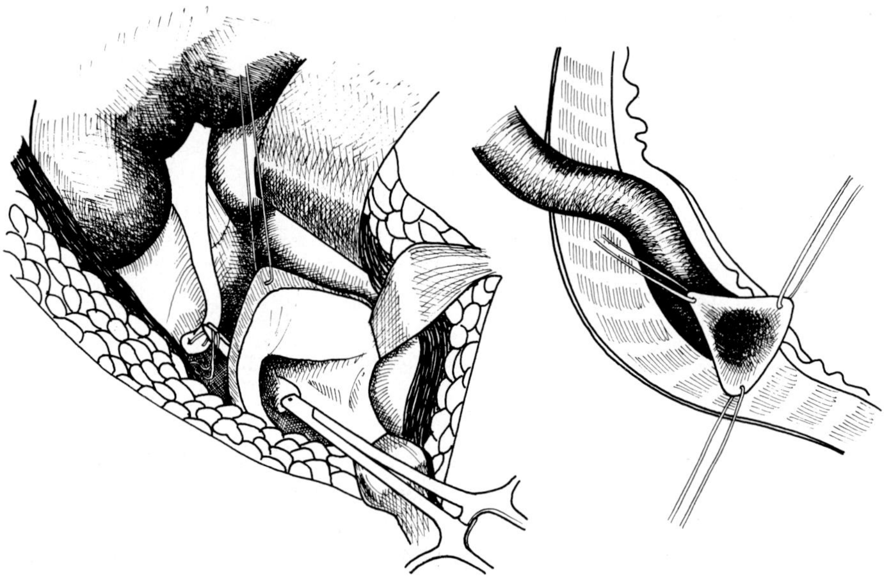

Fig. I.10. Kidney transplantation in the right iliac fossa. Antireflux implantation of the ureter into the bladder; on the *right*, a detail of the intramural course of the ureter.

wall and the submucous tunnel are wide enough to avoid constricting the lower end of the ureter. The bladder is then closed in two or three layers[33, 34] and a catheter is left in place.

The extravesical ureteroneocystostomy according to Gregoir[9] and favored by Konnak et al[15] does not require a large bladder opening and avoids cystotomy dehiscence. The muscle layer is incised 3 to 4 cm to make the ureteral tunnel. The mucosa is opened 1 cm at the lower end of the incision. The ureter is then anastomosed from outside the bladder to the mucosal opening. The muscle layer is then repaired by interrupted catgut sutures over the terminal ureter (Fig. I.11).

Contrary to the practice in most centers, we prefer to use the recipient ureter. In our view, ureterovesical anastomosis should be used only when the patient's own ureter is not suitable for anastomosis.

End-to-end ureteroureteral anastomosis is preferable, in our view, whenever the recipient ureter can be used (Fig. I.12).

This method of re-establishing continuity of the urinary tract combines maximum simplicity with minimum risk of infection. Using the patient's own ureter protects the transplanted kidney from the risk of reflux and does not necessarily require removal of the homolateral kidney. We have abandoned concomitant nephrectomy since January 1979: whenever the recipient has no appreciable diuresis and is not severely hypertensive, his own kidney is left in place with its ureter simply ligated; its function

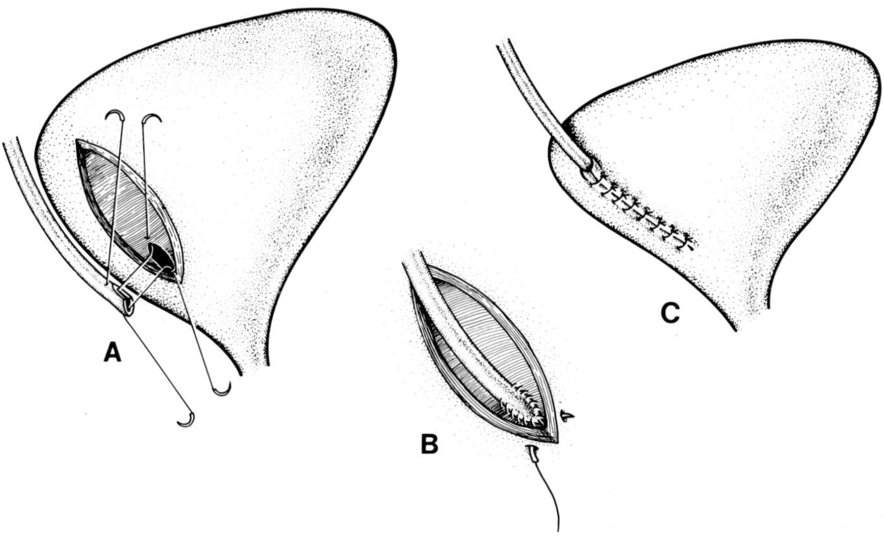

Fig. I.11. Kidney transplantation in the right iliac fossa. Extravesical ureteroneocystostomy. *A* and *B*, ureter to mucosa anastomosis; *C*, operation completed.

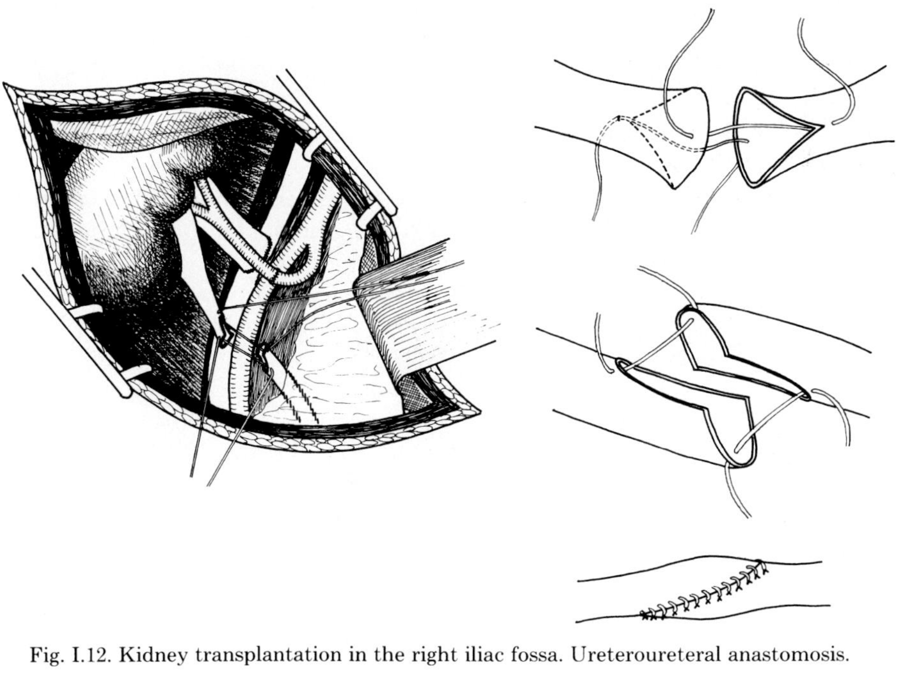

Fig. I.12. Kidney transplantation in the right iliac fossa. Ureteroureteral anastomosis.

ceases quickly if the transplant functions well. Small vesicoureteral reflux is not an absolute contraindication to ureteroureteral anastomosis provided that the recipient ureter has good peristalsis and is not greatly widened.

This type of anastomosis is not always possible. When the patient's own ureter is severely hypoplastic, atonic, fibrotic or grossly widened, a ureterovesical anastomosis is certainly preferable.

The particular complication of ureteroureteral anastomosis is fistula. The risk of fistula is greatly lessened, although not avoided completely, by an atraumatic and minutely accurate technique (using unabsorbable sutures and working with a magnifying loupe). Stricture and lithiasis are not common.

Although it requires great care, this technique presents no difficulties. The donor ureter is divided at a distance below the pelviureteral junction and slit longitudinally to give wider anastomosis; bleeding from the cut end is evidence of adequate blood supply. The recipient ureter is prepared in a similar fashion; in order to avoid interfering with the blood supply of this ureter, only the shortest possible segment should be freed, the mesoureter must be left intact and the ureter should not be separated from the peritoneum; coagulation near the ureter must be avoided, and hemostasis of the ureteral vessels is made with fine stitches. Stay sutures are placed at each end of the anastomosis which is then completed with a single layer of fine interrupted sutures. For years, we have been using very fine unabsorbable sutures; using 6/0 monofilament nylon instead of catgut has drastically reduced the incidence of fistulas, which does not exceed 3% at the present time.

Pyeloureteral anastomosis[38] is but a variant of the preceding technique (Fig. I.13).

When the donor renal pelvis is largely extrarenal, when there is a great discrepancy in caliber between donor and recipient ureters (the latter being wider) or when the transplanted kidney presents congenital pyeloureteral junction obstruction, this type of anastomosis is an elegant solution to the problem of re-establishing continuity of the urinary tract.

The renal pelvis is freed of fibrofatty tissue and divided immediately above the pyeloureteral junction. If necessary, the opening may be enlarged by a vertical slit. The recipient ureter is prepared as in the preceding technique and the anastomosis is performed with very fine unabsorbable sutures.

This type of anastomosis has the same advantages as end-to-end ureteroureteral anstomosis; in theory it should be even better both because the renal pelvis always had a good blood supply so there is no danger of necrosis, and because the wall of the renal pelvis is thicker and easier to suture. This type of anastomosis seems very safe, but its

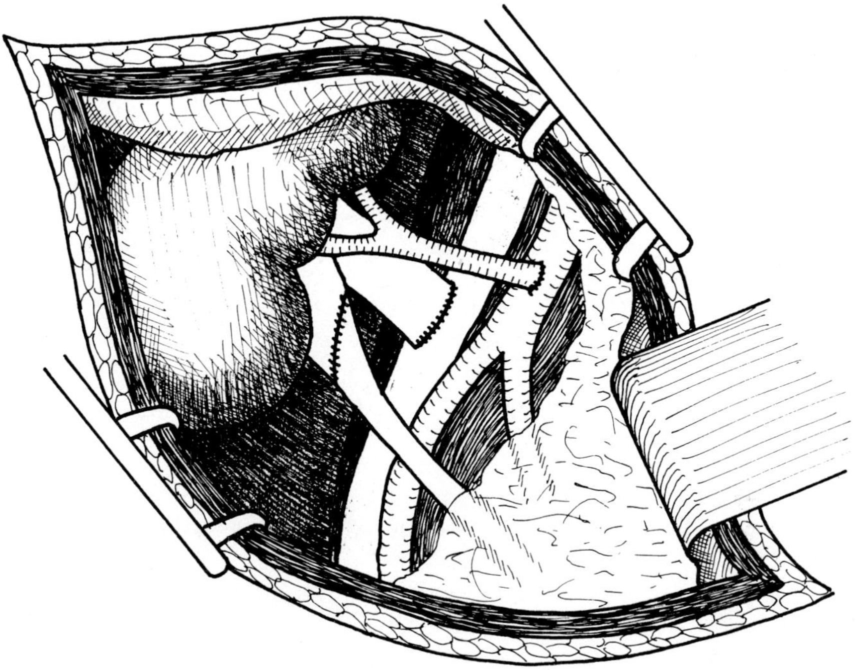

Fig. I.13. Low lumbar kidney transplantation. Vessels anastomosed to the common iliac vessels, pyeloureteral urinary anastomosis.

disadvantage is that any breakdown is serious because the upper part of the pelvis may retract within the renal hilum and the resulting fistula is very difficult to close.

Pelvis-to-pelvis anastomosis is advocated by Gil-Vernet.[8] The pelvis of the recipient's right kidney is used to re-establish continuity of the urinary tract.

Technically, this procedure requires great care. The donor renal pelvis is prepared as above. It must be opened widely, and stay sutures are placed at the upper and lower ends on each side. The recipient's right kidney has to be removed, the renal pelvis being divided at the hilum of the kidney close to the parenchyma. The pelvis and ureter are then freed from above downward and the pelvis is passed down to meet the transplant kidney. Great care must be taken to preserve the blood supply which is derived from the gonadal vessels that run alongside the ureter in the lower lumbar region. When the recipient renal pelvis has been brought down in this fashion, the ureter runs in a hairpin course, with the apex of the bend held up by the ureteral vascular pedicle. Anastomosis is performed with a continuous over and over fine catgut suture; a binocular loupe should be used for the anastomosis.

The advantages of this technique are the large anastomosis with no risk of stricture and the thickness of the walls of the renal pelvis which allows easier and better suture. The only blood supply to the recipient renal pelvis is by retrograde flow from the gonadal vessels but it is adequate if care is taken to preserve the ureteral pedicle. The hairpin course of the ureter causes no functional problem. Gil-Vernet, who developed this technique, had excellent results and found no complications (neither fistula nor stricture), but other groups did not adopt it as a routine procedure.

Whatever procedure is chosen to restore urinary tract continuity, it is essential to ensure perfect vascularization on both sides of the anastomosis.[24, 25]

The choice of technique depends primarily on individual circumstances; for example, ureterovesical anastomosis may be necessary because of disease in the recipient ureter. Thereafter, it depends on the preference and experience of the surgeon. In any given case, the best technique is that with which the surgeon is most familiar and with which he is most expert.

4. *The question of urinary drainage* has given rise to much controversy.

In all cases we use an indwelling catheter to drain the bladder. In the postoperative period it permits measurement of urinary output from the transplant kidney to guide rehydration of the patient. If the bladder has not been opened, the catheter may be removed as early as 24 hours after surgery. If the bladder has been opened (for ureterovesical implantation), it is essential to keep a catheter in place until the cystotomy has healed, that is, for at least 10 days. Before removing the catheter, healing of the bladder should be verified by retrograde cystography.

On the contrary, a ureteral catheter, passed up to the pelvis of the transplant kidney, is seldom necessary. Reasons for use of a ureteral catheter are that transplant urine output can be quantitated, that postoperative obstruction from edema of the anastomosis is prevented and that urinary obstruction can easily be ruled out if anuria occurs postoperatively. On the other hand, placing a ureteral catheter lengthens the surgical procedure because of the need for cystoscopy and makes subsequent nursing care more complex; the catheter is also a major source of external contamination. For all these reasons we have now abandoned the use of a ureteral catheter and have found no difference in the postoperative course or in the incidence of postoperative complications. However, if a urinary fistula requires reoperation, the use of a ureteral catheter is necessary. The catheter may be brought out through the urethra or across the bladder and through the abdominal wall in the suprapubic region.

Because of the incidence of fistula after ureteral anastomosis, even with an indwelling ureteral catheter, the Boston group has recommended nephrostomy drainage with a fine silastic tube.[23] Despite the absence of published complications, we believe that this type of drainage is dangerous. Transplanted kidneys are sometimes very fragile, and nephrostomy entails the risk of bleeding or even rupture of the parenchyma. From this point of view, pyelostomy would be preferable to nephrostomy.

Whatever their advantages, all tubes are a possible source of infection and should be removed as soon as possible.

The total operating time is approximately 3 hours. Attempts to fix the kidney are pointless. The abdominal wound is closed with one or two suction drains.

Special Surgical Techniques

Special surgical techniques are frequently necessary. They may be indicated at each stage of the operation.

Special Techniques for Arterial Anastomosis. *End-to-side anastomosis of the renal artery* to the common iliac artery is a valid alternative to the renohypogastric anastomosis. The technique is easier and quicker because less dissection of the iliac arteries is necessary. The recipient arteriotomy is usually made by excising an ellipse of common iliac artery while the renal artery is cut obliquely to enlarge the anastomosis. As far as possible the renal artery must take off from the common iliac obliquely in the direction of the arterial flow; acute angled implantations with retrograde flow must be avoided in order not to create disturbed hemodynamics which possibly lead to late stenosis.[22]

Some surgeons[8, 16] consider this type of implantation the procedure of choice and use it routinely. Circumstances sometimes make it necessary:

1. When the vessels are short, either on donor or recipient sides: renohypogastric anastomosis often creates an acute angulation at the origin of the internal iliac artery and implantation on the common iliac artery seems preferable;
2. In children who are receiving an adult kidney: the renal artery must be implanted on the common iliac artery or even on the terminal aorta because the volume of the kidney makes the low iliac position impossible and because the caliber of pelvic vessels may be too small compared to the renal artery;
3. When the kidney has two renal arteries taken with a patch of aorta: implanting the patch on the common iliac artery is the procedure of choice; and
4. The recipient vessels are not always in good condition: even in young patients, the internal iliac artery may have one or more atheromatous plaques. Rather than have recourse to endarterectomy, we prefer in such

cases to perform end-to-side anastomosis to the common iliac artery; atheroma may involve this artery also and on several occasions we have had to remove calcified plaques from the posterior wall before making the arterial anastomosis above the endarterectomized zone.

The presence of two renal arteries is the most common problem. Various methods of solving this problem have been suggested (Fig. I.14).

If a patch of aorta has been taken, including the origin of both renal arteries, this patch is placed on the side of the common iliac artery.

If the two arteries have been taken separately, various techniques may be used. The two renal arteries, especially when their caliber is approximately the same, may be double barreled to form a single trunk that is then anastomosed end-to-end to the internal iliac artery. Each renal artery may be anastomosed to a branch of the internal iliac artery; or one renal artery may be anastomosed end-to-end to the internal artery, the other being implanted end-to-side into the common iliac artery, into the external iliac artery or into the trunk of the internal iliac artery. When one of the two arteries is a small independent polar artery, it may be implanted end-to-side into the main trunk or anastomosed end-to-end to the inferior epigastric artery.[6] We have also used the latter as a free autograft to repair a polar artery cut close to the parenchyma. Use of the inferior epigastric artery must be kept in mind as a valuable means of revascularizing small polar arteries.

The donor artery may also present many problems. The renal artery is often slender, friable or of small caliber and contrasts with the internal iliac artery which is wide and thick. Technique must then be meticulous: careful dilatation of the renal artery, oblique cutting of its end and the use of small shallow bites can overcome these difficulties. If the renal artery is short and branches early, great care must be taken to arrange the anastomosis so that none of the branches is twisted or kinked.

Special Techniques for Venous Anastomosis. *A short renal vein*, especially with a right donor kidney, makes venous anastomosis difficult. Division of the internal iliac vein may release the iliac venous axis so that the latter can be brought up to meet the renal vein. It is probably simpler to place the kidney higher and implant the vein directly into the vena cava or common iliac vein.

The presence of two renal veins is more common on the right side. If a patch of vena cava including the orifice of both veins has been taken, this patch is implanted on the side of the common iliac vein or the inferior vena cava. Two separate veins, of approximately the same caliber, may be double barreled to form a single trunk that is then anastomosed in the usual manner; if the two veins are too far from one another, separate implantations are advisable. If the caliber of one of the two veins is less than 5 mm, this vein is simply tied.

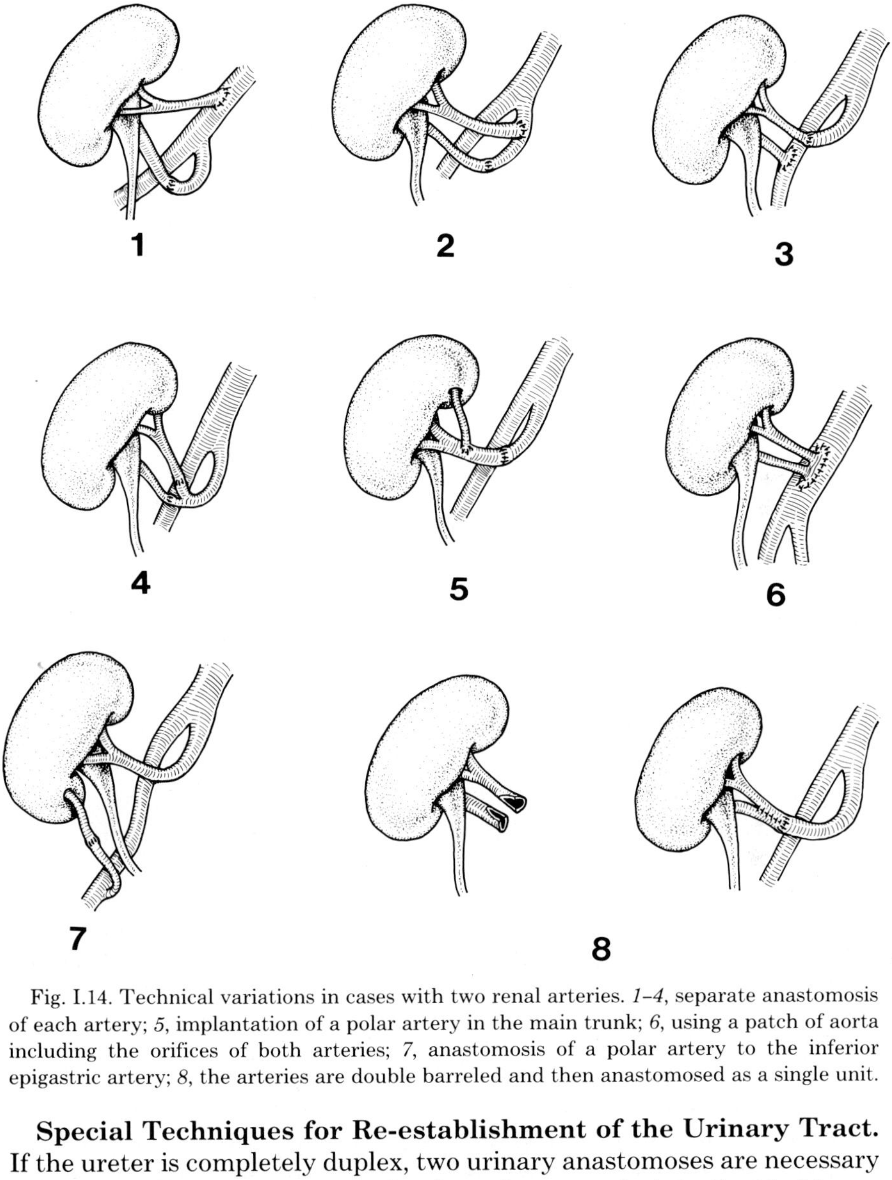

Fig. I.14. Technical variations in cases with two renal arteries. *1–4*, separate anastomosis of each artery; *5*, implantation of a polar artery in the main trunk; *6*, using a patch of aorta including the orifices of both arteries; *7*, anastomosis of a polar artery to the inferior epigastric artery; *8*, the arteries are double barreled and then anastomosed as a single unit.

Special Techniques for Re-establishment of the Urinary Tract. If the ureter is completely duplex, two urinary anastomoses are necessary (Fig. I.15). The ureters may be implanted separately into the bladder or they may be anastomosed to the recipient ureter, either in a double barreled manner or separately, one end-to-end and the other end-to-side. Another possibility is to anastomose the smallest of the two ureters to the other end-to-side, the latter being dealt with as described for the standard procedure.

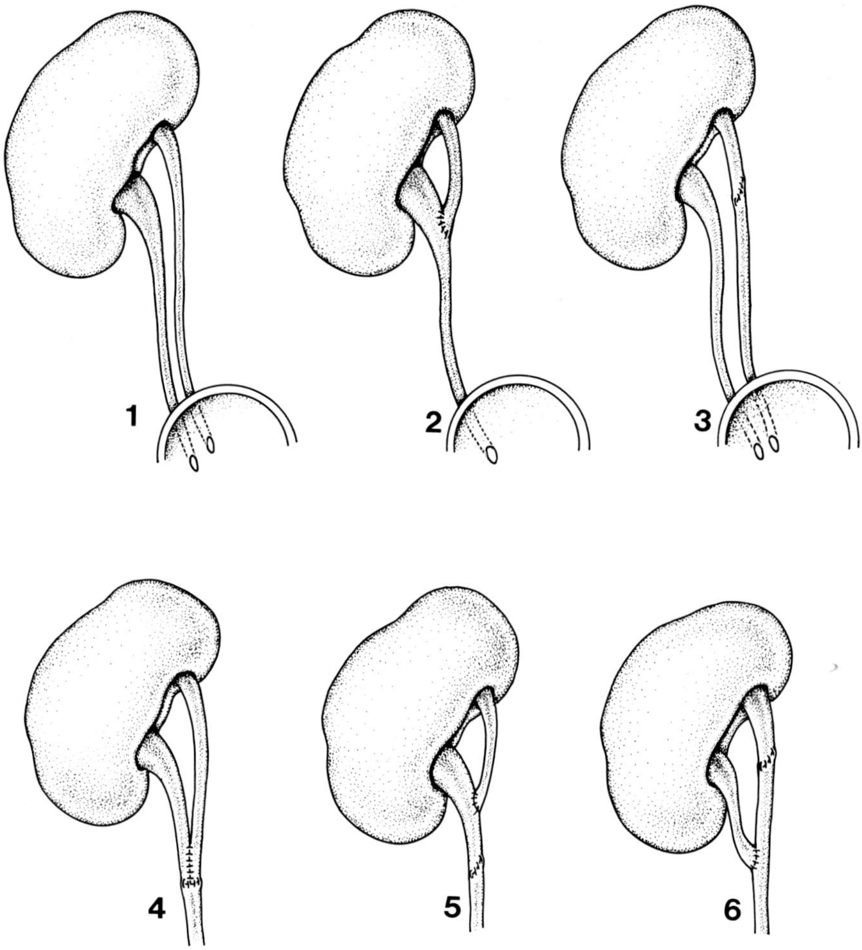

Fig. I.15. Technical variations in cases with two ureters. *1*, two separate implantations into the bladder; *2*, anastomosis of one ureter into the other and the latter into the bladder; *3*, anastomosis of one ureter to the recipient ureter and implantation of the other into the bladder; *4–6*, anastomoses with the recipient ureter only.

Patients with disease or malformation of the lower urinary tract were until recently excluded from transplantation, but in some cases urinary diversion by an isolated intestinal loop is a possible solution. Kelly et al[13] have reported good results in six patients in whom the donor renal pelvis was anastomosed to an isolated intestinal loop. The loop should be prepared at least 6 weeks before transplantation, and this procedure may be combined with recipient nephrectomy; the distal end of the isolated loop is brought out in the right iliac fossa half way between the umbilicus and the anterior superior iliac spine. The subsequent transplantation is performed transperitoneally; the pelvis of the donor kidney is divided and anastomosed to an opening in the side of the isolated loop, or the donor ureter may be implanted into the loop.

Other Special Techniques. Transplantation en bloc of two kidneys into one recipient is also unusual (Fig. I.16). In this case, the donor kidneys are removed with a segment of abdominal aorta and vena cava, and these vessels are joined end-to-side to the common iliac vessels or to the aorta and vena cava of the recipient. The two ureters are handled as just described for duplex ureters. This technique was formerly used for heterotransplantation from primates to man. Presently, its only indication is the transplantation of pediatric kidneys into an adult.[16]

Surgical Tactics

The standard technique described above concerns renal transplantation performed alone without any other associated surgical procedure.

Often, however, the transplantation is associated with nephrectomy on the same side so that the recipient ureter can be used for the urinary anastomosis. The nephrectomy is then performed first through the same

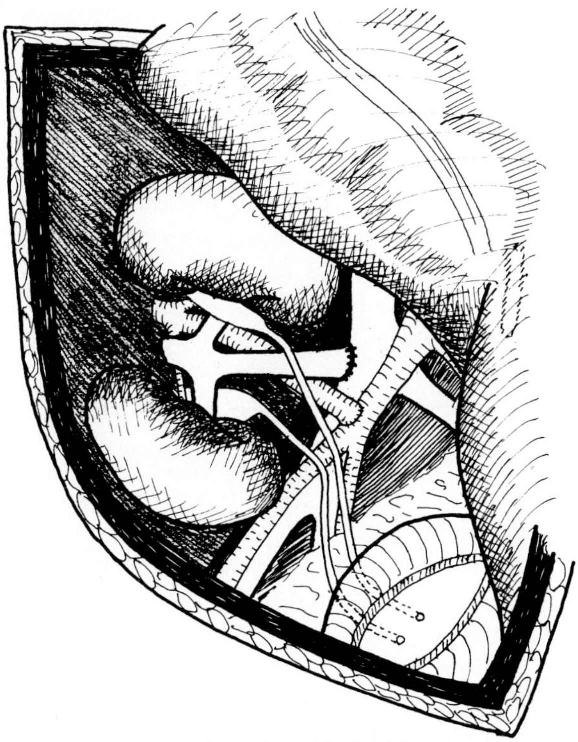

Fig. I.16. Transplantation of both kidneys en bloc.

approach, but the incision is made a little longer. In fact, with increasing experience, nephrectomy does not appear always necessary when ureteroureteral anastomosis is planned. When patients have no appreciable diuresis and are not severely hypertensive we have for several years been leaving the kidney in place with its ureter ligated without adverse effect. Possible subsequent embolization of that kidney could be considered if any unexpected complication occurs.

The transplantation may be associated with bilateral nephrectomy. The indications for this procedure are severe hypertension not responsive to hemodialysis and medical treatment and urinary infection of renal origin. Usually, bilateral nephrectomy is performed at another session. If it is to be carried out in the same session as the transplantation, the surgical approach is by a midline incision from the xiphoid to the pubis. The kidneys are removed through this anterior approach after reflecting the flexures of the colon; the transplantation is then performed in the usual way after reflecting the cecum and right colon (or the sigmoid and left colon if the left iliac fossa has been chosen). In these circumstances, if the local anatomic conditions were favorable, transplantation in situ might be considered. Splenectomy is also easy by this approach, but removal of the spleen has been abandoned by our group, as by many others. The postoperative course of major procedures when splenectomy is associated with binephrectomy and transplantation is often difficult: for that reason, they have been abandoned by our group.

During recent years our personal tendency has been toward simplification of the surgical procedure in order to ensure a smooth postoperative course. Thus, we have progressively abandoned concomitant bilateral nephrectomy and more recently homolateral nephrectomy; during surgery we try to reduce dissection of the vessels and exposure of the retroperitoneal and pelvic spaces to a minimum. Renal transplantation thus now appears a safe procedure.

Technique for Reoperation on the Artery of Transplant

Stenosis of the artery supplying a grafted kidney is a well recognized complication of renal transplantation.[19] At the present time, surgical correction of this complication has been necessary in about 6% of our patients. Difficulties presented by the reoperation depend on the interval between the initial procedure and the reoperation: within 6 months, difficulties are great because of local postoperative changes; after 6 months, difficulties are less. In all cases, they can be overcome by a well planned technique.

The surgical approach is a median transperitoneal incision. This route is always preferable because it gives direct access to the iliac vessels and avoids passing through the previous operative site, where freeing of adhesions is always painful. The small bowel is retracted superiorly and protected with moist packs. The parietal posterior peritoneum is incised along the iliac vessels and the course of the ureter of the transplant is identified.

The dissection of the vessels (Fig. I.17) is the most difficult stage of the operation. The common iliac artery is dissected first at a distance from the origin of the transplant artery. The external iliac is then similarly

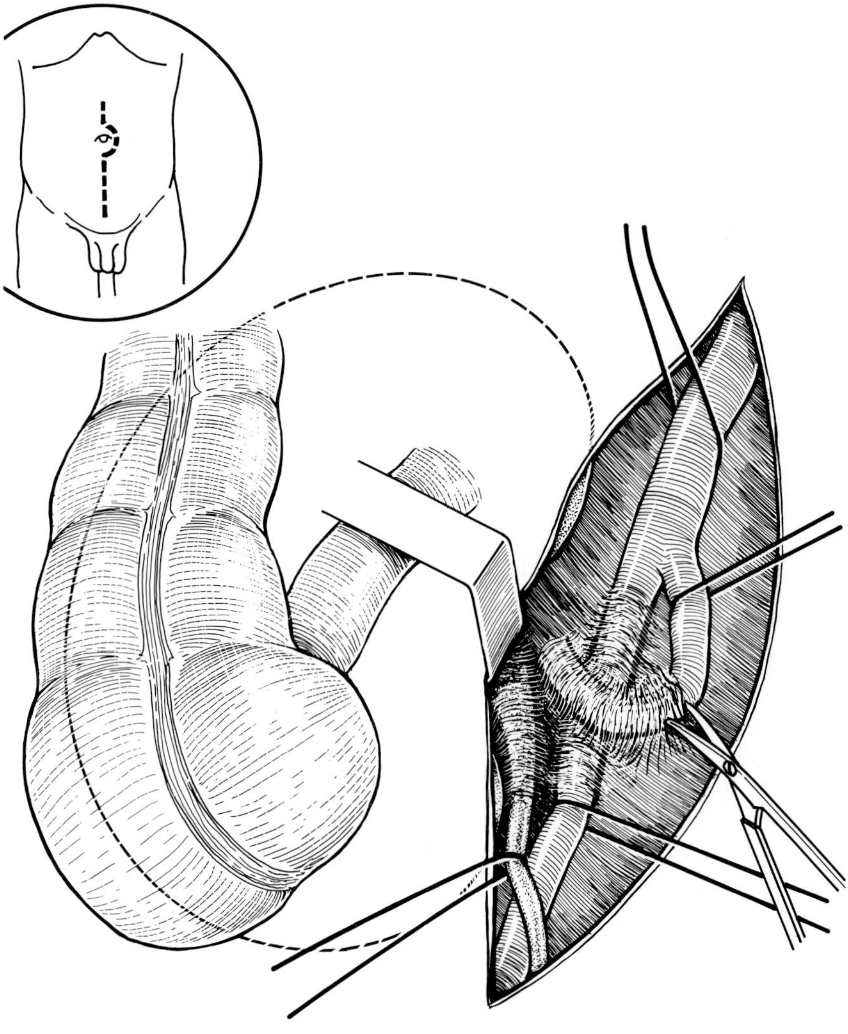

Fig. I.17. Reoperation for stenosis of the artery of the transplant. *Above right*, the incision; *below*, dissection of the artery.

freed at a distance from the previous operative site. Control of these two vessels avoids massive hemorrhage if an incidental arterial injury occurs during a difficult dissection.

From these two sites, the dissection progresses towards the origin of the renal artery. When this vessel has been implanted on the common iliac artery, the internal iliac artery must be controlled before dissecting the renal artery; when it has been anastomosed end-to-end to the internal iliac artery, the latter vessel is dissected downward from its origin.

The arteries are encased in scar tissue and, using sharp dissection, a groove is dissected between the artery and the fibrous tissue, first on one side of the artery and then on the other. Traction to the artery and countertraction to the surrounding fibrous tissue help to identify the dissection plane. Circumferential dissection of the artery can be accomplished by alternating sides. Difficulties are maximum in the area of the previous suture; sometimes, the segments adjacent to it must first be mobilized before completing the dissection of the suture area where the artery must be carved out of the fibrous tissue. Dissection of the renal artery becomes easier near the hilum of the kidney. Finally, all vessels must be completely mobilized up to the branches of the renal artery.

Vascular repair can now be undertaken. Several techniques are advisable: resection of the stenotic area with end-to-end anastomosis, implantation of the renal artery into the common iliac artery, either directly or with interposition of a venous or arterial autograft or transposition of the iliac arteries,[20] selected according to operative findings.

Protection of the kidney against ischemia by the clamping of its artery is mandatory since, under normothermic conditions, circulatory arrest for more than 50 min causes irreversible alterations of the kidney. Whenever the vascular repair is presumed to be difficult and the clamping to be of long duration, special protective measures are necessary. General hypothermia (by a cold bath) is, in our view, the safest procedure because the kidney is cooled homogeneously; when body temperature reaches 30°C, the time for which circulatory arrest can be permitted is about twice that possible at 37°C. Local hypothermia by application of ice around the kidney is far less satisfactory because it predominantly affects the renal cortex; it should not be used as the only protective measure. Perfusion of a cold solution through the artery is a valuable and simpler alternative to general hypothermia; its efficiency is greater when the perfusion is associated with application of ice around the kidney and with clamping of the renal vein (to avoid reflux of warm blood). In our experience, general hypothermia and cold fluid perfusion gave equally satisfying results and were very safe procedures in complex cases.

REFERENCES

1. Alexandre, G. P., Morelle, J., Kestens, P. J., Pillen, E., Michielsen, P., and Van Ypersele, C. Les méthodes de prélèvement du rein en transplantation rénale et leur influence sur

le fonctionnement immédiat du greffon. In *Proceedings of the European Dialysis and Transplant Association, 1965,* vol. 2, p. 232. Excerpta Medica, Amsterdam, 1966.
2. Barra, J. A., Kermarrec, J. Y., Cledes, J., and Doutriaux, M. Prélèvement des reins chez l'homme sous réfrigération "in situ" par canulation aorto-cave. Technique, premiers résultats. J. Chir., *116:*357, 1979.
3. Baue, A. E., Tragus, E. T., Anstadt, G. L., and Blakemore, W. S. Circulating support by mechanical cardiac massage in potential donors for organ transplantation. In *Organ Perfusion and Preservation*, edited by J. C. Norman, p. 425. Appleton-Century-Crofts, New York, 1968.
4. Calne, R. Y. In *Renal Transplantation*, Arnold, London, 1963.
5. Denis, L. J. L'homotransplantation rénale humaine. Acta Urol. Belg. *34:*101, 1966.
6. Dubernard, J. M., Pin, J., Gignoux, N., and Perrin, J. Utilisation de l'artére épigastrique en transplantation. J. Urol. Néphrol., *82:*469, 1976.
7. Garcia-Rinaldi, R., Lefrak, E. A., Defore, W. W., Feldman, L., Noom, G. P., Jachimcyk, J. A., and De Bakey, M. E. In situ preservation of cadaver kidneys for transplantation: Laboratory observations and clinical application. Ann. Surg., *182:*576, 1975.
8. Gil-Vernet, J. M. Le remplacement du rein: Technique chirurgicale. J. Urol. Néphrol., *75:*221, 1969.
9. Gregoir, W. Le reflux vésico-urétéral congénital. Acta Urol. Belg., *30:*286, 1962.
10. Hume, D. M. Kidney transplantation. In *Human Transplantation*, p. 110. Grune and Stratton, New York and London, 1967.
11. Hume, D. M., Lee, H. M., Prout, G. R., Jr., Bower, J. D., Wolf, J. S., and Slapak, M. Renal homotransplantation in man: Studies in 63 cases. Monograph on the kidney. In *Proceedings of International Academy of Pathology.* Williams & Wilkins, Baltimore, 1965.
12. Hume, D. M., Magee, J. H., Kauffman, H. M., Jr. Rittenbury, M. S., and Prout, G. R., Jr. Renal homotransplantation in man in modified recipients. Ann. Surg., *158:*608, 1963.
13. Kelly, W. D., Merkel, F. K., and Markland, C. Ileal urinary diversion in conjunction with renal homotransplantation. Lancet, *i:*222, 1966.
14. Kinne, D. W., Spanos, P. K., McGrade, D. E., Shazo, M., Simmons, R. L., and Najarian, J. S. Double renal transplants from pediatric donors to adult recipients. Am. J. Surg., *127:*292, 1974.
15. Konnak, J. W., Herwig, K. R., Finkbeiner, A., Turcotte, J. G., and Freier, D. T. Extravesical ureteroneocystostomy in 170 renal transplant patients. J. Urol., *113:*299, 1975.
16. Küss, R., Camey, M., Poisson, J., and Chatelain, C. Aspects chirurgicaux de l'homotransplantation rénale chez l'homme. Mém. Acad. Chir., *92:*22, 1966.
17. Küss, R., and Poisson, J. A propos du prélèvement de reins de cadavre. Mém. Acad. Chir., *93:*859, 1967.
18. Küss, R., Poisson, J., Auvert, J., and Denis, M. Expérience française sur la transplantation rénale. In *XIV Kongress der Internationalen Gesellschaft für Urologie*, vol. 1, p. 181. Munich, 1967.
19. Lacombe, M. Arterial stenosis complicating renal allotransplantation in man. A study of 38 cases. Ann. Surg., *181:*283, 1975.
20. Lacombe, M. Correction of renal transplant artery stenosis by transposing iliac arteries. Urology, *XIII:*21, 1979.
21. Leadbetter, G. W., Jr., Monaco, A. P., and Russell, P. S. A technique for reconstruction of the urinary tract in renal transplantation. Surg. Gynecol. Obstet., *123:*839, 1966.
22. Morris, P. J., Yadav, R. V. S., Kincaid-Smith, P., Anderton, J., Hare, W. S. C., Johnson, N., Johnson, W., and Marshall, V. C. Renal artery stenosis in renal transplantation. Med J. Austr., *1:*1255, 1971.
23. Murray, J. E., Merrill, J. P., Dammin, G. J., Dealy, J. B., Alexandre, G. W., and Harrison, J. H. Kidney transplantation in modified recipients. Ann. Surg., *156:*337, 1962.

24. O'Conor, V. J., Jr. The role of the ureter in renal transplantation. II. A full length ureteral transplant. J. Urol., *86:*51, 1961.
25. O'Conor, V. J., Jr., and Dawson-Edwards, P. The role of the ureter in renal transplantation. I. Studies on the denervated ureter with particular reference to uretero-ureteral anastomosis J. Urol., *82:*566, 1959.
26. Paquin, A., Jr. Ureterovesical anastomosis. The description and evaluation of a technique. J. Urol., *82:*573, 1959.
27. Poisson, J. Le remplacement du rein. Transplantation rénale. J. Urol. Néphrol., *75:*5, 1969.
28. Politano, V. A., and Leadbetter, W. F. An operative technique for the correction of vesicoureteral reflux. J. Urol., *79:*932, 1958.
29. Rampal, M., Menguy, P., Melchior, G., and Giudicelli, R. Le Leadbetter facilité. J. Urol. Nephrol., *79:*942, 1973.
30. Reemtsma, K., McCracken, B. H., Schlegel, J. U., Pearl, M. A., Pearce, C. W., de Witt, C. W., Smith, P. E., Hewitt, R. L., Flinner, R. L., and Creech O., Jr. Renal heterotransplantation in man. Am. J. Surg., *160:*384, 1966.
31. Salvatierra, O., and Belzer, F. O. Pediatric cadaver kidneys. Their use in renal transplantation. Arch. Surg., *110:*181, 1975.
32. Shackman, R., Dempster, W. J., and Wrong O. M. Kidney homotransplantation in the human. Br. J. Urol., *35:*222, 1963.
33. Starzl, T. E. In *Experience in Renal Transplantation.* Saunders, Philadelphia, 1964.
34. Starzl, T. E. Marchioro, T. L., Dickinson, T. C., Rifkind, D., Stonington, O. G., and Waddell, W. R. Technique of renal homotransplantation. Experience with 42 cases. Arch. Surg., *89:*87, 1964.
35. Starzl, T. E., Marchioro, T. L., Morgan, W. W., and Waddell, W. R. A technique for use of adult renal homografts in children. Surg. Gynecol. Obstet., *119:*106, 1964.
36. Starzl, T. E., Marchioro, T. L., Peters, G. N., Kirkpatrick, C. H., Wilson, W. E. C., Porter, K. A., Rifkind, D., Ogden, D. A., Hitchcock, C. R., and Waddell, W. R. Renal heterotransplantation from baboon to man: Experience with six cases. Transplantation, *2:*752, 1964.
37. Veith, F. J., Attai, L., Panossian, A., Bogartz, L., Swain, B., Dougherty, J., Buchberg, A., and Gliedman, M. L. Perfusion techniques for lung, liver and kidney transplantation with immediate functional adequacy. In *Organ Perfusion and Preservation,* edited by J. C. Norman, p. 453. Appleton-Century-Crofts, New York, 1968.
38. Whelchel, J. D., Cosimi, A. B., Young, H. H. II, and Russell, P. S. Pyeloureterostomy reconstruction in human renal transplantation. Ann. Surg., *181:*61, 1975.
39. Woodruff, M. F. A., Robson, J. S., Ross, J. A., Nolan, B., and Lambie, A. T. Transplantation of a kidney from an identical twin. Lancet, *i:*1245, 1961.

SURGICAL TECHNIQUES IN ANIMALS

Kidney Homotransplantation in Dogs

The technique we have adopted[2] is derived from that of Calne.[1]

Preparation of Animals

Dogs of either sex may be used. After premedication with acepromazine (12.5 mg/kg, intramuscularly) various types of anesthesia are possible: Nembutal (initial dose of 15 mg/kg), pentobarbital sodium perfusion or gas anesthesia. The animals are always intubated.

Removal of Donor Kidney

The donor kidney may be removed via the lumbar approach or, better still, by a midline approach. On the left side the renal pedicle is longer, but there is a higher incidence of double arteries. The vessels and ureter are dissected. The dissection should not be carried close to the ureter so as to avoid damage to its accompanying vessels. The ureter is divided low in the pelvis. Then the artery and vein are clamped with bulldog clamps to avoid loss of blood from the kidney. Before clamping, we usually inject the artery with 5 mg of heparin diluted in 2 ml of isotonic saline, but this is not essential.

If the ischemia time is short (30 min or less) the kidney can be grafted immediately. If there is a longer ischemia time, it is better to cool the kidney. Simple surface cooling, by placing the organ in saline at 4° for 7 to 10 min, gives excellent protection against ischemic damage.

Vascular Anastomoses

The kidney may be implanted in the neck, in the abdomen, in the lumbar fossa or in the *iliac fossa*. The last is generally preferred and we shall confine our description to this technique.

The *renal artery* is generally anastomosed to the external iliac artery. Many techniques can be used. We generally use end-to-end anastomosis with an over and over stitch and sometimes an end-to-side anastomosis with an everting stitch. The suture material is 00000 silk. In dogs, it is possible to transplant a kidney into each iliac fossa, with a section of both external iliac arteries, without causing any ischemic problems in the hind limbs.

The *renal vein* is anastomosed end-to-side to the external iliac vein.

Anastomosis of Ureter

If the kidney is transplanted in the neck, the ureter is brought to the skin surface. This permits accurate collection of urine from the graft but runs the risk of ascending infection.

If the kidney is transplanted in the iliac fossa, either ureteroureteral or ureterovesical anastomosis may be used. The former is not recommended because stricture is common. There are two main techniques for ureterovesical anastomosis.

In the technique suggested by Calne, the end of the ureter is slit longitudinally and sutured to the bladder mucosa in a triangular fashion (Fig. I.18*A* and *B*).

Another technique involves making two slits in the end of the ureter. The two "lips" of the ureter are then fixed by sutures passing through

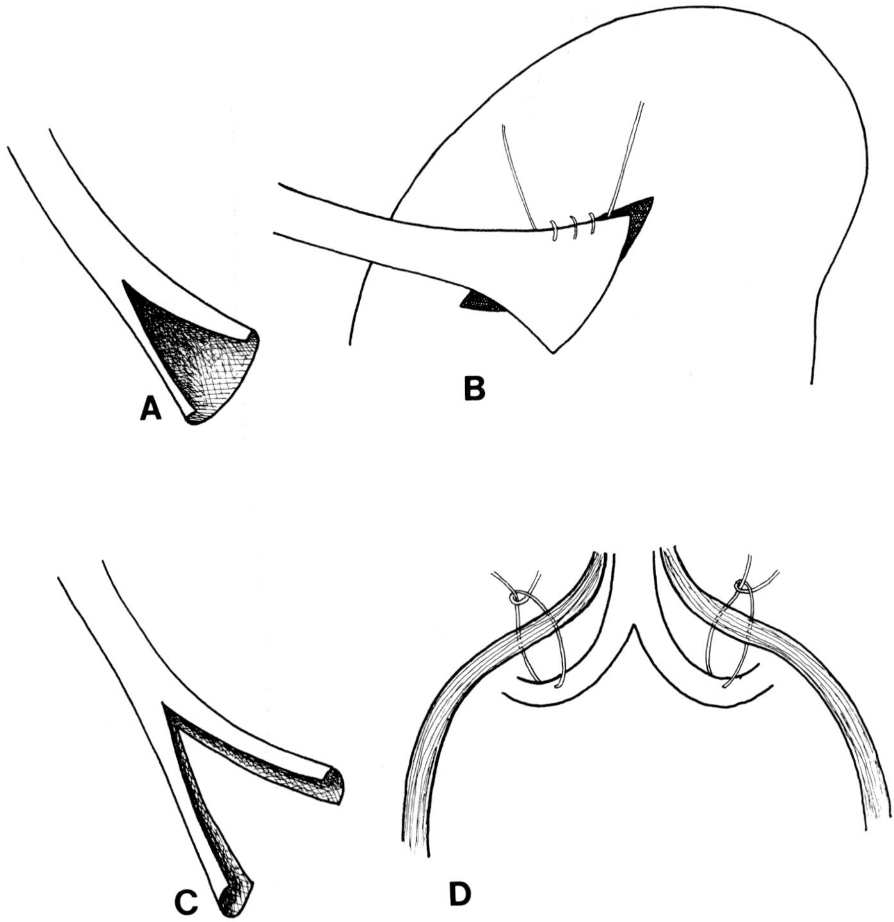

Fig. I.18. Transplantation in dogs. *Above*, ureterovesical anastomosis after Calne. *A*, ureter slit longitudinally; *B*, suture of ureter to bladder mucosa. *Below*, another technique of ureterovesical anastomosis. *C*, ureter fish-tailed; *D*, the two lips of the ureter fixed by transvesical sutures tied on the outer aspect of the bladder.

the bladder and tied on the outer aspect of the bladder (Fig. I.18*C* and *D*).

The suture material for ureterovesical anastomosis is 000 catgut. There is little risk of stricture or fistula in dogs, even with immunosuppressive therapy.

REFERENCES

1. Calne, R. Y. *Renal Transplantation.* Arnold, London, 1963.
2. Dormont, J., Auvert, J., Cukier, J. and Zmerli, S. Autotransplantation rénale chez le chien après conservation prolongée à basse température. Rev. Franç. Etud. Clin. Biol., *9:*1043, 1964.

Kidney Transplantation in Pigs

The advantage of the pig for kidney transplantation is to provide homogeneous material and kidneys of a size similar to normal human kidneys.

We shall describe an original technique which we devised. It allows either auto- or allografting. In our experience, this technique proved simple and safe, with a strikingly low operative risk and low postoperative complication rate.

When a median transperitoneal approach is used, the operation is difficult; moreover, a high rate of surgical complications occurs in the postoperative period,[1, 2, 3] the most serious being intestinal (ileus due to adhesions, internal hernias, volvulus, intussusception) or vascular (infarction of gut, paraglegia due to aortic clamping). In order to avoid these disadvantages, we devised an extraperitoneal approach and orthotopic transplantation.

Anesthesia

The animals are premedicated with atropine sulfate (0.25 mg) and acepromazine maleate (4 mg/kg) given intramuscularly 90 min before operation.

General anesthesia is induced in starved pigs by snout mask inhalation of a mixture of halothane, nitrous oxide and oxygen and is maintained by varying the percentage of halothane in the mixture with spontaneous ventilation. Endotracheal intubation is not necessary.

Arteriovenous Shunt

A silicone rubber arteriovenous shunt is placed in the recipient between the common carotid artery and the jugular vein 2 to 5 days before transplantation. This shunt allows blood pressure surveillance and the infusion of fluid during the operation as well as repeated blood sampling during the postoperative period.

At the same time, a unilateral nephrectomy may be performed, the other kidney being removed at the time of transplantation.

Removal of Donor Kidney

The easiest access to the kidney is by a lumbar extraperitoneal approach, which is the incision of choice. Approach through a midline incision is far more difficult and we do not recommend it.

The incision lies along the last rib and extends inferiorly for 15 to 20 cm according to the weight of the animal (Fig. I.19). The abdominal muscles are divided and the peritoneum reflected medially.

The kidney is surrounded by loose connective tissue without any vessel, and blunt digital dissection frees the kidney in a few seconds. The vessels are dissected with venous tributaries being tied and cut. The ureter is dissected and divided 5 cm distal to the hilum of the kidney. The vessels are tied and cut so as to preserve the greatest possible length of artery and vein with the transplant. The kidney is then cooled by perfusion of Collins' solution at 4°C.

Transplantation

The surgical approach in the recipient is exactly the same as in the donor. The kidney of the animal, its vessels and ureter are dissected as described above for the donor.

The ureter is cut near the kidney. The renal vessels are clamped together in a single vascular clamp which must not grasp the aorta. They

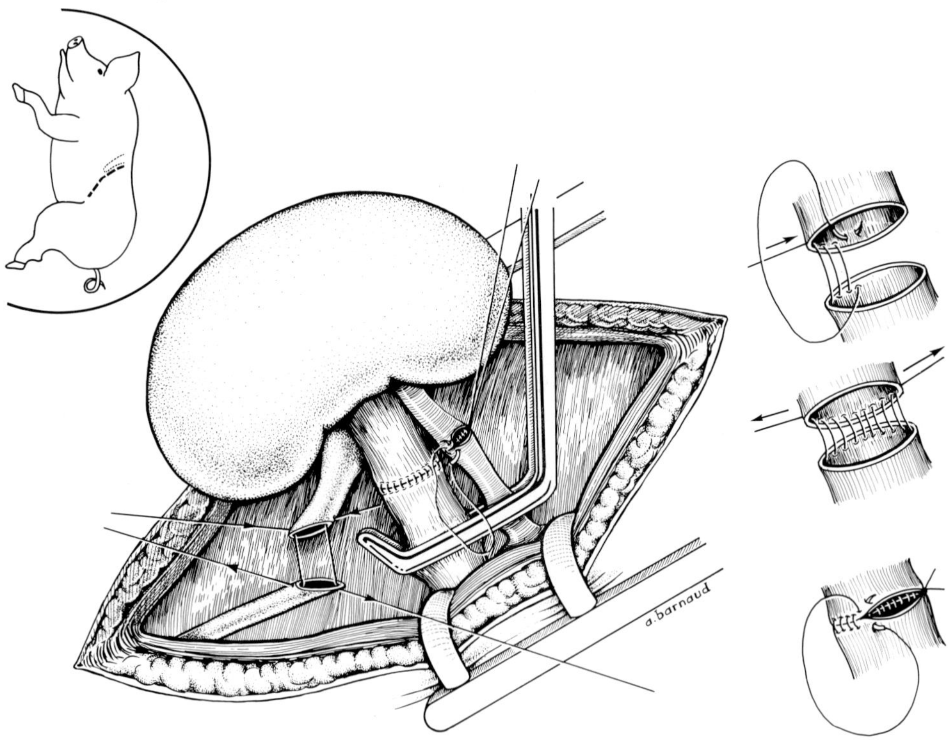

Fig. I.19. Transplantation in pigs. *Left*, the incision; *middle*, general view showing the disposition and making of the anastomoses; *right*, details of the venous anastomosis.

are cut near the hilum of the kidney and the latter is removed. Thus, the maximum length of the vessels is preserved in the recipient.

Venous anastomosis is done first. The vein of the transplant is anastomosed end-to-end to the renal vein of the recipient. The posterior layer is done with an everting Blalock continuous mattress suture, whose stitches are placed with the kidney lying outside the lumbar fossa, on the abdominal wall. Drawing the suture taut approximates the posterior layer of the vessels. The anterior layer is then sutured in the usual way with a continuous over and over suture (Fig. I.19).

Arterial anastomosis comes next. The ends of the donor and recipient arteries are carefully dilated and an end-to-end anastomosis is done with a continuous over and over suture (Fig. I.19).

Anastomosis of the ureter completes the procedure. The ends of the donor and recipient ureters are cut obliquely and spatulated. An end-to-end anastomosis is performed either with a continuous suture or with separate stitches.

The suture material for all three anastomoses is 6/0 monofilament nylon.

No drainage is used.

The contralateral kidney of the recipient would have been removed at the time of arteriovenous shunting. If not, it may be removed at the same session through a contralateral lumbar approach.

We have used this technique extensively for auto and allografts with excellent results. A possible procedure for autografts includes removal of one kidney and transplantation of that kidney in the opposite lumbar fossa, the other kidney being simultaneously removed.

REFERENCES

1. Golby, M., and White, H. J. O. The operation of orthotopic renal allografting in the pig and its complications. Br. J. Surg., *58:*287, 1971.
2. Mazzoni, G., Di Martino, C., Demofonti, A., Valli, A., Pellegrini, S., Gentili, B., and Melis, M. Simultaneous allografts of both kidneys in pigs with different portal and caval venous drainage. Am. J. Surg., *124:*39, 1972.
3. Nerstrøm, B., Gyrd-Hansen, N., Hansen, R. I., and Løkkegaard, H. Renal autotransplantation in the pig: Surgical aspects. Scand. J. Urol. Nephrol., *6:*151, 1972.

Kidney Transplantation in Rats

The principal advantage of the rat for organ transplantation is the possibility of using pure strains. In addition, the operation is performed by a single surgeon, and large series of experiments are possible.

In 1964, Gonzalez et al[2] suggested a technique of placing the kidney in the neck with cutaneous ureterostomy. In 1965, Fisher and Lee[1] described a technique of placing the graft in the abdomen with re-establishment of continuity of the urinary tract. With several modifications,[3, 4, 5, 10] this technique has been adopted by most centers. We shall describe the modified Lee technique with particular emphasis on the re-establishment of continuity of the urinary tract.

General Considerations and Preparation of Animals

Young adult rats of either sex, weighing some 200 g, are chosen. Heavier rats have the disadvantage of excess adipose tissue and their blood vessels are not larger. Donor and recipient should be of the same sex because, in some strains, sex-linked incompatibility (antigen carried on chromosome Y) is significant, as shown by the fact that in the female isogenic grafts from the male are rejected.[6]

Anesthesia with a short acting barbiturate, such as Nembutal (2.5 mg/100 g) given intraperitoneally, is usually employed.

The instruments are those used in ophthalmic surgery.[1] A microscope allowing 4 × to 10 × magnification is necessary for precise placement of the stitches during the vascular sutures.

The operation is carried out without strict asepsis but cleanly, with minimum contamination.

After operation, neither rehydration with fluids nor antibiotics is required.

Removal of Donor Kidney (Fig. I.20)

1. Removal of the right kidney is advised by Sakai.[7] The abdomen is opened and the intestines reflected to the left. The right kidney is freed completely from neighboring tissues and the dissection is continued to the aorta and vena cava. The superior mesenteric artery is tied with 6/0 silk and divided. Using the stump of this artery for traction, the aorta is freed from its surrounding connective tissue and from the celiac adrenal and spermatic arteries. The dissection between the renal artery and vein is carried as far as possible to facilitate subsequent venous anastomosis.

The right ureter is dissected and freed from the genital organs at the base of the bladder. If half of the donor bladder is to be removed, the left ureter and the region of the bladder neck are tied close to the bladder and divided; the bladder is then transsected into equal halves. If only a patch of bladder is to be removed, it is cut widely around the ureteral orifice.

It remains to divide the vascular pedicle. The aorta is tied and divided below the origin of the renal artery. The proximal part of the aorta is clamped and divided below the clamp. The renal vein is taken with a patch of vena cava. The kidney is now completely free. The renal artery

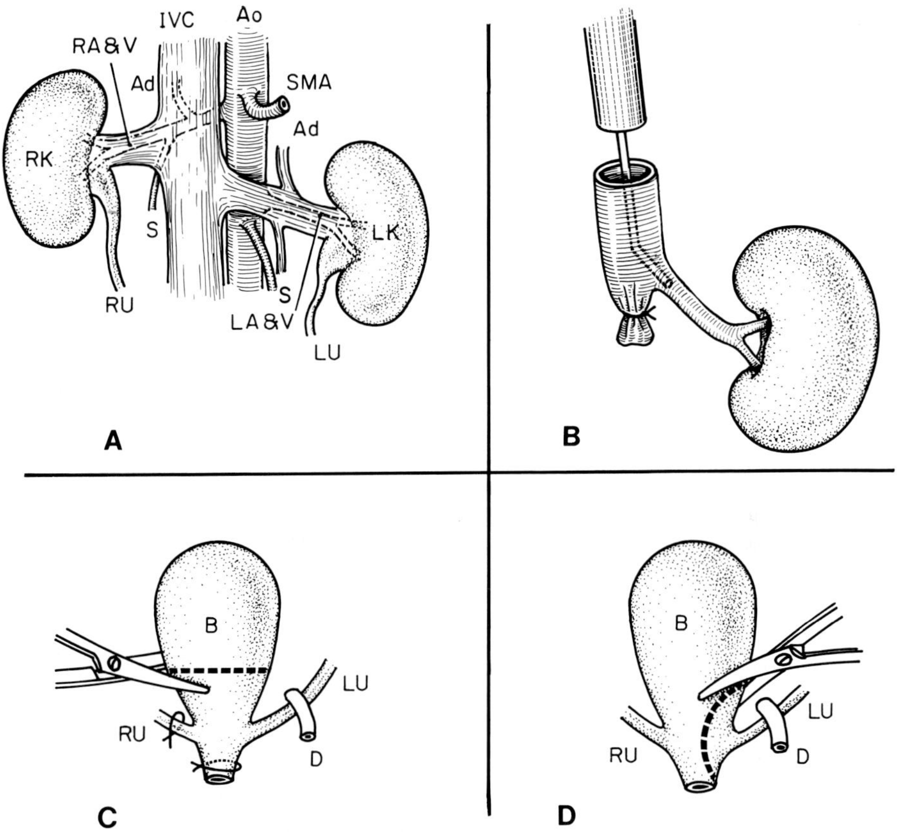

Fig. I.20. Kidney transplantation in the rat. Removal of kidney and ureter. *A*, anatomic arrangement of the kidneys and of their vessels. *B*, perfusion of the artery with cold fluid. *C*, taking half of the bladder. *D*, taking a patch of bladder around the ureter. *RK*, right kidney; *LK*, left kidney; *Ao*, aorta; *IVC*, inferior vena cava; *Ad*, adrenal vessels; *S*, spermatic vessels; *SMA*, superior mesenteric artery; *RA&V*, vessels of the right kidney; *LA&V*, vessels of the left kidney; *RU*, right ureter; *LU*, left ureter; *B*, bladder; *D*, deferent duct.

is cannulated with a microcannula and Collins' solution cooled to 4°C is injected into it, care being taken to avoid too high a pressure during the injection. When the kidney has been washed out, it is placed in saline solution cooled to 4°C.

The entire dissection takes about 30 min.

2. Removal of the left kidney is far easier, and we recommend it as the routine choice. The kidney is freed from the neighboring tissues. The renal vein is dissected; the adrenal vessels are tied and divided at its upper border and the spermatic vessels at its lower border. The aorta is then dissected from the surrounding tissue above and below the renal vein. The latter vessel is separated from the aorta. The aorta is then tied

and divided below the renal vein. According to the site of its origin, the superior mesenteric artery is not necessarily tied and divided. A lumbar artery frequently has to be tied and cut.

The remaining stages of the dissection are the same as for the right kidney. Division of the vessels is performed as follows. The aorta is clamped as high as possible and cut above the origin of the renal artery; the renal vein is cut at its junction with the vena cava, along the right border of the aorta. Cooling of the kidney is performed as previously described.

Transplantation

Vascular Anastomoses (Fig. I.21). The recipient aorta and vena cava are dissected in their subrenal part. The two vessels are clamped together with two microvascular clamps.

The right lateral wall of the inferior vena cava is opened longitudinally

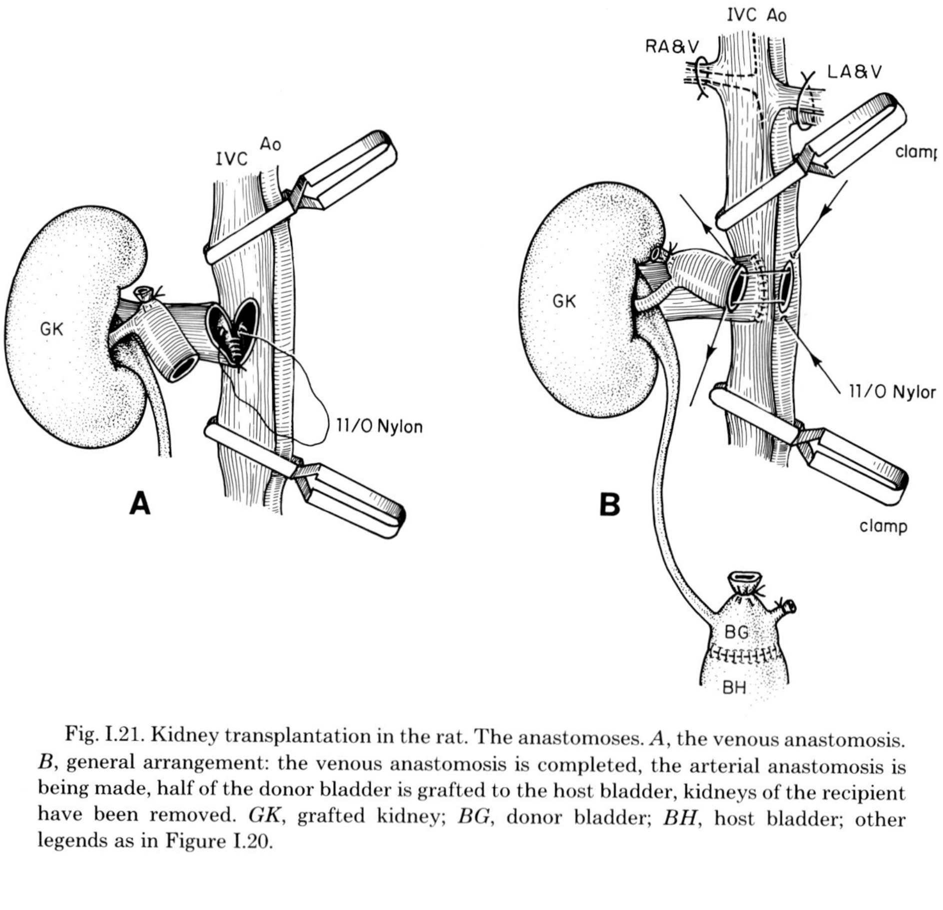

Fig. I.21. Kidney transplantation in the rat. The anastomoses. *A*, the venous anastomosis. *B*, general arrangement: the venous anastomosis is completed, the arterial anastomosis is being made, half of the donor bladder is grafted to the host bladder, kidneys of the recipient have been removed. *GK*, grafted kidney; *BG*, donor bladder; *BH*, host bladder; other legends as in Figure I.20.

with fine scissors, the length of the incision being the diameter of the renal vein (or of the caval patch). The vessel is freed from clot by injecting heparinized saline into the lumen. The renal vein, or the caval patch, is sutured to the recipient vena cava with a continuous suture of 11/0 monofilament nylon; the posterior layer of the anastomosis is done from within the venous lumen and the anterior layer from the outside.

The aortic anastomosis comes next. A longitudinal incision is made with fine scissors on the anterior wall of the recipient aorta. The lumen of the vessel is flushed with saline. The donor aorta is anastomosed end-to-side to the recipient aorta with a continuous suture of the same 11/0 monofilament nylon. The layer of the anastomosis facing the venous anastomosis is made from within the aortic lumen, the other layer from the outside.

When the anastomoses are complete, the vascular clamps are removed; pressure is maintained on the anastomoses for a short while with a cotton-wool pad. An additional stitch is rarely necessary.

The total ischemia time is about 40 min. Peristalsis returns in the ureter as soon as the circulation is re-established.

Re-establishment of Continuity of the Urinary Tract (Fig. I.22). This is the most delicate and the most important part of the procedure for obtaining long-term survival without hydronephrosis.[8, 9] Cutaneous ureterostomy[2] and implantation of the ureter into the bladder[1] are not satisfactory. Stricture often develops in the first postoperative week. Ureteroureteral anastomosis is difficult and often complicated by stricture.

Early hydronephrosis can be avoided by anastomosing half of the donor bladder to half of the recipient bladder,[4, 5] but a study of isogenic grafts has shown that this procedure is not entirely satisfactory. In the 1st month after transplantation, the grafted bladder is thin-walled and atrophic and does not contract, probably due to defective blood and/or nerve supply.

It remains distended during contraction of the recipient bladder below the anastomosis. This can lead to bladder stasis and the formation of stone (present in most cases after 2 months), infection, reflux into the grafted kidney (and the rat's own kidney if this has been left in place) and pyelonephritis. The consequences of the pyelonephritis may be difficult to distinguish from chronic rejection.

The best method is to use a small patch of donor bladder around the ureter and to anastomose this patch to the recipient (Fig. I.22*E*), as recommended by Sakai.[7] This method avoids infection, reflux and stone, even many months after grafting.

Recipient Nephrectomy. It is desirable to remove the two recipient kidneys at the same time as the graft is done. Nephrectomy prolongs the operation for only 3 to 5 min.

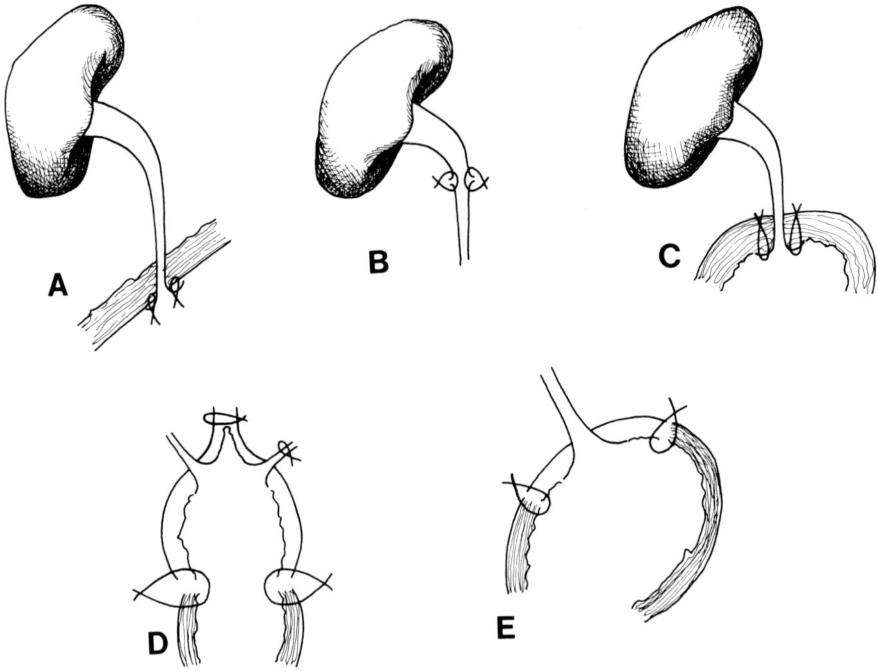

Fig. I.22. Various techniques of transplantation of the ureter in rats. *A*, ureteroureterostomy (Gonzalez 1964); *B*, end-to-end anastomosis (Sakai, 1966); *C*, implantation into the bladder (Fisher, Lee and Sakai, 1965); *D*, vesicovesical anastomosis (Sakai, 1967); *E*, patch technique (Sakai, 1968).

Xenografts

Xenografts have been developed in the rat to study immunologic phenomena and hyperacute rejection. Three types of renal xenograft have been developed: dog to rat (using 1 to 3-week-old puppies), rabbit to rat (using 2 to 3-week-old rabbits) and guinea pig to rat (using adult guinea pigs).

The technique used for these xenografts is similar to that of allografting. The kidneys are removed with the adjacent segments of aorta and vena cava from which the renal vessels originate. The vascular anastomoses are made end-to-side to the aorta and vena cava of the recipient rat as described above for allografts. The ureter is implanted into the bladder.

REFERENCES

1. Fisher, B., and Lee, S. Microvascular surgical techniques in research, with special reference to renal transplantation in the rat. Surgery, *58:*904, 1965.
2. Gonzalez, E. E., Nathan, P., and Miller, B. F. A method for transplantation of the rat kidney. Ann. NY Acad. Sci., *99:*795, 1962.

3. Guttmann, R. D., Lindquist, R. R., Parker, R. M., Carpenter, C. B., and Merrill, J. P. Renal transplantation in the inbred rat. I. Morphologic, immunologic and functional alterations during acute rejection. Transplantation, *5:*668, 1967.
4. Lee, S. An improved technique of renal transplantation in the rat. Surgery, *61:*771, 1967.
5. Sakai, A. Rat kidney transplantation. I. Technique and results of 232 cases. Jpn. J. Transplant., *2:*191, 1967.
6. Sakai, A. Antigenicity of skin and kidney in the rat, as studied in a transplantation model. Transplantation, *8:*882, 1968.
7. Sakai, A. Kidney transplantation in the rat. In *Renal Transplantation, Theory and Practice*, edited by J. Hamburger, J. Crosnier, J. Dormont and J. F. Bach, p. 273. Williams & Wilkins, Baltimore, 1972.
8. Sakai, A., Festenstein, H., and Simonsan, M. Does syngeneic preference operate in kidney transplantation? In *Advances in Transplantation*, edited by J. Dausset, J. Hamburger and G. Mathé, p. 269. Munksgaard, Copenhagen, 1967.
9. Sakai, A., Simonsen, M., and Jensen, E. Kidney transplantation in siblings. Transplantation, *7:*444, 1969.
10. Taguchi, Y., MacKinnon, K. J., and Dossetor, J. B. Renal allograft modification by donor antigen in the rat: evidence for significance of this principle in man. In *Advances in Transplantation*, edited by J. Dausset, J. Hamburger and G. Mathé, p. 393. Munksgaard, Copenhagen, 1967.

Kidney Transplantation in Rabbits

Because of our very limited experience in kidney grafting in rabbits, we shall merely cite certain references to the literature on this technique.

REFERENCES

1. Bayuk, J. M., and Schmidlapp, C. J. Kidney transplantation in the rabbit. A method for the study of transplantation immunology. Invest. Urol., *4:*378, 1966.
2. Heron, I. Kidney transplantation in the rabbit. Acta Pathol. Microbiol. Scand. Section A, *78:*90, 1970.
3. Klassen, J., and Milgrom, F. The role of humoral antibodies in the rejection of renal homografts by rabbits. Transplantation, *8:*566, 1969.
4. Lund, B. Renal transplantation in the rabbit. Acta Pathol. Microbiol. Scand. Section A, *78:*85, 1970.
5. McDonald, J. C., and Fukuda, A. Rabbit renal homografts. I. Technique for grafts to the neck. Surgery, *59:*1156, 1966.
6. Nathan, P., Gonzalez, E. E., Fowler, R., Jr., Pescovitz, H., and Miller, B. F. A method for the transplantation of the rabbit kidney. Proc. Soc. Exp. Biol. Med., *107:*51, 1961.
7. Owen, E. R., Slome, D., and Waterston, D. J. Prolongation of rabbit kidney allograft survival by desensitization. In *Advances in Transplantation*, edited by J. Dausset, J. Hamburger and G. Mathé, p. 385. Munksgaard, Copenhagen, 1965.

APPENDIX II

Immunologic Techniques

HLA TYPING AND CROSS-MATCHING PROCEDURE USING THE LYMPHOCYTOTOXICITY MICROTECHNIQUE

Jacques-Henri Hors

The determination of human leukocyte A (HLA) antigens is based on the property of the corresponding specific antibodies to be cytotoxic in the presence of complement.

The lysis of the target cell can be measured by chromium release[10] or by using fluorochromasia[2, 3] or ATP loss,[4] all of which will permit automation of the reading in the near future.

However, in the great majority of laboratories, reading is presently made by staining with dyes, utilizing the micromethod designed by Terasaki and McClelland[15] 16 years ago which has been somewhat modified since then.[11, 14] We will describe one of the variants of the National Institute of Health two-step reference technique in Falcon trays. However, many other techniques, such as the use of coverslip trays as described by Kissmeyer-Nielsen and Thorsby[9] or other procedures,[1] are currently being used.

For further details, see the NIAID Manual of Tissue Typing Techniques[13] and the excellent reference manual entitled *Histocompatibility Techniques*, edited by Dick and Kissmeyer-Nielsen.[5]

The principle of the typing test is to bring together, in a two-step process:

1. The lymphocytes, carrying the HLA antigen on their membrane, and the previously distributed serum, containing the specific antibodies.
2. The complement rabbit serum and the reading of the lysis.

HLA-A, B, C Typing

Preparation of the Lymphocyte Suspension

1. **From Peripheral Blood.** The procedure is based on that of Harris and Ukaejiofo.[7] Ten milliliters of blood are collected on dry heparin (Liquemin, Roche, 200 IU) and mixed by several inversions. The blood is

diluted to 1:4 in phosphate-buffered saline [PBS:KH_2PO_4 (0.20 g), Na_2HPO_4 (1.44 g), KCl (0.20 g), NaCl (8.00 g), double distilled water (1000 ml), pH 7.2]. Then, using a Pasteur pipette, it is gently layered onto the surface of an equal volume of Ficoll-Isopaque mixture which is obtained by mixing 24 volumes of 9% Ficoll (9 g diluted in 100 ml of distilled water) with 10 volumes of 33.9% Isopaque (20 ml of 75% Isopaque added to 24.8 ml of distilled water).* The sterilized mixture may be stored at +4° for a maximum period of 1 month.

The tube is centrifuged for 20 min at 1000 × g at 18°.

The layer of lymphocytes and platelets at the interface between the colored plasma above and the colorless Ficoll-Triosil mixture below is aspirated until the junction of the two layers is linear (Fig. II.1).

The suspension is placed in a hemolysis tube, mixed and centrifuged for 8 min at 1000 × g at +4°.

The supernatant is discarded; the sediment is resuspended in 3 ml of autologous plasma and centrifuged at low speed (6 min, 225 g, +4°). The platelet rich supernatant is decanted and the lymphocyte pellet resuspended in 0.20 ml of Hanks' solution.

The degree of platelet contamination is checked by counting. If the preparation contains more than 10% platelets, it is centrifuged again at low speed.

The lymphocyte suspension is counted and adjusted to a concentration of 1800 to 2000/μl in Hanks' solution (Institut Pasteur, Paris).

2. **From Cadaver Donor Lymph Nodes.** Because of intensive care treatment and anoxia, the cell suspension obtained from peripheral blood of a cadaver donor is often in a state of poor viability and not suitable for typing. On the contrary, lymph nodes can provide a quickly prepared suspension of 90% pure T lymphocytes. They are taken at the time of kidney removal and put into a saline solution in an isothermic container, without refrigeration. Using scissors they are separated from the surrounding fatty tissue, which is yellow and shapeless, while the lymph nodes are firm and round.

They must not be sliced but are multiperforated with a needle, and several millimeters of Hanks' solution is injected into the center. The perfusion liquid which drains from the holes is collected, counted, concentrated if necessary, and adjusted at 2000 cells/μl. This cell suspension generally consists of more than 90% pure viable T lymphocytes and constitutes the ideal target cells for A, B, C typing and cross-match.

---

* Final specific gravity must be checked and adjusted to 1.077. Ficoll is obtained from Pharmacia, Uppsala, Sweden; Isopaque (Triosil) 440 from Njegaard, Oslo, Norway. It may be replaced by sodium diatrizoate: Hypaque, from Winthrop, New York.

Test Sera

The test sera are derived from subjects immunized mainly by multiparity but also by blood transfusions or kidney grafts. They are selected and prepared to present three ideal characteristics: 1) Specificity (monospecificity if possible) with (ideally) neither extra nor missing reaction, after screening against the cells of a reference panel (+/+, +/−; −/+; −/− observed/expected reactions). Barely 3 to 10% of the positive sera studied are good reagents for practical use. 2) Reproducibility of the results. 3) Strength and clearly defined reaction: tests clearly negative, or totally positive. The test sera are stored in aliquots at −30°, or at −80° if they are to be used over a period of many months.

In preparation for typing, the test sera are placed in Terasaki plates (Falcon Plastic, Los Angeles, California: microtest culture plate 3034) previously covered with 4 ml of mineral oil (Merck or Fisher Scientific Company: Saybolt viscosity 335/350).

All subsequent manipulations are made with a micromanipulator and microsyringe [micromanipulator PB 600-1 and microsyringe (50 μl) 705: Hamilton Company, Whittier, California] calibrated to 1 μl. (Fig. II.2).

The volume of serum added to each of the 60 wells of the plate is 1 μl, diluted or not.

The plates ready for use are stored at −80°, or at −30° if they are to be used within 2 months. The plates should be closed carefully and placed in a hermetically sealed box.

The distribution of oil and/or sera can be performed automatically (Oil Dispenser, Seromat) (Greiner ZIP 67240, Bischwiller, France).

Preparation of Rabbit Complement

Complement is the reagent which tends to have the greatest influence on the sensitivity of the technique. It is thus necessary, in order to improve reliability, to standardize it as carefully as possible. If it is too weak, some antigens will not be detected, whereas if it is too strong, extra reactions will appear due to cross-reaction and might result in false positive, "triplet" antigens.

The rabbit should be free of parasites and unvaccinated. Blood is taken from the carotid artery.

A minimum of 50 or 100 rabbits is required in order to obtain homogeneity among batches of complement.

The blood of each rabbit is collected separately and only when the clot has retracted are the sera mixed together.

Retraction is carried out at room temperature and can be accelerated by squeezing the clot in gauze.

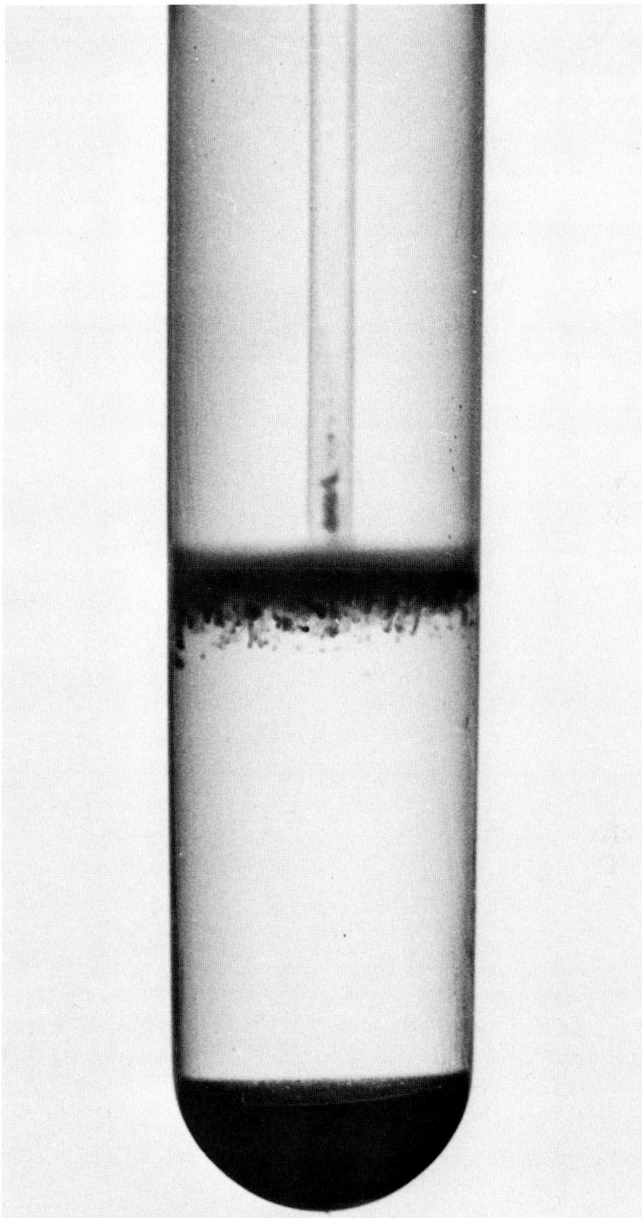

Fig. II.1. Separation of lymphocytes by Ficoll-Triosil gradient.

The rabbit sera mixture is stored on crushed ice until it is centrifuged at 0° for 15 min, at 2000 × g, and is placed in aliquots in small volume rhesus tubes.

The tubes are stored at −80°. They are warmed to +4° only once

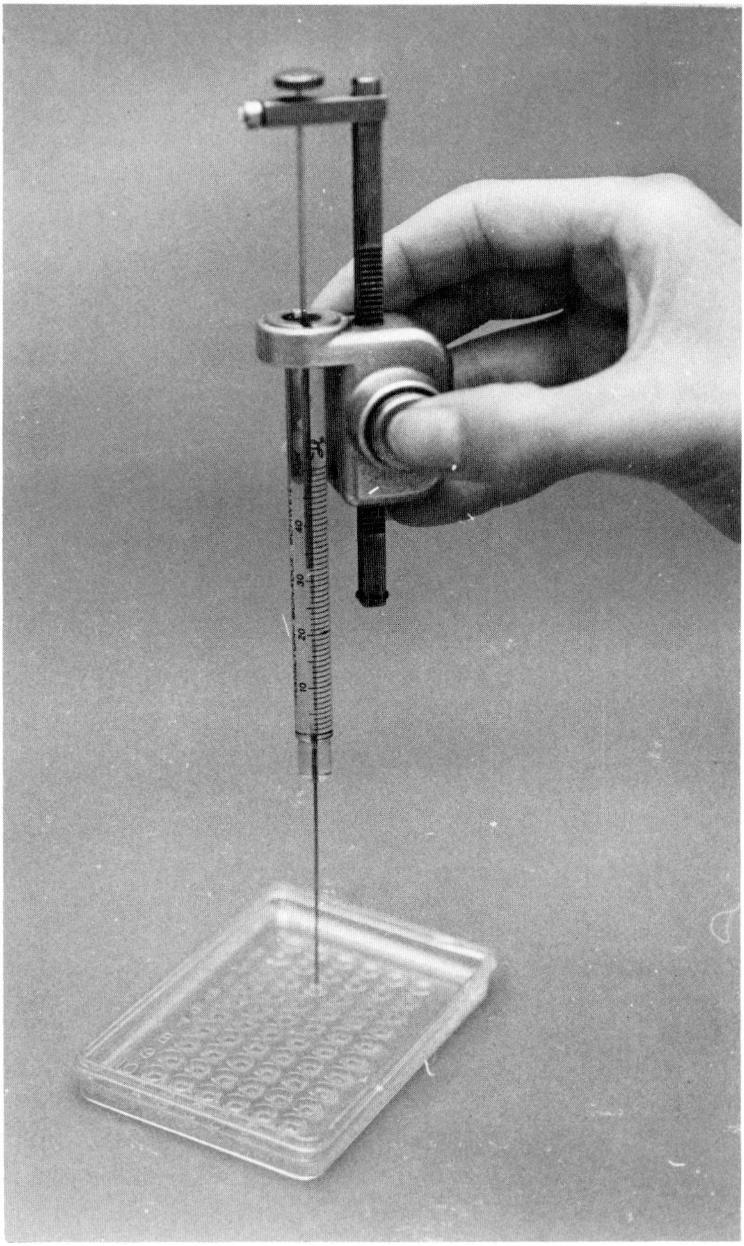

Fig. II.2. Distribution of sera or cells into a Terasaki plate, under oil, using micromanipulator and 1 μl microsyringe.

immediately before use. If they are stored for longer than 1 month they must be kept in liquid nitrogen.

Each lot of complement must be tested. 1) It must not itself be cytotoxic for human lymphocytes in the presence of inactivated AB sera. 2) It must have adequate complement activity, verified by preliminary titration in a lymphocytotoxicity test using several weak sera.

However, the best method is to type in parallel five different lymphocyte suspensions of A and O/ABO groups with a reference complement and a new batch of complement.

Test

The test is carried out as follows: 1) mix serum, 1 μl, and lymphocytes (2000/μl in Hanks' solution), 1 μl; 2) incubate for 30 min at 22°; 3) add rabbit complement, 5 μl; and 4) incubate for 1 hour at 22°.

The lymphocyte lysis can be read with the aid of trypan blue or eosin.

Trypan Blue. The supernatant is removed from each well by flicking.

To each well is added 1 μl of trypan blue (BDH Ltd. Laboratory Chemical Group, England), prepared, just before use, by mixing 3 volumes of 0.3% blue in distilled water, with 1 volume of hypertonic Hanks' solution (Hanks' solution with 2.55 g of NaCl added to each 100 ml).

The test can be read with an inverted microscopic (ocular 10, objective 25) or a direct microscope (ocular 10, objective 15).

If the cells do not absorb the trypan blue, they remain refractile (vary the focus) and are of normal size, they are alive and do not carry the antigen against which the antibody is directed. If they take up the blue dye and are swollen and lackluster, they are dead and this indicates that they carry the antigen against which the antibody is directed. They swell to several times their normal size before being lysed.

The test must be read within an hour after the end of incubation.

Eosin. To read the test with eosin and formaldehyde, a phase contrast microscope is required; it has the advantage of allowing several hours' delay in reading and obviating the need for preliminary decanting.

One microliter of eosin (RAL, Prolabo, Paris) (3 volumes of 5% eosin mixed with 1 volume of hypertonic Hanks' solution) is added to each well. After 2 min, 2 μl of formaldehyde (40% formaldehyde; the pH must be adjusted to 6.7 by adding KOH) are added.

The living cells are brilliant and of normal size (keep adjusting the focus). The dead cells are lysed, lackluster, dark and increased in size.

Interpretation of Results. The percentage of dead cells reflects the strength of the reaction.

0–20%	–
21–30%	+
31–50%	++
51–80%	+++
81–100%	++++

HLA-DR Typing

Although the HLA-A, B and C antigens are present on the membrane of all nucleated cells, the D-related (DR) antigens are only carried by B lymphocytes (and monocytes) and lack on platelets.

Precautions to Take Prior to DR Typing

1. Absorb the test sera on a pool of platelets in order to remove the possible anti-HLA-A, B, C contaminating antibodies (10–20.10^9 platelets/ml of sera).

2. Obtain an enriched lymphocyte B suspension (≥70%):

a. From the recipient's peripheral blood, either by using columns of nylon fibers upon which the B lymphocytes attach themselves[6] or by removing the T lymphocytes forming rosettes with 2-amino-ethyl isothiouronium bromide (AET)-treated sheep red cells,[12] from the original suspension obtained after Ficoll-Isopaque separation.

In the latter technique, 3 ml of lymphocytes (3.10^6/ml) are mixed with 0.3 ml of AET-treated sheep red cells and centrifuged at 1,000 g at 4°C on a Ficoll-Isopaque gradient. The nonrosetting lymphocytes, recovered from the interface, are washed and resuspended in Hanks' solution and adjusted to 2,500–3,000/μl.

An interesting technique described by Van Rood et al[16] does not include B lymphocyte separation and bicolor fluorescence is used to distinguish both between dead and living and between B and T cells.

b. From the donor's spleen. Spleen lymphocytes have the advantage of being numerous and contain a considerable percentage (40–70%) of B lymphocytes. The slice of spleen is gently scraped with the use of a scalpel. The splenic pulp thus obtained is diluted in Hanks' solution, the debris are sedimented and the supernatant is placed on a Ficoll-Isopaque gradient and centrifuged in order to eliminate the contaminating red cells.

Although the percentage of B lymphocytes thus obtained is quite high, it is advisable to carry out a further B enriching process using one of the techniques described above.

Test Procedure

The incubation period for DR typing has been discussed by many investigators. When fresh cells are tested, there is an incubation period of 3 hours (1 before and 2 after the addition of complement), whereas with previously frozen cells, the time of incubation can be reduced to 2 hours (30 and 90 min, respectively).

Most of the other parameters are the same as in the standard ABC technique described above, with the exception of cell concentration, which is higher—2,500 to 3,000/μl. The purity of the B cell enriched suspension must be checked by lymphocytotoxicity using an anti-T and a polyspecific anti-DR sera.

Cross-Match Procedure

Before any transplantation, it must be verified that the recipient is devoid of preformed cytotoxic antibodies against the T cells of the donor; if not, they would give rise to a hyperacute rejection.

The cross-match must therefore be performed using the most sensitive technique and the widest spectrum of antibodies. It should be remembered that an antibody may have diminished or disappeared from the serum, while sensitization remains in the immunologic memory.

Serum Testing in Dialyzed Patients

Since antibodies vary in strength, titre and width of spectrum against the panel, a 15-ml serum sample must be tested 8 to 15 days (10 days average) after each blood transfusion; this period corresponds to the peak of positivity of the antibody.

The sera are distributed into small aliquots and stored at −30°C. They are kept so as to be easily located in an emergency, and each microtube is thawed only once.

Serum is screened against the lymphocytes of 30 members of the reference panel, chosen because they bear all of the known specificities and some blanks.

It is necessary to specify the exact spectrum of the antibodies; computer programs are often helpful, especially in cases of multispecific antibodies.

Target Cell Selection

The only valid T cell suspensions are lymph node lymphocytes from the donor, easily and quickly obtained as described above.

Peripheral blood cells are often unsuitable due to poor viability, and since spleen lymphocytes contain variable proportions of T, B and nul lymphocytes, the reaction might express those of other cells than T lymphocytes.

Cross-Match Test

The standard two-step technique of microlymphocytotoxicity is commonly used. Longer periods of incubation have not provided proof that greater positivity was correlated with a greater risk of rejection.

If the recipient had developed antibodies, the widest possible panel of sera must be tested against the donor lymphocytes, and in case of absence of antibodies, the most recent sera are used.

In order to avoid prozone phenomena which are often due to anticomplement activity, different volumes of sera must be used: 5, 4, 3, 2, 1, ½ μl (diluted in inactivated noncytotoxic AB sera). The percentage of killed cells is evaluated and compared to the nonspecific background; when the difference exceeds 30%, results are considered positive.

Freezing Lymphocytes in Liquid Nitrogen

Freezing offers the incomparable advantage of allowing delayed typing—provided the lymphocytes are separated and frozen within 24 hours—and especially of retyping stored cells, using new sera defining new specificities or splits.

Moreover, freezing permits studying patient immunization in favorable conditions. Using 30 different chosen frozen cell suspensions, one can define the spectrum of antibodies within a serum in 1 day. It also allows serial study of post-transplantation specific immunization sequences against donor cells, thawed only once, using retrospective cross-match with all the recipient's sera.

Although many techniques have been described, one of the most frequently used involves freezing of the cell suspension in plastic straws (Instruments de Médecine Vétérinaire, Etablissements Cassou, Laigle, 61300 France).

The lymphocytes are prepared in autologous sera at a concentration up to 20,000/μl. The cell suspension is mixed volume by volume with a 20% dimethyl sulfoxide (DMSO) solution in phosphate-buffered saline, prestored at 4°C, added drop by drop, just before freezing, and used as a protective agent.

For details, see the previously published description of the technique.[8] It consists (Fig. II.3) in placing the straws (*G*) on metal tray (*A*), 20 cm from the level of liquid nitrogen (*C*), in container (*B*) (RBC 60, Air Liquide, 92 Plessis Robinson, France) for 20 min. The metal tray is then lowered to the level of the liquid nitrogen. After 5 min the straws are arranged in plastic tubes (*F*), beakers (*D*) and canister (*E*).

The cells can be kept in excellent condition for years. Thawing is performed by quickly immersing the straws in a 40°C water bath for 20 sec. Viability is generally ⩾88%, provided the DMSO has been quickly removed as follows: The cell suspension is collected in a conical tube. Two millimeters of a mixture composed of one-half phosphate-buffered

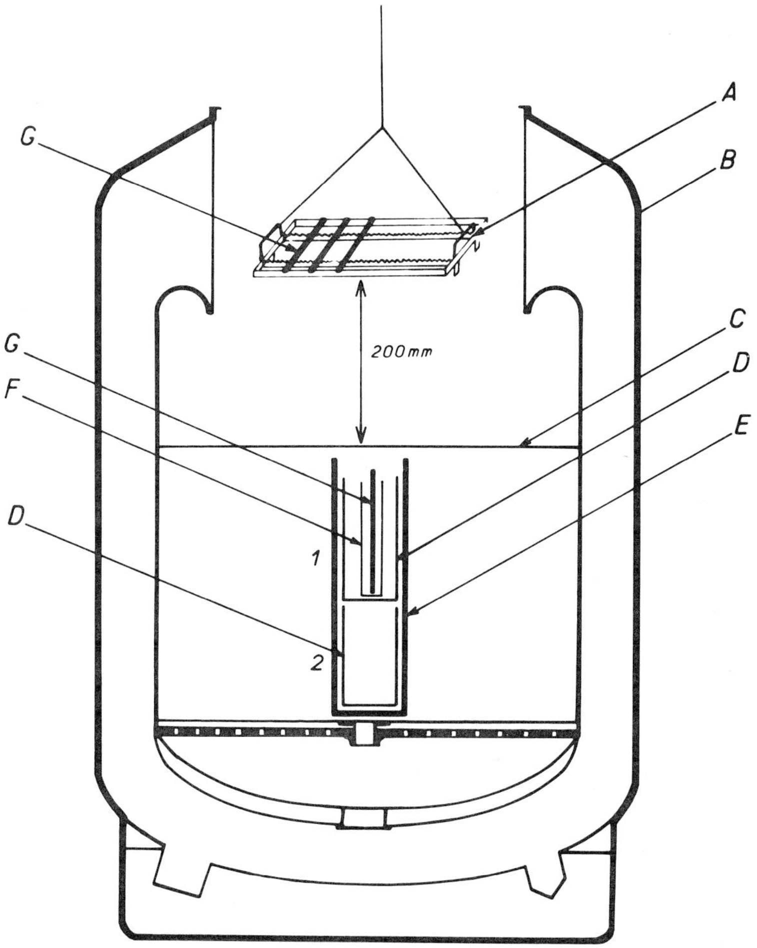

Fig. II.3. The lymphocyte suspension in the straws (*G*) are frozen on a metal tray (*A*) in a container (*B*) at 200 mm above the level of liquid nitrogen (*C*). The straws are stored in tubes (*F*), beakers (*D*) and canisters (*E*).

saline (PBS) and one-half AB nontoxic sera are added, drop by drop, with gentle agitation. The suspension is centrifuged at 200 g for 6 min, resuspended in Hanks' solution, and adjusted to 2,000/μl.

Although empirical, the above technique is extremely reliable, has been used for a number of years and remains one of the quickest and least expensive.

Other techniques use sophisticated machinery and still others include simple freezing of ampoules or Beckman tubes, containing both the cell suspension and the DMSO protective agent in PBS, directly placed into freezers at −80°C overnight and immersed the following day in liquid nitrogen.

REFERENCES

1. Amos, D. B., Bashir, H., Boyle, W., Mac Queen, M., and Tiilikaineu, A. A simple microcytotoxicity test. Transplantation, *7:*220, 1969.
2. Benajam, A., Poirier, J. C., Beraud, L., Marcelli-Barge, A., and Dausset, J. Qualitative and quantitative study of the antigens and antibodies of the HLA system. Automatic fluorochrome method. Vox Sang., *28:*337, 1975.
3. Bodmer, W. F., Tripp, M., and Bodmer, J. G. Application of a fluorochromatic cytotoxicity assay to human leukocyte typing. *Histocompatibility Testing, 1967,* edited by E. S. Curtoni, P. L. Mattiuz and R. M. Tosi, p. 341. Munksgaard, Copenhagen, 1968.
4. Descamps, B. Determination of intracellular ATP for detecting anti-HLA antibody mediated cytolysis. Introduction to a new method for HLA typing. Transplantation, *29:* 295, 1980.
5. Dick, H. M., Kissmeyer-Nielsen, F. (Ed). *Histocompatibility Techniques.* Elsevier/ North Holland, Biomedical Press, Amsterdam, 1979.
6. Eisen, S. A., Wedner, H. J., and Parker, C. W. Isolation of pure human peripheral blood T lymphocytes using nylon wool columns. Immunol. Commun. *1:*571, 1972.
7. Harris, R., and Ukaejioho, E. O. Tissue typing using a routine one step lymphocyte separation procedure. Br. J. Haematol., *18:*229, 1970.
8. Hors, J., Preud'homme, J. L., Tolze-Zapateria, M. T., Guillet-Bigot, J., Roy, J. P., and Dausset, J. A simplified method for freezing lymphocytes in nitrogen vapors. Transplantation, *15:*417, 1973.
9. Kissmeyer-Nielsen, F., and Thorsby, E. Human transplantation antigens. Appendix: Current methods in histocompatibility testing. *Transplantation Review, 1970,* 4. Munksgaard, Copenhagen, 1970.
10. Lightbody, J., Bernoco, D., Miggiano, V. C., and Ceppellini, R. Cell mediated lympholysis in man after sensitization of effector lymphocytes through mixed leucocyte cultures. J. Bact. Virol. Immunol., *64:*243, 1971.
11. Mittal, K. K., Mickey, M. R., Singal, D. P., and Terasaki, P. I. Refinement of microdroplet lymphocyte cytotoxicity test. Transplantation, *6:*913, 1968.
12. Pellegrino, M. A., Ferrone, S. and Theofilopoulos, A. N. Isolation of human T and B lymphocytes by rosette formation with 2-aminoethyl iso thiouronium bromide (AET) treated sheep red blood cells and with monkey red cells. J. Immunol. Methods, *11:*273, 1976.
13. Ray, J. G. NIAID manual of Tissue Typing Techniques. DHEW Publication NO (NIH) 80-545, 1979.
14. Terasaki, P. I., Bernoco, D., Park, M. S., Ozturk, G., and Iwaki, Y. Microdroplet testing for HLA-A, B, C and D antigens. Am. J. Clin. Pathol., *69:*103, 1978.
15. Terasaki, P. I., and MacClelland, J. D. Microdroplet assay of human serum cytotoxins. Nature, *204:*998, 1964.
16. Van Rood, J. J., Van Leeuwen, A., and Ploem, J. S. Simultaneous detection of two cell populations by two colour fluorescence and application to the recognition of B cell determinants. Nature, *262:*795, 1976.

DETECTION OF DONOR SPECIFIC ANTIBODY- OR CELL-MEDIATED CYTOTOXICITY IN ALLOGRAFT RECIPIENTS

Béatrice Descamps

Many techniques have been proposed for detecting both humoral and cellular sensitization of allograft recipients against their respective donors. Those used in our center include the complement-dependent cytotoxicity (CDC) assay, the antibody-dependent cell-mediated cytotoxicity (ADCC) assay and the lymphocyte-mediated cytotoxicity (LMC) assay. These three cytotoxicity assays are performed at various intervals after transplantation. Donor lymphocytes, either fresh (in case of living donors) or cryopreserved (in case of cadaver donors), are used as target cells. The technique for measuring cytotoxicity is based on the release of ^{51}Cr by target cells previously labeled with this radioactive isotope, as described by Cerottini and Brunner.[2]

Preparation of Components for Cytotoxicity Reactions

Target Cells

Separation from Peripheral Blood. The procedure is based on the Ficoll gradient sedimentation described by Boyum.[1] Venous blood is collected on 200 IU heparin (Liquemine, Roche). Heparin preparations containing preservative agents such as phenol, which might be toxic for the cells, should not be used.

The blood is then diluted in twice its volume of Hanks' BSS (Institut Pasteur) and gently layered onto the surface of a 10 ml volume of Ficoll-Angiocontrix mixture in a 40 ml plastic tube with a round bottom. The Ficoll-Angiocontrix mixture is obtained by mixing 24 volumes 9% Ficoll (Pharmacia) and 10 volumes 30% sodium iothalamate (Guerbet). After an 800 g centrifugation for 20 min at 22°C, cells layering at the interface are removed, transferred into a 40 ml plastic tube with a conic bottom and washed twice by centrifugation at +4°C (8 min at 1000 g, then 8 min at 400 g) in Hanks' BSS.

Separation from Lymphoid Organs. *Spleen.* A 10 to 20 g fragment of the whole spleen is sufficient. It is placed in approximately 15 ml of cold Hanks' BSS in a Petri dish and cut into 2 to 3 mm fragments with sharp scissors. These fragments are carefully teased so as to gently disrupt splenic structures. The large aggregates can be partly dissociated by repeated up and down sucking into a Pasteur pipette. Cell debris and clumps are removed either by passing the suspension through a loose strainer or by sedimentation in a 10-cm column for 10 min. The cell suspension thus obtained is heavily contaminated with erythrocytes, but these may be removed by sedimentation on a Ficoll gradient, as described above.

Lymph Nodes. The lymph nodes are carefully freed of surrounding fatty tissue. They are then pricked many times with a medium-sized intramuscular needle. Approximately 40 ml of Hanks' solution is then injected into the lymph node under slight pressure, and the lymphocyte suspension which drains from the punctures is collected and washed twice (200 g for 5 min at +4°C).

Techniques for freezing and thawing cell suspensions are described on p. 348.

^{51}Cr Labeling Technique. Target cells are labeled with ^{51}Cr according to the technique of Cerottini and Brunner.[2]

Approximately 10^7 cells are resuspended in 0.1 ml Eagle's medium (MEM) supplemented with 10% heat-inactivated (60 min at 56°C) fetal calf serum (iFCS) and then incubated with 150 μ Ci of Na2 ^{51}Cr04 in a water bath at 37°C for 60 min. Cells are then washed three times in 40 ml of MEM + 10% iFCS by centrifugation (400 g for 8 min), counted and adjusted to a final concentration of 5×10^5 cells/ml.

Effector Cells

Effector cells are separated from heparinized blood by a two-step technique consisting of filtration over nylon wool followed by Ficoll gradient sedimentation. The method used for nylon wool filtration is based on that described by Greaves and Brown.[4] A 1.5 × 15-cm glass column or a 25-ml plastic seringe is filled with 1-g nylon fibers Fenwal leukopak (LP-1, Fenwal Laboratories), previously washed with 0.2N HCl, rinsed with distilled water and dried. The column is washed with 50 ml of a 0.9% NaCl solution prewarmed to 37°C. Twenty-five milliliters of prewarmed (37°C) heparinized blood is then allowed to incubate and filter through the column during approximately 20 min. The eluate is diluted in twice its volume in Hanks' BSS and layered on the Ficoll gradient as described above. After the two washings, the cells are resuspended at a concentration of 2×10^7/ml in MEM with 10% iFCS.

Serum

Ten milliliters of venous blood is drawn into a nonheparinized test tube and left to clot at room temperature. After removal of the clot, the tube is centrifuged (2000 g, 10 min). The serum is then gently removed with a pipette and placed in a 10-cc test tube which is incubated in a 56°C water bath for 30 min in order to inactivate serum complement.

When serum is to be stored, it is distributed into 0.5-ml aliquots in 1-ml plastic tubes and kept at −80°C.

Complement

Preparation of complement is described on p. 348.

Measurement of ^{51}CR Release and Expression of Results

In all three assays described below, 1 ml of cold Hanks' medium is added to each tube at the end of incubation. Cells are separated from supernatant by centrifugation (800 g at 4°C for 7 min) and the respective radioactivity of supernatant and cells is counted in a well-type Packard Gamma Spectrometer. Percent release (*R*) of ^{51}Cr is expressed as:

$$R = \frac{1.2\ (\text{Sample} - \text{Bgd})}{\text{Sample} + \text{Residual} - 2\ \text{Bgd}}$$

where *Bgd* represents the background of the Gamma Spectrometer. The coefficient 1.2 is used to take into account the ratio between the total assay volume and the volume of the sample. The mean percent release (*R*) is obtained from triplicate experiments.

The CI is then calculated from Brunner's formula:

$$CI = \frac{\bar{R}\ (\text{experimental}) - \bar{R}\ (\text{control})}{\bar{R}\ (\text{maximum}) - \bar{R}\ (\text{control})} \times 100$$

where $\bar{R}$ (maximum) represents the mean percent of ^{51}Cr released from 50 μl of target cells incubated with distilled water in the place of serum (for CDC) or effector cells (for ADCC and LMC).

Experiments can be considered to be interpretable only when $\bar{R}$ (control) is below 25%. It is usually below 10% in CDC and between 15 and 25% in ADCC or LMC.

For all three techniques, results can be considered positive only when the following conditions are met: 1) $\bar{R}$ is significantly greater ($P < 0.01$ according to Student's t test) in experimental than in control combinations; and 2) cytotoxicity index (CI) value is above 5%.

Tests For Measuring Cytotoxicity

Complement-Dependent Cytotoxicity

The technique we use for the evaluation of CDC is that described by Rogentine and Plocinik.[5] The ^{51}Cr labeled target cell suspension (50 μl, i.e., 2.5×10^4 cells) is distributed into 15 × 40 mm plastic tubes containing 0.05 ml of 10^{-1} diluted control or recipient serum. Tubes are prepared in triplicate for both control and test combinations. Target cells and serum are incubated for 15 min at 22°C before the addition of 50 μl of 1:3 diluted rabbit serum. In order to eliminate occasional noncomplement-dependent cell lysis, an additional control replacing the normal rabbit serum by heat-inactivated rabbit serum is also included for both control and recipient serum samples. At the end of a 2-hour incubation period at 22°C, the ^{51}Cr release from labeled target cells is measured as described above.

Antibody-Dependent Cell-Mediated Cytotoxicity

Details of the technical conditions necessary for the ADCC technique have been described elsewhere.[3] The ^{51}Cr labeled target cell suspension

(50 μl, i.e., 2.5×10^4 cells) is distributed into 15 × 40-mm plastic tubes containing 50 μl of 10^{-1} diluted control or recipient serum. For both control and test combinations, tubes are prepared in triplicate. Target cells are incubated with serum for 45 min at 37°C and then washed once in Hanks' BSS medium. The effector cell suspension (50 μl, i.e., 10^6 cells) are added to each tube, with an effector to target cell ratio of 40 to 1. The mixture is then incubated for 4 hours at 37°C in an atmosphere of 5% CO_2. At the end of incubation, the ^{51}Cr release from labeled target cells is measured as described below.

Lymphocyte-Mediated Cytotoxicity

The technique we use is that described by Cerottini and Brunner.[2] The ^{51}Cr labeled target cell suspension (50 μl, i.e., 2.5×10^4 cells) is distributed into 15 × 40-mm plastic tubes. Tubes are prepared in triplicate for both control and test combinations. One hundred microliters (i.e., 2×10^6 cells) of recipient or control effector cell suspension is then added to each tube, giving an effector to target cell ratio of 80:1. The mixture is gently spun (200 g for 2 min) to provide better contact between target and effector cells. It is then incubated for 4 hours at 37°C in an atmosphere of 5% CO_2. At the end of the incubation period, the ^{51}Cr release from labeled target cells is measured as described above.

REFERENCES

1. Boyum, A. Isolation of mononuclear cells and granulocytes from human blood. Scand. J. Clin. Lab. Invest. 21(Suppl.), *97:*77, 1968.
2. Cerottini, J. C., and Brunner, K. T. In vitro assay of target cell lysis by sensitized lymphocytes. In *In Vitro Methods in Cell-Mediated Immunity*, edited by B. Bloom and P. Glade, p. 369. Academic Press, New York, 1971.
3. Decamps, B., Gagnon, R., Van Der Gaag, R., Feuillet, M. N., and Crosnier, J. Antibody-dependent cell-mediated cytotoxicity (ADCC) and complement-dependent cytotoxicity (CDC) in 229 sera from human renal allograft recipients. J. Clin. Lab. Immunol., *2:*303, 1979.
4. Greaves, M. F., and Brown, G. Purification of human T and B lymphocytes. J. Immunol., *112:*420, 1974.
5. Rogentine, G. N., and Plocinik, B. A. Application of the ^{51}Cr cytotoxicity technique to the analysis of human lymphocyte isoantigens. Transplantation, *5:*1323, 1967.

MIXED LYMPHOCYTE REACTION AND CELL-MEDIATED LYMPHOLYSIS TECHNIQUES

Catherine Fournier

When lymphocytes from two genetically different individuals are mixed together and cultured in vitro, they transform into lymphoblasts and proliferate. This proliferation can be evaluated in the mixed lymphocyte reaction (MLR) by enumerating the transformed cells or, better still, by measuring thymidine incorporation into DNA. We have applied this technique to the selection of donors in kidney transplantation.

Moreover, cytotoxic cells specifically directed against the relevant antigens are generated during the MLR. This cytotoxicity can be evaluated by the cell-mediated lympholysis (CML) test.

Preparation of Cell Suspensions

All the procedures are carried out in a sterile fashion. Mononuclear cells are isolated from heparinized venous blood using Ficoll gradient sedimentation as described in Appendix II, "Detection of Donor-Specific Antibody- or Cell-Mediated Cytotoxicity in Allograft Recipients" and then suspended in complete medium. This medium consists of RPMI 1640 supplemented with 2 mM glutamin, 100 U/ml penicillin, 100 μg/ml streptomycin (Flow Laboratories) and 20% heat-inactivated human AB serum (pool of 3 to 5 donors).

Allogeneic Mixed Lymphocyte Reaction

The microtechnique used is derived from that described by Hartzman et al.[4] Both the two-way and the one-way cultures are carried out in quadruplicate, using flat bottomed microplates (Falcon No. 3040) and all the cells are suspended in complete medium at a concentration of 2×10^6 cells/ml. In each well, 0.1 ml of responding cells is mixed with 0.1 ml of stimulating cells. For the one-way culture, the stimulators are either irradiated (2000 rads) or mitomycin-treated (incubated at 37°C for 20 min with 25 μg/ml of mitomycin C and then washed twice).

Different mixtures of cells are set up in culture and their stimulation is compared with that of background cultures containing the responding cells alone. In practice, when the cells from the recipient (R) are incubated with the cells from the potential donor(s) (D) or from an unrelated individual (X), we use the following scheme:

Background cultures	R + Ri	D + Di	X + Xi
Experimental cultures	R + Di	D + Ri	X + Ri
	R + Xi	D + Xi	X + Di

After a 5-day incubation at 37°C in a humidified 5% CO_2 atmosphere, the cultures are pulsed with 1 μCi-tritiated thymidine (specific activity = 1 Ci/mM) and incubated for an additional 18 hours at 37°C. The cells are then harvested with an automated sample harvester (Microbiological Associates, U.S.A.) and the radioactivity incorporated in the cells is determined by liquid scintillation counting.

The results are expressed in Δcpm obtained as follows: Δcpm = cpm of experimental culture − cpm of background culture. In some cases, an index can be calculated by dividing the cpm of experimental culture by the cpm of background culture.

Allogeneic Cell-Mediated Lympholysis

The ^{51}Cr release test was originally reported in the mouse by Brunner et al.[2] It was then extensively used in man and proved itself as a tool for the characterization of the major histocompatibility complex.[3] The technique we describe here is derived from that of Bonnard et al.[1]

The generation of cytotoxic cells is obtained by mixing 1×10^7 responding cells with 1×10^7 irradiated cells either from an allogeneic donor or autologous to the responder. Cells are co-cultured in plastic flasks (Falcon No. 3013) in a total volume of 20 ml for 7 days at 37°C in the conditions described above for the micro-MLR test.

At the end of the incubation, cells are harvested by vigorous pipetting, washed once in Hanks' medium and resuspended in fresh culture medium.

Target cells are phytohemagglutinin (PHA)-blasts derived from the donor of the stimulator cells. For this purpose, on day 0 of the culture, 1×10^7 cells are cultured in 10 ml of complete medium, and 3 days later PHA is added at a concentration of 100 μg/ml. Finally, at the end of the whole culture period of 7 days, the PHA blasts are collected and washed twice in medium. Five million cells are then labeled by incubating 1 hour at 37°C with 100 μCi of ^{51}Cr as described on p. 358.

The cytotoxicity test is conducted in triplicate in round bottomed microplates:10,000 chromium-labeled target cells are distributed in each well and varying amounts of educated or noneducated lymphocytes are added. The term "noneducated" cells refers to the cells cultured for 7 days in the presence of autologous irradiated cells. The effector/target cell ratio ranges from 100:1 down to 12.5:1 in a final volume of 0.2 ml.

The plates are then incubated at 37°C in a 5% CO_2 humidified atmosphere for 6 hours, at the end of which they are centrifuged at 600 g for 5 min at 4°C. 100 μl of supernatant are removed from each well and the radioactivity measured in a Packard Autogamma counter.

Maximum chromium release is measured after addition of detergent to the same amount of target cells. Spontaneous release from target cells incubated alone must not exceed 20% of the maximum chromium release. The specific release is calculated according to Brunner's formula:

$$\frac{\text{educated lymphocytes (cpm)} - \text{noneducated lymphocytes (cpm)}}{\text{maximum release (cpm)} - \text{spontaneous release (cpm)}} \times 100$$

REFERENCES

1. Bonnard, G. D., Lemos, L., and Chappuis, M. Cell-mediated lympholysis after sensitization in unidirectional mixed lymphocyte culture in man. Scand. J. Immunol., *3:*97, 1974.
2. Brunner, K. T., Mauel J., Cerottini, J. C., and Chappuis, B. Quantitative assay of the lytic action of immune lymphoid cells on ^{51}Cr labeled allogeneic target cells in vitro: Inhibition by isoantibody and by drugs. Immunology, *14:*181, 1968.
3. Eijsvoogel, V. P., Du Bois, M. J., Melief, C. J., De Groot-Kooy, M. L., Koning, C., Van Rood, J. J., Van Leeuwen A., Du Toit, E., and Schellekens, P. T. Position of a locus determining mixed lymphocyte reaction (MLR) distinct from the known HL/A loci, and its relation to cell-mediated lympholysis (CML). In *Histocompatibility Testing 1972*, edited by J. Dausset and J. Colombani, p. 501. Munksgaard, Copenhagen, 1973.
4. Hartzman, R. J., Segall, M., Bach, M. L., and Bach, F. H. Histocompatibility matching. VI. Miniaturization of the mixed leukocyte culture test: A preliminary report. Transplantation, *11:*268, 1971.

ENUMERATION OF HUMAN T CELLS (E ROSETTE FORMATION)

Marie-Anne Bach

T cells have been shown to form rosettes with sheep erythrocytes (E rosettes).† This T cell-specific property is commonly used to enumerate T lymphocytes among human peripheral blood cells.[2] Rosettes can be formed either with normal or neuraminidase-treated sheep red blood cells (SRBC). The latter method gives higher figures due to the detection of an additional T cell subpopulation.[1]

Rosette Formation with Normal Sheep Erythrocytes

Lymphocytes are separated from the peripheral blood using a mixture of Ficoll and Triosil as described in Appendix II, "Detection of Donor-Specific Antibody- or Cell-Mediated Cytotoxicity in Allograft Recipients." Lymphocytes (washed twice) and SRBC (washed three times) are resuspended in Hanks' medium in a hemolysis tube. Fifty microliters of a 10^7/ml lymphocyte suspension are mixed with 100 μl of a 2×10^8/ml SRBC suspension and 120 μl fetal bovine serum previously absorbed with SRBC and human red blood cells. Two hundred microliters of Hanks' medium are added to the mixture and the tubes are incubated for 30 min at 37°C. The preparation is centrifuged for 5 min at 200 g. The pellets are kept overnight at 4°C and then resuspended gently for 2 min. The reading

† The rosette technique is now widely used for several purposes. In the human, two main techniques are commonly employed. *E rosettes* (E for Erythrocytes) are formed by human lymphocytes with SRBC; as hereabove mentioned, they are commonly regarded as identifying T lymphocytes (normally 65 to 75% of blood lymphocytes). *EAC rosettes* (Erythrocyte-Amboceptor-Complement) use erythrocytes coated with IgM antibody and complement deficient in C_5 (to avoid cell lysis) in order to detect cells bearing receptors for complement (mainly B cells, monocytes and polymorphs).

is made in a hematocytometer (1 μl chamber). The lymphocytes and the rosettes are counted separately and the number of rosettes is compared with the number of lymphocytes. For each tube, the content of at least two chambers is counted (or 6,000 lymphocytes). The percentage of lymphocytes forming E rosettes is then calculated (60 to 80% in normal subjects).

Rosette Formation with Neuraminidase-Treated Sheep Erythrocytes

Five milliliters of a 2% SRBC suspension is incubated for 30 min at 37°C with 150 μl neuraminidase (Behring) and then washed three times in Hanks' medium. After the third washing the pellet is resuspended in 5 ml Hanks' medium and this neuraminidase-treated SRBC suspension may be stored for a week at 4°C.

Fifty microliters of a 10^7/ml lymphocyte suspension is mixed with 100 μl of the neuraminidase-treated SRBC suspension and 50 μl of fetal bovine serum previously absorbed with SRBC in a 5-ml hemolysis tube. The preparation is then centrifuged for 5 min at 200 g and left for 60 min at room temperature. The pellets are gently resuspended for 2 min and the reading is made as described above. The range of E rosette percentages obtained with this method is 70 to 85% in normal subjects.

REFERENCES

1. Hoffmann, T., and Kunkel, H. G. The E-rosette test. In *In Vitro Methods in Cell-Mediated and Tumor Immunity*, edited by B. R. Bloom and J. R. David. Academic Press, New York, 1976.
2. Jondal, M., Wigzell, H., and Aiuti, F. Human lymphocyte subpopulation: Classification according to surface markers and/or functional characteristics. Transplant. Rev., *16:*163, 1973.

INHIBITION OF MIGRATION OF HUMAN PERIPHERAL LEUKOCYTES[1, 6]

Michel Dy and Monique Debray-Sachs

Twenty milliliters of blood are taken in sterile fashion on calcium heparinate (Calciparine, Choay, Paris). The blood is allowed to sediment for 90 min at 37°C. The buffy coat is washed three times in Hanks' medium (7 min, 200 g). The cells are resuspended in 2 ml of medium 199, the final concentration of cells being adjusted to 30,000/cu mm.

Twenty siliconized capillary tubes (external diameter 1.4 mm) are then filled with the cell suspension and sealed with Seal-Ease (Clay-Adams Inc., New York, New York). The tubes are centrifuged (10 min, 1200 g) and cut at the leukocyte-supernatant interface. The tubes are then placed in small plastic chambers, one per chamber, and fixed with a silicone adhesive (silicone lubricant, high vacuum grease, Dow Corning, Midland, Michigan). The chambers are filled with medium 199 to which has been added 10% human serum and the test antigen in various dilutions. The chamber is closed by a cover slip and incubated for 24 hours. At the end of this time, the area of migration is measured by planimetry, either on a photograph or by projecting a magnified image of the capillary tube onto a screen: the area of a thick sheet of paper covered by the superimposed image of the migration area is weighed. The migration index is defined as the ratio between the mean migration area of the tubes incubated with the antigen to the mean migration area of the control tubes (incubated without antigen).

Sensitization is usually shown by migration inhibition. Our results suggest that a migration index lower than 0.70 is good evidence of sensitization.

In studying rejection, the antigen may be present in the form of donor leukocytes[3] (mixed with donor cells and incubated 2 hours before insertion into the capillary tube) or in the form of soluble preparations of fetal antigens,[2] kidney antigens[4] or specific leukocyte antigens from the donor.[5]

REFERENCES

1. Bendixen, G., and Söborg, M. Comments on the leukocyte migration technique as an *in vitro* method for demonstrating cellular hypersensitivity in man. J. Immunol., *104:*1551, 1970.
2. Eddleston, A. L. W. F., Williams, R., and Calne, R. Y. Cellular immune response during rejection of a liver transplant in man. Nature, *222:*674, 1969.
3. Falk, R. E., Thorsby, E., Möller, E., and Möller, G. *In vitro* assay of cell-mediated immunity: The inhibition of migration of sensitized human lymphocytes by HL-A antigen. Clin. Exp. Immunol., *6:*445, 1970.
4. Melnick, H. D., and Friedman, H. Cellular immunity to a purified kidney antigen assessed by macrophage migratory inhibition and MIF release by human leukocytes. Third International Congress of the Transplantation Society, The Hague, 1970. Transplant. Proc., *3:*465, 1971.
5. Smith, M. G. M., Eddleston, A. L. W. F., Dominguez, J. A., Evans, D. B., Bewick, M., and Williams, R. Changes in leucocyte migration after renal transplantation. Br. Med. J., *4:*275, 1969.
6. Söborg, M. *In vitro* detection of cellular hypersensitivity in man: Specific migration inhibition of white blood cells from brucella-positive persons. Acta Med. Scand., *182:* 167, 1967.

APPENDIX III

Other Techniques

RENAL BIOPSIES IN TRANSPLANT RECIPIENTS

Dominique Droz and Laure-Hélène Noël

Open biopsies remain the best method for carrying out histologic study of transplanted kidneys. In order to obtain a representative cortical specimen, a needle technique should be used. Surgical biopsies are too superficial and thus do not give useful results.

Percutaneous methods using a Vim Silverman needle are often well tolerated by transplant recipients who may undergo repeated biopsies. However, certain investigations must always precede the biopsy. Ultrasonography of the transplant should be performed to determine the size and thickness of the renal parenchyma and to detect any perirenal collection or pyelocalyceal distention. Coagulation should also be normal.

Two points should be underlined. 1) Percutaneous biopsy is particularly hazardous in patients who have undergone previous repeated abdominal surgery, because of cicatricial changes. 2) This method should not be employed during the 3 initial post-transplantation months since complications are more frequent during that period.

In our own experience, percutaneous needle biopsy provides a representative specimen in 70% of cases.

RADIOLOGIC INVESTIGATION OF THE RENAL TRANSPLANT

Jean-François Moreau

The development of ultrasonographic methods has modified the strategy of radiologic investigations of the transplanted kidney, partly decreasing the use of intravenous urography and angiography.

Plain Film and Intravenous Urography

There is no problem in making plain films of the renal graft with an anteroposterior view, except when the purpose is to detect stones. In that case films taken in oblique incidence or with local compression may be necessary to avoid superimposition with sacroiliac bone images.

Contrast media are no more nephrotoxic on a grafted kidney than normally. During the first weeks following transplantation, however, they may contribute to the functional damage of an already poorly functioning renal graft.[6]

Urography is mainly useful in detecting urologic complications (excretory obstruction, fistulae or lymphocele). This may require high dosage of contrast medium if glomerular filtration is low (0.60 to 0.80 g iodine/kg body wt, instead of 0.20 or 0.40 g). In our experience this high dosage does not result in acute renal failure when glomerular filtration is low because of urologic obstruction. Conversely, nonobstructive renal insufficiency may be aggravated. In this regard, safety has been increased with the extensive use of ultrasonography, allowing the distinction between obstructive and nonobstructive renal insufficiency in many cases.

When the chosen dosage is 0.40 to 0.80 g iodine/kg body wt, for example, urography may be performed without using the whole amount of contrast medium at once, but rather completing the dose in a second stage if necessary.

Urography should always include a cystography and a micturating uretrocystogram. Recent low osmolarity contrast media[7] (ioxaglic acid or iopamidol, not yet fully commercialized) are less nephrotoxic and give better contrast than usual contrast media (diatrizoic or iothalamic acids).

Arteriography

Arteriography is performed using the Seldinger method.[4] Needles and catheters used for femoral puncture and catheterization should be as small as permitted by the injection flow required (usually 1.6 mm diameter) because of the frequent fragility of the arterial wall in these patients. We commonly puncture the femoral artery on the side of the transplant, contrary to the technique used by some other groups.[3] The advantages of this homolateral technique are: 1) limitation of the amount of contrast medium; 2) easier selective catheterization; and 3) injection closer to the ostium of the artery, an important point particularly for tests using vasoactive substances. In our experience, injection on the side of the transplant does not increase the rate of local complications.

For nonselective arteriography, 30 ml of contrast medium is injected at 2 ml/sec (approximately 3 sec for the whole injection). Since 1978, we have used the precited newer contrast media (Iopamidol and Ioxaglic acid) which do not induce pain, contrary to usual media. Twelve exposures are taken during the first 4 sec. This gives a satisfactory estimation of the transit time, hence of the arterial blood flow. Thereafter, two films per second are taken during 10 sec.

For selective arteriography, specially precurved Kifa's catheters are used. The amount and flow of contrast medium are chosen on the basis of the hemodynamic data suggested by the nonselective films. With a normal circulatory state, 12 ml are injected at 4 to 5 ml/sec. The amount and rate of injection are reduced in proportion to the reduction in renal blood flow. In some cases of acute rejection with cortical necrosis, as little as 0.5 ml/sec may be injected. The schedule for exposures is similar to that used for nonselective arteriography.

The main artery of a renal transplant is rarely parallel to the film in the anteroposterior position. Oblique views should be taken, generally with the patient at 45° or more and the side where the transplant is located closest to the film.

The dopamine test[5] is performed by perfusing intravenously 100 mg in 10 min (less than 2.5 μg/kg body wt/min). At the 5th min of this perfusion, 40 mg furosemide are injected through the femoral catheter. At the 10th min, arteriography is resumed, following exactly the same schedule as previously used in the control arteriography.

Contraindications and local complications do not differ from those generally described for other arteriography. The renal graft tolerates arteriography at least as well as intravenous urography.

The nephrographic phase of arteriographic films usually permits visualization of the renal veins, especially on films taken during the dopamine test. Selective *phlebography* is never used in our center. A few cases, however, may require phlebographic examination of the vena iliaca when thrombosis is suspected—a rare complication, since we have observed only one case in 10 years.

Ultrasonography

Ultrasonography has now assumed a major role in the field of renal transplantation and is often the first investigation used, replacing invasive radiologic examinations. Its use is especially easy because of the superficial placement of the renal transplant in the iliac fossa. High frequency transducers (5 MHz) are preferable since they allow satisfactory corticomedullary differentiation and accurate study of the renal sinus. Differential diagnosis of the various types of obstructive or not acute renal failure of the graft may be suggested on the basis of ultrasonographic data alone.[1, 2]

Another advantage of ultrasonography is that it provides the possibility of exploring perirenal and perivesical spaces. This may require multidirectional scanning, easier with real time ultrasonographs.

Computerized Tomography

At the present time, computerized tomography provides fewer objective data than does ultrasonography with regard to the state of the parenchyma of the graft, the urinary tract and the perirenal space. Densitometric studies require the injection of contrast media. Although recently developed equipment permits a significant decrease in iodine dosage, its use remains almost always necessary, entailing a nephrotoxic risk.

REFERENCES

1. Hillman, B. J., Birnholz, J. C., and Busch, G. J. Correlation of echographic and histologic findings in suspected renal allograft rejection. Radiology, *132:*673, 1979.
2. Hricak, H., Toledo-Pereya, L. H., Eyler, W. R., and Adrazo, B. L. Role of ultrasound in renal transplantation. A review of clinical and experimental observations. Dial. Transplant., *8:*818, 1979.
3. Kaude, J. V., and Hawkins, I. F. Angiography of renal transplant. Radiol. Clin. North Am., *14:*295, 1976.
4. Moreau, J. F., Kleinknecht, D., Grünfeld, J. P., Reboul, F., Sabto, J., and Michel, J. R. Angiographic patterns of renal cortical necrosis. J. Radiol. Electrol. Med. Nucl., *55:*1, 1974.
5. Moreau, J. F., Baillet, P., Kreis, H., Descamps, J. P., Dana, A., Crosnier, J., and Michel, J. R. Dopamine-frusemide pharmaco angiography of human transplanted kidneys (submitted for publication).
6. Moreau, J. F., Kreis, H., Barbanel, C., and Michel, J. R. Effets des produits de contraste iodés sur la fonction des reins transplantés. Nouv. Presse Méd., *4:*2643, 1975.
7. Sovak, M., Ranganathan, R., Lang, J. H., and Lasser, E. C. Concepts in design of improved intravascular contrast agents. Ann. Radiol., *21:*283, 1978.

TRANSPLANT SCANNING WITH RADIONUCLIDES

Toong See Ngeh

After adequate hydration whenever possible, 0.15 m Ci/kg of diethylenetriamine pentaacetic acid (DTPA)-Technetium 99m is injected intravenously as a bolus, and serial images in the anterior projection are recorded every 2 sec over the kidney and the external iliac artery for a minimum of 8 min using a minicomputer and a gamma camera with a low-energy, high-sensitivity collimator.

Information on renal blood flow is obtained by analysis of the normalized time activity curves corresponding to the first pass of the radioactive bolus through the kidney and the external iliac artery, using this artery as a reference and thus taking into account possible variations due to injection and to absorption by overlying tissues. The following "perfusion indices" can be calculated: 1) the ratio of the heights of the vascular peaks of the kidney and the iliac artery (normally >0.50); 2) the ratio of their mean vascular transit times (normally < 2.0); 3) the ratio of the

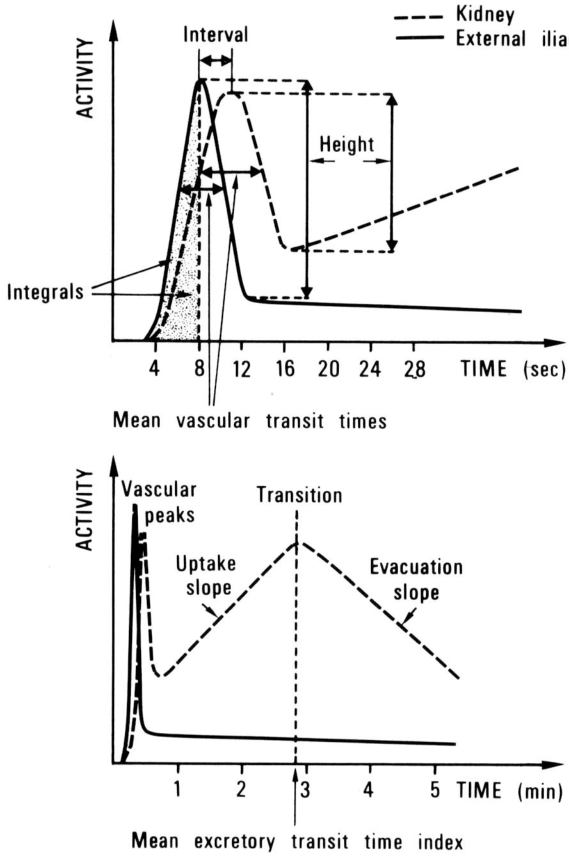

Fig. III.1.

integrals of the up-slope of their vascular peaks to a point limited by the maximum activity of the peak of the iliac artery (normally >0.65); 4) the interval between the peaks of the iliac artery and the kidney (normally <5 sec). In normal renal transplants, in acute tubulonephritis without other complications and in the early stage of acute ureteral obstruction, these indices remain within the normal range. In rejection, when blood flow deteriorates, the indices move into the abnormal zone. In the very early stages of rejection, however, blood flow could still be within the normal range. In renal artery stenosis, indices are subnormal. In arterio-venous fistula, images during the vascular phase show a localized area of increased activity within the kidney. The kidney is not seen when blood flow is absent or in cortical necrosis (Fig. III.1).

During the uptake phase, the ascending slope of the renal curve, divided by the radioactivity injected, is proportional to the glomerular filtration rate.

During the evacuation phase, the descending slope (relative to the ascending slope of the uptake phase) is proportional to the rate of urine evacuation from the kidney.

The mean excretory transit time is proportional to the time corresponding to the transition of these two slopes (normally <3.5 min). In ureteral stenosis and in stenosis of the renal artery, urine excretion is reduced and mean excretory transit time increased. When both the uptake and the urine radioactivity are sufficient, images during the evacuation phase can indicate the precise site of ureteral stenosis and can detect any urinary extravasation.

Complete stenosis of a branch of the renal artery with segmental infarction is best diagnosed using DMSA-Technetium 99m, whereas incomplete stenosis of a branch of the renal artery is difficult to detect.

Index